PEDIATRIC PULMONOLOGY

Edited by

Brittany Heitkamp

ALLIED
HEALTH
PRESS

Pediatric Pulmonology

Editor: **Brittany Heitkamp**

Allied Health Press
4164 Lakeshore Road
Burlington ON L7L 1A4
Canada
www.alliedhealthpress.com
Email: orders@arclereducation.com

ISBN: 978-1-77956-266-1

Allied Health Press publishes wide variety of books and eBooks. For more information about Allied Health Press and its products, visit our website at www.alliedhealthpress.com

ABOUT THE EDITOR

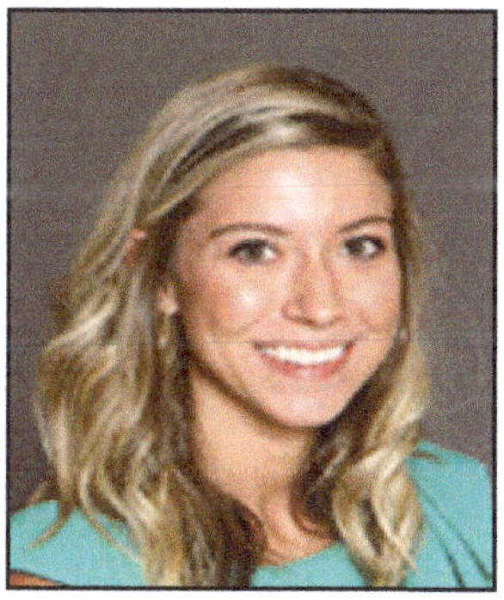

Brittany Kenney is a certified pediatric nurse practitioner with a diverse background in pediatric neurosurgery, pediatric intensive care, and neonatal intensive care. She graduated magna cum laude from Saint Louis University with a Bachelor of Science in Nursing with certifications in family nursing and interprofessional education. She then worked at Vanderbilt Children's Hospital in the pediatric intensive care unit, and then at St. Thomas Midtown Hospital in the neonatal intensive care unit. After a few years, she went back to school and graduated summa cum laude from Emory University with a Master of Science in Nursing. She specialized as a pediatric primary care nurse practitioner. She worked as a pediatric neurosurgery nurse practitioner at Children's' Healthcare of Atlanta and then relocated back to St. Louis and worked as a pediatric neurosurgery nurse practitioner through Washington University St. Louis. She currently works as an adjunct clinical professor teaching undergraduate nursing students. She is also a data abstractor who completes research on oncological diseases and treatment protocols.

Word Roots, Prefixes, and Suffixes by Chapter

Chapter 1 Pediatric Pulmonology: An Introduction

ad- at, increase, on, toward adduction, addition

aden- of or relating to a gland adenocarcinoma, adenology, adenotome

adip-of or relating to fat or fatty tissue adipocyte

brachi(o)- of or relating to the arm brachium of inferior

Chapter 2 Allergic Conditions

pulmon-, pulmo- of or relating to the lungs

rhin(o)- of or pertaining to the nose

dermat(o) , derm(o)- of or pertaining to the skin

myc(o)- fungus

asthmat/o- related to the lung

Chapter 3 Anatomical Disorders

Anatom-: Root referring to anatomy, the structure of organisms.

-al: Suffix indicating "pertaining to."

Dis-: Prefix meaning "apart" or "away."

-order: Suffix indicating a state of disarray or dysfunction.

Patho-: Prefix indicating disease or abnormality.

Chapter 4 Upper and Lower Airway Infections

-ar, –ary Pertaining to

-capnia Carbon dioxide

-centesisSurgical puncture with needle to aspirate fluid

-ectasis Stretching or expansion

-gram Record

-graphy Process of recording

-itis Inflammation

Chapter 5 Pediatric Asthma

ach- pain

card-, cardi-, cardio- heart

cata- heart

-derm- skin

-emia blood

Chapter 6 Noninfectious Pulmonary Disorders

cancer/o cancer cancerization, cancerogenic, cancerous

celi/o abdomen celiac artery, celiocentasis

cyan/o blue cyanosis, hemocyanin, cyanocobalamine

leuk/o white leukocytc, lcukemia, leukoplakia

nephr/o kidney nephron, nephropathy, nephrosclerosis

Chapter 7 Pediatric Sleep Medicine

cardio-, kardia, relates to the heart or the cardiovascular system

poly-, many or multiple

Somno-, refers to sleep

narc(o)-, numb, sleep

somn(o), somnus, Sleep

Chapter 8 Genetic Disorders

dys- Bad, abnormal, painful, difficult

endo- Within, in

epi- On, upon, over

hyper- Above, excessive

hypo- Below, deficient

inter- Between

Chapter 9 Lung Disease Associated with Systemic Disorders

Auto- Self Autocrine

Bio- Life Biology

Chem/o- Chemistry Chemotherapy

Contra- Against Contraception

Cyt/o- Cell Cytokine

Chapter 10 Treating and Managing Pulmonary Disease

-pnea (breathing)

-thorax (chest, chest cavity)

-emia (in the blood)

-algia (pain)

Word Roots, Prefixes, and Suffixes by Chapter

Table of Contents

7 Pediatric Sleep Medicine 245

8 Genetic Disorders 281

LIST OF FIGURES

LIST OF TABLES

PREFACE

Respiratory illnesses are a major cause of sickness and death in children. Healthy lungs are crucial for children's overall well-being. When lungs are obstructed or infected, children can suffer serious health issues. Preventing respiratory diseases and improving the health of infants, children, and young adults with respiratory illnesses can be achieved through research, education, and clinical care.

Recent advances in pediatric pulmonology research have provided new insights into this field. This Special Issue aims to showcase recent developments and emerging trends in pediatric pulmonology, focusing on advancements in disease definitions and classification, identification of new biomarkers, effective lung function tests, and advancements in respiratory endoscopy.

It is noteworthy that many adult pulmonary diseases seem to originate from early life events, underscoring the importance of early prevention and therapy. Understanding how early-life factors impact the development of pulmonary diseases is crucial for improving long-term outcomes. Respiratory illnesses have become more common, partly due to improved survival of preterm infants, early diagnosis and management of chronic respiratory diseases, and the availability of better diagnostic tools.

Accurate diagnosis of lung diseases is critical, and pathology plays a central role in this. Techniques like bronchoalveolar lavage, which is like a liquid biopsy of the lungs, require specialized training for pathologists and careful interpretation by clinicians. Specialized training in interpreting findings from small tissue samples is also crucial. Collaboration between pathologists and clinicians can significantly improve diagnostic accuracy in challenging cases.

Children with neuromuscular problems and developmental delays often have significant respiratory issues and may require pulmonary rehabilitation and other supportive care. Pulmonologists need to work closely with neurologists and adult pulmonologists, especially in the evolving field of sleep medicine.

Pediatric pulmonologists also play a crucial role in diagnosing and managing opportunistic infections in immunocompromised children. Airway malformations, including tumors and malacias, may require surgical intervention and close collaboration with pediatric surgeons and otolaryngologists.

This book aims to provide a comprehensive overview of recent advancements and current trends in pediatric pulmonology. It seeks to address the needs of a broad audience, including pediatricians, pulmonologists, respiratory therapists, pediatric surgeons, otolaryngologists, pathologists, and other healthcare professionals involved in the care of children with respiratory diseases. Additionally, medical students, residents, and fellows interested in pediatric respiratory medicine will find this book to be a valuable resource.

The primary objective of this book is to highlight the latest research findings, clinical guidelines, and technological innovations in pediatric pulmonology. It covers a wide range of topics, including the diagnosis, management, and prevention of respiratory diseases in infants, children, and adolescents. Special emphasis is placed on the impact of early-life events on the development of respiratory illnesses and the importance of early intervention and therapy.

Furthermore, this book aims to enhance the understanding of the pathophysiology of pediatric respiratory diseases and the role of pathology in their diagnosis. It provides insights into the use of advanced diagnostic tools and techniques, such as bronchoalveolar lavage and respiratory endoscopy, in the evaluation of lung disorders in children.

The book also addresses the multidisciplinary nature of pediatric pulmonology, emphasizing the importance of collaboration between different specialties, such as neurology and pediatric surgery, in the management of complex respiratory conditions. It discusses the role of pulmonary rehabilitation and supportive care in improving the quality of life of children with neuromuscular problems and developmental delays.

This book serves as a comprehensive reference for healthcare professionals involved in the care of children with respiratory diseases, providing them with up-to-date information and practical insights to enhance their clinical practice and improve patient outcomes.

Chapter

PEDIATRIC PULMONOLOGY: AN INTRODUCTION

1

Contents

Introduction

A subspecialty of pediatric medicine called pediatric pulmonology is concerned with the identification, care, and treatment of respiratory conditions in newborns, kids, and teenagers. It includes a broad spectrum of diseases that impact the respiratory system, such as congenital lung abnormalities, pneumonia, bronchiolitis, asthma, and cystic fibrosis. Pediatricians, respiratory therapists, nurses, and other medical professionals collaborate closely with pediatric pulmonologists to provide comprehensive and individualized care for young patients with respiratory symptoms, breathing difficulties, or lung diseases. Pediatric pulmonologists are trained to assess and treat these patients. Optimizing lung function and respiratory health in children is one of the main objectives of pediatric pulmonology. This helps to promote normal growth and development while reducing the negative effects of respiratory diseases on quality of life. To determine the underlying cause of respiratory symptoms or abnormalities, a comprehensive evaluation and diagnosis utilizing imaging studies, pulmonary function testing, clinical assessment, and other diagnostic modalities are required. Additionally, pediatric pulmonologists are essential in the management of long-term respiratory disorders because they create customized treatment regimens based on the unique requirements, symptoms, and severity of each child's ailment.

To relieve symptoms, lower inflammation, or stop respiratory disease exacerbations, pharmacotherapy in pediatric pulmonology may involve bronchodilators, corticosteroids, mucolytics, or antibiotics. In addition, non-pharmacological interventions like oxygen therapy, respiratory therapy, airway clearance techniques, or pulmonary rehabilitation may be recommended for children with respiratory compromise or chronic lung diseases in order to optimize oxygenation, strengthen the respiratory muscles, and improve lung function. Additionally, to fully address the needs of children with complex respiratory conditions, pediatric pulmonologists work closely with multidisciplinary teams. This includes providing nutritional support, psychosocial interventions, genetic counseling, and, when necessary, surgical interventions. To maximize long-term results, they also offer patients and their families education and support, equipping them with the information and abilities necessary to properly manage respiratory disorders, identify early warning signs, and follow treatment plans.

A key component of pediatric pulmonology is preventive care and health promotion, which emphasizes the value of immunizations, environmental controls, quitting smoking, and lifestyle changes to lower the risk of respiratory infections, exacerbations, and complications in kids with underlying lung diseases or risk factors. Pediatric pulmonologists work to improve overall well-being, maximize functional capacity, and improves the quality of life for children with respiratory disorders by promoting respiratory health and disease prevention. This helps to foster optimal growth, development, and participation in daily activities.

Orientation and Directional Terms

Term	Definition	Illustration
Pharmacotherapy	Defined as medical treatment that utilizes one or more pharmaceutical drugs to improve ongoing symptoms, treat the underlying condition, or act as a prevention for other diseases.	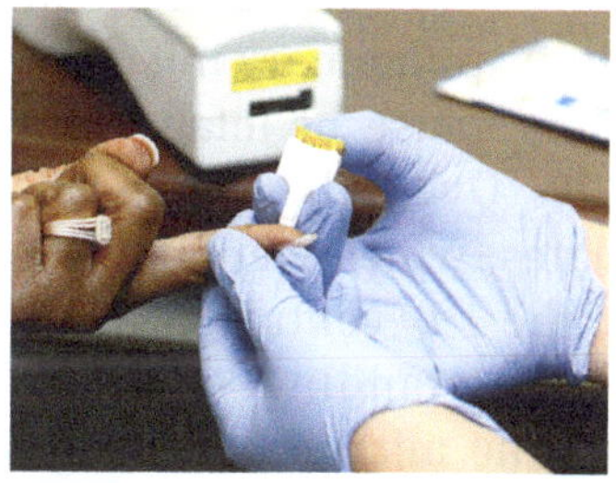
Respiratory syncytial virus (RSV)	A contagious virus that causes infections of the respiratory tract. It is a negative-sense, single-stranded RNA virus. Its name is derived from the large cells known as syncytia that form when infected cells fuse.	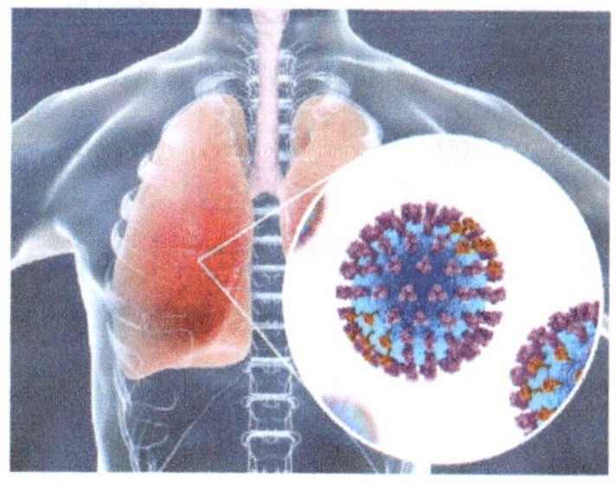
Rhinovirus	A positive-sense, single-stranded RNA virus belonging to the genus Enterovirus in the family Picornaviridae.	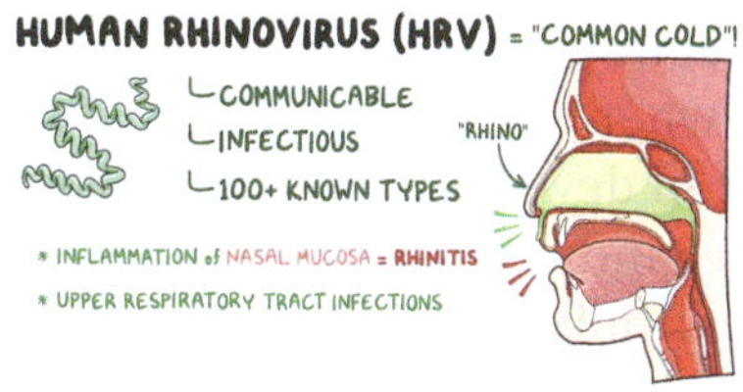
Microbiome	Collection of all microbes, such as bacteria, fungi, viruses, and their genes, that naturally live on our bodies and inside us.	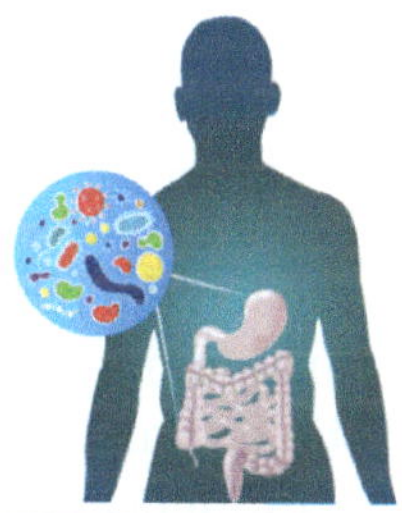
Computed tomography	A medical imaging technique used to obtain detailed internal images of the body. The personnel who perform CT scans are called radiographers or radiology technologists.	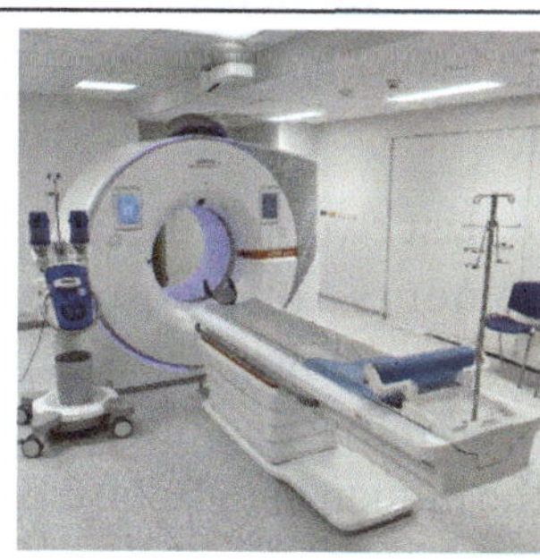

1.1. Pediatric Respiratory Infections

In addition to causing a significant burden of morbidity, pulmonary infections continue to be a leading cause of infant and child mortality globally. Over the past 125 years, Koch's postulates, which were developed in the latter half of the 19th century, have greatly influenced our understanding of infectious diseases. Finding the microbes causing serious illnesses like meningococcal meningitis, pneumococcal pneumonia, influenza, and tuberculosis was made possible thanks in large part to this method. Consequently, these discoveries paved the way for the creation of targeted treatments, such as antibiotics for bacterial infections and immunization programs for many of the more dangerous organisms. But as we pass from a time when infectious respiratory diseases frequently resulted in childhood deaths to one where mortality is now extremely low, at least in developed nations, the focus is shifting more and more toward the effects of more chronic infectious diseases and the mechanisms underlying acute but treatable infectious diseases. The shortcomings of the conventional Koch one-organism/one-disease model have been brought to light by the identification of the significance of biofilms in long-term illnesses like persistent bacterial bronchitis, chronic otitis media, and chronic sinusitis, the bacterial–viral interactions linked to even the most common cold, and the influence of complex microbiota in the gut and airways on a range of chronic diseases.

The past two decades have seen enormous advancements in sequencing and other technologies, which are beginning to have a substantial impact on our understanding of the role of the human body as an environmental niche colonized by a vast number of microorganisms that can have a variety of effects on the host's health, all of which are influenced by the host response and other environmental factors. Moreover, the epidemiology of infectious disease outbreaks and the evolution of organisms in response to environmental stressors like the availability of nutrients, antibiotics, and the introduction of novel organisms from the environment or other humans are now being better-understood thanks to the application of this technology.

1.1.1. Contrasting Impacts of Acute Respiratory Infections in Developing and Developed Countries

The disparities in the difficulties that the various healthcare systems face are illustrated by contrasting data on hospitalizations for "radiologically proven pneumonia" from North America with data on infant and child mortality from rural Kenya. While infant mortality nearly halved over the 8 years (2003–2010) of the study, childhood mortality (60 and 20 per 1000 live births, respectively) in rural Kenya remains very high when compared to that seen in developed countries. While respiratory infections were the most common cause of death during the entire period, by 2010 infant mortality from malaria had surpassed respiratory infections, accounting for the majority of the reduction in mortality. On the other hand, a study conducted in the United States of America found that the rate of hospital admission for pneumonia with radiological proof was only 6.2 per 1000 for infants and 1.6 per 1000 for children. There were only three fatalities among the 2358 children admitted to the hospital. It's interesting to note that 33% of study participants had a diagnosis of "asthma" or "reactive airways disease." The low rates of respiratory infection-related death in developed countries are likely the result of many factors, including better sanitation, low exposure to biofuel combustion, nutrition, easy access to antibiotics, and vaccination.

1.1.2. Diagnosis of Pneumonia and Acute Lower Respiratory Tract Infections

The well-established conclusion that no single sign, or even combination of signs, reliably identified infants with pneumonia was confirmed by a systematic review of numerous papers addressing the usefulness of a wide range of signs in accurately identifying infants with pneumonia. The World Health Organization's (WHO) respiratory rate-based approach, as pointed out in an editorial, significantly overestimates the incidence of pneumonia; however, it was created to guarantee the early administration of antibiotics in low-resource nations in an attempt to reduce the high mortality rates. The editorial continues by highlighting the importance of immunization and the demand for more accurate point-of-care diagnostics, potentially built around metabolomics techniques. The systematic review's findings call into serious doubt the applicability of recommendations like the pediatric pneumonia guidelines from the British Thoracic Society, which essentially ignore data demonstrating the low specificity of clinical assessment.

1.1.3. Identification of Pathogens and Relationship to Disease and Disease Severity

Only a small percentage of cases had bacterial pathogens identified; the majority had viruses, mainly rhinovirus in older children and respiratory syncytial virus (RSV) in younger subjects. Depending on the age group, 15–30% of cases had multiple viruses or a combination of bacteria and viruses identified. Whenever a "respiratory pathogen" is found in the airways of patients experiencing an acute illness, there is an inevitable temptation to attribute a causal relationship. Potential bacterial pathogens like *Haemophilus influenzae* species, *Moraxella catarrhalis*, and *Streptococcus pneumoniae* are frequently found in the nose and nasopharynx of seemingly asymptomatic individuals, as has long been known. The same is true for viruses, as demonstrated by several studies, which show that asymptomatic individuals are less likely than symptomatic ones to have certain "respiratory" viruses detected. The type of rhinovirus (A, B, or C) did not significantly affect the likelihood of symptoms in conjunction with a positive swab (19% for the upper respiratory tract and/or 14% for the lower respiratory tract). Not a single baby was admitted to the hospital. In a related study using a panel of viruses, 795 (or 39%) of the samples had a virus identified, and 228 of these samples had two or more viruses. The most often discovered virus was, predictably, the rhinovirus. Of the 53% of positive samples, a virus was found in 28% of the asymptomatic infants. Of the asymptomatic subjects who had experienced upper respiratory symptoms in the previous week, an additional 75 (51%) samples tested positive. The odds ratio between an asymptomatic infant with RSV and a positive viral identification in a symptomatic subject (again, all relatively mild community infections) was determined by the authors to be 11.7. RSV, hMPV, influenza, and adenovirus were found in significantly higher concentrations in community-acquired pneumonia cases compared to healthy controls; however, rhinovirus, and other viruses, including bocavirus, were not detected in the same proportions. These results were essentially corroborated by a more comprehensive systematic review of published literature on acute lower respiratory tract infections, which found strong evidence for the causative attribution of RSV (OR 9.8), influenza (OR 5.0), parainfluenza (OR 3.4), and hMPV (OR 3.8).

A close relationship between the quantity and duration of respiratory symptoms and the levels of interleukin (IL)-8 and neutrophils in the upper airway is relevant to the discussion of both symptomatic and asymptomatic infections. This finding supports previous research that highlighted the role of IL-8, neutrophils, and their products in the development of symptoms brought on by "respiratory" viruses. The interplay of bacteria and viruses in the respiratory system has long been known. A significant amount of the deaths in the 1919 pandemic were caused by staphylococcal pneumonia, which followed an influenza infection; chickenpox predisposes to severe group A streptococcal pneumonia and infection at other sites; and more recently, research has focused on the role of viruses in changing the behavior of biofilms during exacerbations. The load of potentially pathogenic bacteria in the nose and nasopharynx seems to be a bigger factor influencing the severity of even a simple "cold" than the mere presence of a respiratory virus, which, as previously mentioned, may not even cause any symptoms. Research conducted in South Africa employing the conjugate pneumococcal vaccine revealed decreases in admissions attributed to apparent "viral-induced lower respiratory tract infection," thereby underscoring the impact of bacteria on the consequences of viruses. More and more, we are realizing that a microbe needs to compete and/or work with other microbes in addition to interacting with the host and its defenses. The host response, which is primarily mediated by neutrophils (whose products not only drive symptoms but also provide the coloration of the nasal discharge), will determine the Sino-Nasal Outcome Test score of a cold. The type of virus, viral load, and presence of potentially pathogenic bacteria are likely to drive the magnitude of this response.

1.1.4. Microbiome

The capacity to perform in-depth genetic sequencing is revealing more about the residing populations, which seem to view any bodily niche as a possible home. Research utilizing 16S ribosomal RNA sequencing to ascertain bacterial populations has demonstrated the immense quantity and variety of organisms present in the mouth and nose, as well as the significant distinctions between them. Populations are dynamic and subject to sudden changes. These populations are both relatively resilient, often returning to pre-disruption patterns relatively quickly in many cases, and susceptible to disruption from interventions such as contracting a virus or being exposed to antibiotics. Although the existence of a pulmonary microbiome remains somewhat uncertain, well-conducted studies indicate that even in healthy individuals, the lower airway is most likely colonized. According to two recent studies, the main method by which organisms establish themselves in the lower airway appears to be micro-aspiration rather than inhalation. Owing to the extreme sensitivity of these techniques, these studies must be carried out with extreme caution, both in terms of sample collection and quality control during the processing of the samples. This is because there have been instances where seemingly significant results have been entirely explained away by contamination, either in the sample itself or in the reagents used to process the samples. Data interpretation needs to be done cautiously because of issues like these and the dynamic, ever-changing populations.

1.1.5. Imaging

To improve the usefulness of images as an end-point in clinical trials, a group from Perth, Australia, and their partners in the Netherlands have published a more sensitive computed tomography (CT) scoring system for use in cystic fibrosis. The most notable aspect is probably the extremely low radiation doses needed, which, when combined with the best scanners available, allay previous worries about using CT to track the progression of cystic fibrosis. In fact, the evidence indicates that it is unethical to fail to ensure that imaging is optimized to guarantee the use of such low radiation levels, rather than that employing this strategy is unethical. MRI is useful for pulmonary imaging in cystic fibrosis patients, but it is not as sensitive as CT imaging—at least not in their hands. They did, however, suggest doing more research on its applicability.

1.1.6. Acute Bronchiolitis

The Cochrane review's findings that hypertonic saline may help treat acute bronchiolitis were not supported by many studies, which added another ineffective intervention to the long list. The effect of giving arbitrary oxygen dosages on hospital stay length in a carefully planned, randomized, double-blind study with more than 500 infants. Patients who had their oxygen therapy stopped when their room air saturations stayed above 90% were released from the hospital much faster and without any negative side effects. However, since the focus of this study was oxygen weaning, the findings should not be construed as supporting the safe discharge of infants at an early stage of illness if their saturation is greater than 90%.

1.1.7. Maternal Immunization

Several countries have recently implemented routine immunization of pregnant mothers against pertussis to address the rising mortality observed in very young infants who contract the illness before receiving their vaccinations. Numerous studies have examined the effects of this policy change; research from the USA and the UK suggests that the strategy seems safe and effective. However, a very recent study has drawn attention to the influence of maternal immunization on the response to postnatal pertussis vaccination and other vaccines in the routine immunization program that are conjugated with the variant of diphtheria toxin. Some studies show that when pregnant women receive the influenza vaccine, there is a decrease in morbidity in both the mothers and the babies. Given seasonal and annual variations in disease severity and incidence, the effect is not as significant as that seen with pertussis, and the authors acknowledge the difficulties in interpreting the data and making recommendations. The RSV vaccine working group and the minutes of a WHO meeting regarding vaccines for this particularly problematic respiratory virus have long supported the same strategy.

1.1.8. Sequencing as a Clinical and Research Tool

Sequencing and omics platforms are influencing microbiome research and could become increasingly important in diagnostics as metabolomics matures. A report on the application of whole-exome sequencing to improve the identification of the underlying genetic defect in patients with primary ciliary dyskinesia and a study where the results of whole-genome sequencing suggested that the risk of *Mycobacterium abscessus* transmission within a clinical setting appears to be very low (despite the presence of genetically identical organisms in a sibling pair) are two more examples of potent gene-sequencing techniques that have been introduced into the clinical space. Further evidence from sequencing supports the idea that RSV has successfully adapted to survive without significant antigenic shifts or the evolution of numerous subtypes. Sequencing also shows that RSV is subject to comparatively few evolutionary pressures. In summary, studies published in the past year have once again brought attention to the stark differences in respiratory mortality between countries with high and low resources for newborns and young children. As better preventative strategies are sought, the traditional major respiratory pathogens will still receive a lot of attention; however, host-microbiome interactions are becoming more and more important in the development and/or maintenance of chronic illness. This has been made easier by the decade-long rapid advancements in sequencing technology, which will eventually likely result in the development of novel strategies for the management and prevention of acute and chronic respiratory illnesses (Adegbola et al., 1994; Adegbola et al., 1999; Addo-Yobo et al., 2004).

1.2. Acute Respiratory Infections in Children

Both upper and lower respiratory tract infections (URIs) and acute respiratory infections (ARIs) fall under this classification (LRIs). From the nostrils to the vocal cords in the larynx, the upper respiratory tract comprises the middle ear and paranasal sinuses. From the trachea and bronchi to the bronchioles and alveoli, the airways continue to form the lower respiratory tract. Because of the potential spread of infection or microbial toxins, inflammation, and decreased lung function, ARIs are not limited to the respiratory tract and can have systemic effects. In addition to affecting other systems, vaccine-preventable diseases like measles, pertussis, and diphtheria can cause whooping cough and other respiratory tract complications. No matter where they live or their financial status, children under five experience three to six episodes of ARIs on average each year, making them the most common cause of illness and mortality outside of the neonatal period. However, the percentage of mild to severe disease varies between high- and low-income countries. Additionally, the severity of LRIs in children under five is worse in developing countries due to variations in specific etiologies and risk factors, leading to a higher case-fatality rate. Many severe LRIs do not respond to therapy, primarily due to the lack of highly effective antiviral drugs, even though medical care can somewhat mitigate both severity and fatality. Approximately 10.8 million children pass away annually. 1.9 million of them are estimated to have died from ARIs in 2000, with 70% of those deaths occurring in Africa and Southeast Asia. An estimated 2 million children under five pass away from pneumonia every year, according to the World Health Organization (WHO).

1.2.1. Causes of ARIs and the Burden of Disease

ARIs in children take a heavy toll on life, especially where medical care is not available or is not sought.

1.2.1.1. Upper Respiratory Tract Infections

The most prevalent infectious diseases are URIs. These comprise laryngitis, tonsillopharyngitis, sinusitis, ear infections, rhinitis (common cold), and acute pharyngitis or tonsillopharyngitis. Of these, pharyngitis, and ear infections are responsible for the more serious side effects, which include acute rheumatic fever and deafness, respectively. The etiology of the great majority of URIs is viral. 25–30% of URIs are caused by rhinoviruses; the remaining percentage is caused by respiratory syncytial viruses (RSVs), parainfluenza, and influenza viruses, human metapneumovirus, and adenoviruses; 10% are caused by coronaviruses; and the remaining viruses are unknown. The complications of URIs are more significant than the infections themselves because most URIs are self-limiting. Children with acute viral infections are at risk for bacterial infections of the sinuses and middle ear, and lung respiratory infections (LRIs) can arise from aspirating infected secretions and cells.

- **Acute Pharyngitis:** More than 70% of cases of acute pharyngitis in young children are caused by viruses. Tonsil enlargement and mild pharyngeal redness and swelling are common. Infection with streptococci is more common in older children and rarer in children under five. Poststreptococcal sequelae like acute rheumatic fever and carditis are common in school-age children but can also occur in children under five in countries where living conditions are crowded and populations may have a genetic predisposition. In developing nations, *Corynebacterium diphtheriae* almost invariably causes acute pharyngitis along with the formation of a membrane on the throat. However, diphtheria is rare now that infants are almost universally vaccinated against diphtheria, tetanus, and pertussis (DTP).

- **Acute Ear Infection:** Up to 30% of URIs result in an acute ear infection. It may result in perforated eardrums, chronic ear discharge in later childhood, and eventually hearing impairment or deafness in developing nations with inadequate medical care. In developing nations, 2–6% of school-age children suffer from chronic ear infections, which develop from recurrent episodes of acute ear infections. The resulting hearing loss could be incapacitating and have an impact on education. Mastoiditis, which can result from recurrent ear infections, can transmit infection to the meninges. Approximately 5% of ARI deaths globally are caused by mastoiditis and other URI complications.

1.2.1.2. Lower Respiratory Tract Infections

Pneumonia and bronchiolitis are the prevalent LRIs in children. When a child is coughing and breathing quickly, the respiratory rate is a useful clinical indicator for identifying acute lung injury (LRI). More information is revealed by the lower chest wall indrawing. RSVs are currently the most frequent cause of viral LRIs. Unlike parainfluenza viruses, which are the next most common cause of viral LRIs, they are typically highly seasonal. Since safe and effective vaccines are available, the epidemiology of influenza viruses in children in developing countries warrants immediate investigation. The measles virus was the primary viral cause of respiratory tract-related morbidity and mortality in children in developing nations prior to the widespread use of the measles vaccine.

- **Pneumonia:** Pneumonia can be brought on by viruses or bacteria. *Haemophilus influenzae*, primarily type b (Hib), or *Streptococcus pneumoniae* (pneumococcus) are the most common causes of bacterial pneumonia. *Staphylococcus aureus* or other streptococci can also occasionally cause bacterial pneumonia. Most cases of bacterial pneumonia are caused by just 8 to 12 of the numerous varieties of pneumococcus, though the exact types can differ between adults and children as well as between different geographical areas. Atypical pneumonias are caused by other pathogens, including *Chlamydia pneumoniae* and *Mycoplasma pneumoniae*. It is unclear how they contribute to serious illness in children under five in developing nations. The amount of LRIs brought on by *S. pneumoniae* is challenging to identify because the sensitivity and specificity of current methods for determining bacterial etiology are lacking. Pharyngeal culture findings don't always identify the pathogen causing the LRI. Although lung aspirate specimen bacterial cultures are frequently regarded as the gold standard, they are not useful in the field.

  An estimate of the disease burden that

can be prevented by vaccination is provided by lower levels of clinical or radiological pneumonia in clinical trials of a nine-valent pneumococcal conjugate vaccine (valency denoting the number of serotypes against which the vaccine offers protection; conjugate refers to conjugation of polysaccharides to a protein backbone). 37% of radiological pneumonia cases were avoided in a study conducted in The Gambia, which indicates the extent of *S. pneumoniae* illness, and there was a 16% decrease in mortality. Aspiration of contaminated secretions and colonization of the upper respiratory tract by potentially pathogenic organisms have been linked to the pathophysiology of bacterial pneumonia in young children. It has been demonstrated that upper respiratory tract infections with influenza viruses or RSVs increase the binding of both *H. influenzae* as well as *S. pneumoniae* to the nasopharyngeal lining cells. This discovery could clarify why pneumococcal pneumonia rates rise in tandem with influenza and RSV outbreaks. According to a South African study, vaccination with a nine-valent pneumococcal conjugate vaccine decreased the incidence of hospitalization-causing virus-associated pneumonia by 31%, indicating a significant role for pneumococcus in the pathophysiology of virus-associated pneumonia.

Although the pathophysiology of Gram-negative organisms has also been linked to the entry of gut bacteria that travel through the bloodstream to the lungs, these bacteria are rare etiological agents of pneumonia in children with healthy immune systems. However, Gram-negative pneumonia is not uncommon in newborns and early infants (Quiambao forthcoming). In developing nations, 40–50% of infections in infants and children hospitalized for pneumonia are caused by viruses. The most common causes of viral pneumonia are the measles virus, RSVs, parainfluenza viruses, influenza type A virus, and adenoviruses. It can be challenging to distinguish radiographically between viral and bacterial cases of pneumonia due to the similar appearance of the lesions and the possibility of bacterial superinfection with RSV, measles, and influenza. Children with bacterial pneumonia have a case-fatality rate of 10 to 14%, mixed viral and bacterial infections of 16 to 18%, and viral pneumonia of 1 to 7% in developing nations.

2. **Bronchiolitis**: In the first year of life, bronchiolitis is more common than in the second and third, when it is less common. The symptoms include wheezing, fever in one-third of the cases, rapid breathing, and lower chest wall indrawing. Lung segments collapse due to inflammatory blockage of the small airways, causing hyperinflation of the lungs. Health professionals may find it challenging to distinguish between bronchiolitis and pneumonia because the signs and symptoms of both conditions are similar. The ability to identify wheezing and a description of the seasonality of RSVs in the area are two characteristics that might be useful. During peak season, RSVs can cause up to 70 or 80% of LRIs and are the primary cause of bronchiolitis globally. A bronchiolitis that is identical to RSV disease is also caused by the recently identified human metapneumovirus.

In addition to influenza viruses, parainfluenza virus type 3 is another virus that causes bronchiolitis.

3. **Influenza**: Influenza viruses are known to be a significant cause of lower respiratory infections (LRIs) in children and may be the second most common cause of hospitalization for children with acute respiratory infections (ARIs), even though they typically cause URIs in adults. Even though influenza is thought to be uncommon in developing nations, there is still much to learn about its epidemiology. The extent to which influenza may contribute to child fatalities is uncertain. Type A and type B influenza viruses can cause seasonal outbreaks and sporadic infections, respectively. In a few Asian nations, the avian influenza virus has recently resulted in infection, illness, and death in a small number of people, including children. It is unknown if it will surface in human outbreaks or a pandemic, but it could have disastrous effects on developing nations and be a global health threat. Type A virus strains will most likely mutate to produce new strains, as happened with the Asian and Hong Kong pandemics in the 1950s and 1960s.

1.2.1.3. HIV Infection and Pediatric LRIs

85% of the 3.2 million children living with HIV/AIDS worldwide are in Sub-Saharan Africa. HIV-related LRIs account for 30 to 40% of pediatric admissions in southern Africa, and their case-fatality rate is 15 to 34%, which is significantly higher than the 5 to 10% rate for children who are not HIV-positive. In more than half of infants with HIV, *Pneumocystis jiroveci* and cytomegalovirus are significant opportunistic infections. Gram-negative bacteria play a significant role in over 70% of HIV-positive malnourished children. Studies on patients have confirmed that these bacteria are frequently associated with *S. pneumoniae* in addition to *S. aureus* as significant microorganisms. According to the first South African report on the total burden of invasive pneumococcal disease, the proportion of HIV-positive children compared to uninfected children was 41.7 times higher (Adegbola et al., 1994; Adegbola et al., 1999; Addo-Yobo et al., 2004).

1.2.2. Interventions

Four main categories can be used to classify interventions to control ARIs: environmental safety, early disease detection and treatment, nutrition improvements, and vaccination against particular pathogens. The health system is responsible for the first two, while public health is in charge of the final two, which call for multisectoral participation.

1.2.2.1. Vaccinations

Vaccinations against influenza, Hib, pneumococcus, measles, diphtheria, pertussis, and Hib should be widely used as this could significantly lower the incidence of ARIs in children in developing nations. The effects of vaccinations against measles, diphtheria, and pertussis The scant information on influenza in developing nations prevents a thorough examination of the vaccine's possible advantages. Thus, the focus of this chapter is on how vaccinations against pneumococcal and Hib may affect low-risk infants.

1.2.2.1.1. Hib Vaccine

There are currently three Hib conjugate vaccinations available for use in newborns and early childhood. Numerous studies conducted in developed nations and one in The Gambia have conclusively shown that the Hib vaccine is effective in preventing invasive diseases, primarily meningitis but also pneumonia. Regardless of the vaccine selected, every study demonstrated a protective efficacy of over 90% against invasive disease confirmed in a lab. Because of the immunity that the Hib vaccine confers on recipients and the herd effect that protects the unvaccinated, invasive Hib disease has all but disappeared in industrialized nations thanks to the inclusion of the Hib vaccine in national immunization programs. There is evidence of a similar herd effect in a few developing nations. Although the initial promise of the Hib vaccine and the resulting general perception were that it would protect against meningitis, it is more likely to prevent LRIs in developing nations. The easily quantifiable impact is on invasive illnesses like bacteremic pneumonia. Although there is currently no reliable way to determine the bacterial etiology of non-bacteremic pneumonia, the vaccine most likely has some effect in this regard. However, this effect is difficult to measure. The Hib vaccination has been linked to a 20–30% decrease in hospital admissions for radiographically confirmed pneumonia in Bangladesh, Brazil, Chile, and The Gambia. On the other hand, the Hib vaccine's impact on pneumonia remained unclear based on the findings of a sizable study conducted in Lombok, Indonesia.

1.2.2.1.2. Pneumococcal Vaccines

Pneumococci can currently be prevented with two different vaccines: the 23-valent polysaccharide vaccine (23-PSV), which is recommended for adults rather than children, and the 7-valent protein-conjugated polysaccharide vaccine (7-PCV). The Philippines is currently testing an 11-valent vaccine (11-PCV), while South Africa and The Gambia have conducted clinical trials for a 9-valent vaccine (9-PCV). Research on the polysaccharide vaccine's effectiveness in shielding children in developed nations from ear infections or ARIs has produced mixed findings. Studies in Finland demonstrate a generally protective effect against the serotypes found in a 14-PSV, despite certain studies on this vaccine demonstrating no discernible efficacy. Comparing older children to younger ones, the efficacy was more pronounced in the former group. Papua New Guinea conducted three trials that are the only studies assessing the effectiveness of the polysaccharide vaccine in children from developing nations. Following vaccination, there was a 50% decrease in LRI mortality in children under two and a 59% reduction in LRI mortality in children under five, according to the analysis of the pooled data from these trials. Based on the results of these and additional investigations, the researchers concluded that the vaccine affected severe pneumonia. Due to the higher contribution of adult serotypes that are more immunogenic to pneumonia in Papua New Guinea, these trials' efficacy was higher than anticipated. These days, efforts are focused on developing more immunogenic conjugate vaccines due to the 23-PSV antigens' poor immunogenicity against common pediatric serotypes.

In four trials, the 7-PCV and 9-PCV were tested for their effectiveness against invasive pneumococcal disease. The results showed that the vaccines were effective against the disease at rates of 71.0 to 97.4% (58 to 65% for children who are HIV-positive, whose rates of pneumococcal disease are 40 times higher than those of HIV-negative children). In 2000, vaccinations against the 7-PCV were made routine for infants and children under two years old in the United States. In this age group, the incidence of all invasive pneumococcal disease had decreased by 69% by 2001, and the disease caused by the vaccine's included serotypes and related serotypes had decreased by 78%. A study conducted in northern California confirmed similar reductions. Although there was a small increase in the rates of invasive disease brought on by pneumococcus serotypes that were left out of the vaccine, it was not significant enough to counteract the vaccine's significant reduction in disease. The studies also revealed a noteworthy decline in invasive pneumococcal disease in older unvaccinated age groups, particularly in adults aged 65 and above and in adults aged 20 to 39. These findings imply that immunizing young children had a sizable herd effect in the community. This benefit is probably going to happen even in situations where adult HIV infection is highly prevalent and pneumococcal illness is potentially fatal and recurrent. It is challenging to determine the vaccine's impact on pneumococcal pneumonia in general because of the difficulties in determining the bacterial cause of pneumonia. The vaccine has been shown to reduce radiographically confirmed pneumonia by 20–37% in three studies that assessed its impact on the condition (regardless of the etiological agent). HIV-positive individuals have shown a reduction of 9–10% in radiographically confirmed pneumonia. The effectiveness of PCV in preventing ear infections has been assessed in multiple field trials. Despite the vaccine's notable reduction in culture-confirmed pneumococcal otitis, there was no discernible net decrease in ear infections in children who received the shot. This is likely due to a rise in otitis caused by pneumococci that the vaccine does not cover, such as *Moraxella catarrhalis* and *H influenzae*. Nonetheless, a trial conducted in northern California revealed that the vaccination decreased the need for tympanostomy tube implantation and provided protection against recurrent ear infections. Therefore, clinical trials should be conducted to assess the potential benefits of an ear infection vaccine in developing nations with high rates of conductive hearing loss and chronic otitis. In developing nations, a vaccine's most notable public health benefit would be a discernible drop in mortality. Initially, child mortality was the main outcome of the Gambia trial; however, later on, radiological pneumonia took precedence. However, a 16% (95% confidence level, 3 to 38) decrease in mortality was demonstrated by the trial. In a remote region of eastern Gambia, this trial was carried out where it is challenging to provide access to 24-hour curative care, including case management. This trial shows that immunizations administered through outreach programs will benefit these populations significantly in terms of both health and finances. Results from another study assessing the impact of an 11-PCV on radiological pneumonia are anticipated in the latter part of 2005; the study is currently underway in the Philippines.

1.2.2.2. Case Management

In developing nations with limited access to pediatricians, the systematization and simplification of case management for the early diagnosis and treatment of ARIs have resulted in notable declines in mortality. The two primary clinical indicators used by WHO clinical guidelines for ARI case management are lower chest wall indrawing, which indicates severe pneumonia requiring hospital admission and referral, and respiratory rate, which separates children with pneumonia from those without. Referrals are also necessary for children who exhibit danger indicators of a serious illness, such as the inability to feed, or who exhibit audible stridor when calm and at rest. Without these symptoms, children are diagnosed with an ARI rather than pneumonia. Outpatient antibiotic therapy is used to treat pneumonia in children who are only breathing rapidly. Children who have had a cough for longer than 30 days are referred for additional testing to rule out other chronic infections such as tuberculosis.

1.2.2.3. Pneumonia Diagnosis Based on Rapid Breathing

In the 1970s, Papua New Guinea developed the first guidelines for using rapid breathing to diagnose pneumonia. 72% of children with audible crackles in their lungs had a respiratory rate of 50 or more breaths per minute, compared to only 19% of children without crackles in a study involving 200 consecutive pediatric outpatients and 50 consecutive admissions. As a result, a child with a cough was considered to have pneumonia if their breathing rate was 50 breaths per minute or higher, according to the original WHO guidelines. The main cause for concern was this the comparatively low sensitivity, which could miss 25–40% of pneumonia cases. According to a study conducted in Vellore, India, sensitivity could be increased by reducing the cutoff point for infants aged 2 months to 11 months to 40 breaths per minute, while maintaining the 50 breaths per minute threshold for children aged 1 to 4. Further research revealed that when these thresholds were applied, the specificity decreased from 92 to 80% in Swaziland and from 65 to 77% in the Philippines, but the sensitivity increased from 62 to 79% in both countries. The WHO suggests a respiratory rate cutoff of 50 breaths per minute for infants aged 2 to 11 months and 40 breaths per minute for children aged 12 months to 5 years, based on these and other data.

The World Health Organization defines rapid breathing as a sign that can detect around 85% of children with pneumonia. Using the WHO diagnostic criteria, over 80% of children with potentially fatal pneumonia can be successfully identified and treated. Antibiotic treatment for children showing rapid breathing has been proven to lower mortality rates. However, the downside is that this criterion has low specificity, leading to the unnecessary prescription of antibiotics in 70 to 80% of cases where they may not be needed. Despite this drawback, for primary care workers in need of a simple diagnostic tool, rapid breathing remains the most useful clinical sign (Table 1.1).

1.2.2.4. Pneumonia Diagnosis Based on Chest Wall Indrawing

When medical professionals think that oxygen or parenteral antibiotics—antibiotics given by a method other than oral means—are necessary, or when they don't think mothers will be able to handle the situation, children with severe pneumonia are admitted to the hospital. Parenteral antibiotics are used to increase antibiotic levels and allay worries about oral medication absorption in sick children. The primary indicator of severity in the Papua New Guinea study was chest wall indrawing; however, due to differing definitions, studies conducted globally reveal significant variations in the rates of indrawing. Limiting the term to lower chest wall indrawing—which is defined as an inward movement of the chest wall's bony structures with inspiration—has produced a more accurate and teachable indicator of pneumonia severity. Compared to intercostal indrawing, which frequently happens in bronchiolitis, it is more specific.

For a year, a group of 500 children, aged one to four, received weekly home visits as part of a research study conducted in The Gambia. 222 cases of LRI—which include rapid breathing, any indrawing of the chest wall, nasal flaring, wheezing, stridor, or warning signs—were referred to the clinic during this time. 62% of these cases had chest indrawing, many of which also had intercostal indrawing. The number of hospitalized children with chest in drawings would overwhelm pediatric inpatient facilities. Research conducted in Swaziland and the Philippines revealed that when diagnosing severe pneumonia that necessitates hospital admission, lower chest wall indrawing was more specific than intercostal indrawing. Lower chest wall indrawing accurately predicted 79% of children with an LRI who were admitted to a pediatric hospital in the Vellore study.

1.2.2.5. Antimicrobial Options for Oral Treatment of Pneumonia

Based on the well-established fact that *S. pneumoniae* is the primary cause of most childhood bacterial cases of pneumonia, an antimicrobial drug is selected for treatment. Despite being long-lasting, a single injection of benzathine penicillin is insufficient to eradicate *H. influenzae*. Technical documents from WHO can be used to compare various antimicrobials based on their antibacterial activity, treatment efficacy, and toxicity, as well as to evaluate the pertinent factors in choosing first- and second-line antibiotics. The development of resistance to antibiotics in *S. pneumoniae* in addition to *H. influenzae* is a significant risk. In certain conditions, *in vitro* experiments reveal that over 50% of respiratory isolates of both bacteria are penicillin- and co-trimoxazole-resistant. Pneumonia is starting to cause problems on a global scale. Unlike meningitis, pneumonia does not always result in treatment failure due to the pathogen's *in vitro* resistance. According to reports from South Africa and Spain, penicillin-resistant *S. pneumoniae* may be the cause. Penicillin at high enough dosages is an effective treatment for pneumonia. Amoxicillin is concentrated in tissues and macrophages, and oral dosages and drug levels are positively correlated. Consequently, penicillin-resistant *S. pneumoniae* ear infections are now being successfully treated with higher doses—twice daily—than in the past. Amoxicillin is unquestionably superior to penicillin in treating these infections. It's unclear how co-trimoxazole works, and since co-trimoxazole resistance is common, amoxicillin might be a better option for kids with severe pneumonia.

1.2.2.6. Intramuscular Antibiotics for Treatment of Severe Pneumonia

Although chloramphenicol works against both *S. pneumoniae* in addition to *H. influenzae*, in very sick children, its oral absorption is irregular. Therefore, before an urgent referral of a case of severe pneumonia, the WHO guidelines recommend administering intramuscular chloramphenicol at half the daily dose. Another justification is that critically ill children might have meningitis or sepsis, which is difficult to rule out and needs to be treated right away. While intramuscular chloramphenicol is inferior to intravenous chloramphenicol, the process can increase the cost of treatment and cause a delay in critically needed care. The effectiveness and safety of intramuscular chloramphenicol have been questioned by investigators. The intramuscular route gained widespread acceptance after clinical reports confirmed its efficacy, despite early studies suggesting that adult blood levels after intramuscular administration were significantly lower than those achieved after intravenous administration. Unlike the previous intramuscular preparations, local complications from intramuscular chloramphenicol succinate are uncommon. While aplastic anemia after chloramphenicol is a common concern, very few young children experience this complication. No proof administering chloramphenicol succinate intramuscularly increases the risk of side effects in comparison to other dosage forms and administration methods.

1.2.2.7. Hypoxemia Diagnosis Based on WHO Criteria

Accurately referring sick children to a hospital and appropriately managing LRI with oxygen or antibiotics while they are inpatient are essential components of the ARI case management and integrated management of infant and childhood illness (IMCI) strategies. Hypoxemia, or low blood oxygen levels in children with lung respiratory illness (LRI), is a strong indicator of death; the case-fatality rate in hypoxemic LRI is 1–4 times higher than in nonhypoxemic LRI, and oxygen lowers death. To prevent death, it is crucial to identify hypoxemia in children with LRI as soon as possible. While diagnosing tachypnea is a relatively simple process for acute LRIs, and chest wall indrawing is a common sign of severe LRIs, diagnosing hypoxemia clinically is a more challenging task. Various clinical rule sets have been investigated to predict if hypoxemia will be present in children with LRI. Using these criteria would still miss a significant number of hypoxemic children, even though some clinical tools have a high sensitivity for detecting hypoxemia. The most effective method for promptly identifying hypoxemia in sick children is pulse oximetry. Nevertheless, most district or even referral hospitals in developing nations do not have pulse oximeters available due to their high cost and ongoing probe replacement expenses.

1.2.2.8. Treatment Guidelines

For children with pneumonia, the current recommendations are intramuscular penicillin or chloramphenicol, and co-trimoxazole twice daily for five days. Studies looking into alternatives to the antibiotics currently used in ARI case management have been prompted by issues with growing co-trimoxazole resistance and needless referrals of kids with any kind of chest wall indrawing. According to one study, amoxicillin, and co-trimoxazole work just as well for treating mild cases of pneumonia, but amoxicillin is twice as expensive as co-trimoxazole. Research conducted in Bangladesh, India, and Indonesia suggests that for children with non-severe pneumonia, three days of oral co-trimoxazole or amoxicillin is just as effective as five days of the medication. In a multicenter trial, children with severe pneumonia were treated with intramuscular penicillin rather than oral amoxicillin. This regimen is not suitable for treating severe pneumonia as an outpatient because patients were treated with oxygen when hypoxemia was detected and were moved to other antibiotics if the treatment did not work. The World Health Organization (WHO) advises providing oxygen to children who exhibit severe pneumonia symptoms and signs if there is an adequate supply. If oxygen availability is limited, children should receive oxygen if they exhibit any of the following symptoms: cyanosis, inability to eat or drink, a respiratory rate of 70 breaths per minute or more, or severe chest wall retractions. For children under two months old, the recommended oxygen administration rate is 0.5 liters per minute, while for older children, the rate is 1 liter per minute. Given the high cost and limited availability of oxygen, particularly in remote rural areas of developing nations, the WHO recommends using basic clinical signs to identify and treat hypoxemia. Despite these recommendations, a study conducted in seven developing countries involving 21 first-level facilities and district hospitals revealed that over 50% of hospitalized children with lung disease received inappropriate treatment with antibiotics or oxygen, with oxygen being in short supply in several of these settings. Although no randomized trials have been conducted to support this practice, it is evident that providing oxygen to hypoxemic infants can save lives.

1.2.2.9. Prevention and Treatment of Pneumonia in HIV-Positive Children

Current recommendations of a WHO panel for managing pneumonia in HIV-positive children and for prophylaxis of *Pneumocystis jiroveci* are as follows:

- **Nonsevere pneumonia up to age 5 years***:* Oral co-trimoxazole should remain the first-line antibiotic, but oral amoxicillin should be used if it is affordable or if the child has been on co-trimoxazole prophylaxis.
- **Severe or very severe pneumonia:** For children under two months old, standard WHO case-management guidelines should be applied. Injectable antibiotics, therapy for *Pneumocystis jiroveci* pneumonia, and initiating *Pneumocystis jiroveci* pneumonia prophylaxis upon recovery are advised for children aged 2 to 11 months. Injectable antibiotics and *Pneumocystis jiroveci*

pneumonia therapy are the main forms of treatment for children between the ages of 12 and 59 months. The prophylactic administration of *Pneumocystis jiroveci* pneumonia to infants born to HIV-positive mothers should last for 15 months; sadly, this advice is rarely followed.

Table 1.1. *Samples and Diagnostic Testing in Pneumonia*

Samples and Diagnostic Testing in Pneumonia.				
Condition of Pneumonia	Blood Cultures	Respiratory Samples	Urinary Antigen Test for Legionella/ Pneumococcus	Comments
Outpatient		Sputum culture		Serology test when pathogens are suspected through epidemiological evidence
Hospitalized patients (ward)	×	×	×	Influenza test during influenza season
Hospitalized patients admitted to ICU	×	BAL/BAS in intubated patients	×	Serology test when pathogens are suspected through epidemiological evidence
Failure of outpatient antibiotic treatment		Sputum culture	×	Serology for intracellular pathogens
CAP cases who do not respond to treatment or suspicion of uncommon pathogens	×	BAL Mycobacterial and mycological culture Nasopharyngeal swab for respiratory viruses		
Hospital acquired pneumonia	×	×	×	Influenza test during influenza season
Ventilator associated pneumonia	×	BAS/BAL/mini BAL	×	

Abbreviations: BAL (bronchoalveolar lavage); BAS (bronchoaspirate); ICU (intensive care unit); CAP (community-acquired pneumonia).

Source: Cilloniz C, Martin-Loeches I, Garcia-Vidal C, San Jose A, Torres A. Microbial Etiology of Pneumonia: Epidemiology, Diagnosis, and Resistance Patterns. International Journal of Molecular Sciences. 2016; 17(12):2120. https://doi.org/10.3390/ijms17122120.

1.2.3. Cost-Effectiveness of Interventions

Approximately 5% of the 10.6 million deaths of children under five that occur each year are thought to be caused by pneumonia. Reducing mortality through public health initiatives is a top priority in areas where primary healthcare is inadequate. As previously mentioned, vaccination serves as primary prevention, and early case detection and management serves as secondary prevention. Because global and regional estimates of the pneumococcal pneumonia burden are still being developed and won't be available until later in 2005, research did not attempt to analyze the cost-effectiveness of pneumococcal vaccines. Furthermore, the cost of vaccines is currently quite stable in developed nations; however, when vaccines are acquired through an international tender, low-, and middle-income nations should expect significantly lower costs.

When diagnosing LRIs in children exhibiting respiratory symptoms, healthcare professionals who use case management may rely on certain warning indicators, such as rapid breathing, lower chest wall indrawing, or fast breathing. We combine both bacterial and viral pneumonia, as well as pneumonia and bronchiolitis, under the umbrella term of clinical pneumonia because these conditions cannot be distinguished using this method. The underlying premise of this approach is that a significant percentage of clinical pneumonia is caused by bacteria and that medical professionals can significantly lower case fatality by diagnosing breathing rates and giving antibiotics on time.

The analysis addresses four categories of case management, which are distinguished by the severity of the infection and the point of treatment:

- Nonsevere pneumonia treated by a community health worker.
- Nonsevere pneumonia treated at a health facility.
- severe pneumonia treated at a hospital.
- very severe pneumonia treated at a hospital.

A report on the assumptions and methodology used to estimate the costs of scaling up specific health interventions targeted at children provides information about these case management categories and their results (WHO and Child Adolescent Health forthcoming). Rather than the report's recommended twice-daily follow-ups for 10 days, we assumed a total of three follow-up visits for each patient treated by a community health worker. Additionally, we considered that, contrary to the report's suggestion that only 20% of patients with severe pneumonia receive an X-ray examination, all of them do. Additionally, we used the five-hour workday as the minimum requirement for community health workers under the Child Health and Survival initiative of the U.S. International Development Agency. Regional variations were caused by variations in hospital and health worker costs because we assumed that the prices of tradable commodities, like drugs and oxygen, were constant across regions. The highest treatment costs were found in Latin America, the Caribbean, the Middle East, and North Africa (Adegbola et al., 1994; Adegbola et al., 1999; Addo-Yobo et al., 2004). (Table 1.2)

Using the standard operating procedures for economic analyses, we computed region-specific cost-effectiveness ratios (CERs) for a model population of 1 million in each region. Due to a lack of incidence data, the regions of Europe and Central Asia were left out of this analysis. The scientists assumed consistent intervention effectiveness rates in the absence of region-specific data.

Table 1.2. *Molecular Platforms for Pneumonia*

Platform	Pathogens	Technology	Sensibility/ Specificity	Time	Sample	Advantages	Disadvantages	Approved
Curetis Unyvero P50 Pneumonia	18 bacterial and fungal pathogens 22 antibiotic resistance markers	Multiplex-PCR cartridge system	81%/99%	4 h	Sputum, BAL, BAS	Detection of resistant patterns	Test limited to a two samples test per run. A relatively large amount of hands-on time	Under FDA/ EC/Under Singapore Registration/ Under Chinese Registration
GeneXpertMRSA/ SA	Methicillin-resistant *S. aureus* (MRSA) methicillin-sensitive *S. aureus* (MSSA)	Multiplex-PCR	99%/72%	1 h	Blood, Nasal swabs	Minimal technical expertise	Only detects MRSA/SA	FDA/EC
MALDI-TOF	200 microorganisms	Mass spectrometry, identification of microorganisms directly from colonies of bacteria and fungi	99%–100%/97%–100%	0.5–1 min	Colonies, positive blood cultures, direct samples such as urine	Rapid and accurate approach to detect microorganism	Lack of standardized assay conditions	
GeneXpert Flu Assay	Influenza A/B (A/2009H1)	multiplex-PCR	97%–100%/100%	1 h	Nasopharyngeal swabs, nasal aspirates and washes	Minimal technical expertise	Only detects influenza viruses	FDA/EC
GeneXpert Flu/RSV Assay	Influenza A/B/RSV	Multiplex-PCR	97%–100%/100%	0.5–1 h	Nasopharyngeal swabs, nasal aspirates and washes	Minimal technical expertise	Only detects influenza viruses and RSV	FDA/EC

FilmArray Respiratory Panel	Adenovirus; coronaviruses 229E, OC43, NL63, HKU1; metapneumovirus; influenza A, H3, H1, 2009 H1; parainfluenza viruses 1, 2, 3, 4; RSV; rhinovirus/ enterovirus *B. pertussis, M. pneumoniae, C. pneumoniae*	An unprocessed biologic/ clinical sample is subjected to nucleic acid purification, reverse transcription, a high-order nested multiplex PCR and DNA melting curve analysis	84%–100%/98%–100%	1 h	Nasopharyngeal Swab	Minimal technical expertise required	Test limited to a single patient test per run. Decreased sensitivity for some adenovirus types	FDA/ EC

Abbreviations: PCR = polymerase chain reaction; MSSA = methicillin sensitive *S. aureus*; MRSA = methicillin resistant *S. aureus*; RSV = respiratory syncytial virus; FDA = Food Drug Administration; EC = European Community; DNA = Deoxyribonucleic acid; MALDI-TOF = matrix-assisted laser desorption/ionization time-of-flight.

Source: Cilloniz C, Martin-Loeches I, Garcia-Vidal C, San Jose A, Torres A. Microbial Etiology of Pneumonia: Epidemiology, Diagnosis, and Resistance Patterns. International Journal of Molecular Sciences. 2016; 17(12):2120. https://doi.org/10.3390/ijms17122120.

Reduced treatment-adjusted life years are achieved by shorter illness durations and lower treatment-associated mortality. They calculated an average length of illness of 8 +/− 5 days for those who did not receive treatment and 6 +/− 0 days for those who did. For patients diagnosed based solely on breath rate, we employed a diagnosis specificity of 78.5% and a case-fatality reduction of 36.0% due to treatment. Concurrent with the infection, the disability weight was 0.28 Since it is unknown whether childhood lung rehabilitation induces long-term lung function impairment or whether children who experience lung function impairment are more susceptible to infection, we did not take into account disabilities resulting from chronic LRI sequelae.

The cost-effectiveness of a five-year intervention was determined because a single year of these interventions only produces cotemporaneous benefits, meaning that individuals who are effectively treated may not live to life expectancy because they are likely to contract the illness again the following year. For this time frame, we could examine the scenario where a whole group of infants to four-year-old's benefits from the intervention by living to life expectancy and does not die from early childhood clinical pneumonia. The fixed costs of starting a program where none currently exists were excluded from this analysis, which only took into account long-run marginal costs, which change depending on the number of people treated. Of all the four case-management categories, treating very severe clinical pneumonia in a hospital was the least cost-effective, and treating nonsevere clinical pneumonia at the facility level was more cost-effective than treating it in the community across all low- and middle-income countries. Since treating non-severe clinical pneumonia at a health facility is less expensive than treating the patient over the course of multiple visits from a health worker, treatment provided by the facility was more economical than that provided by the latter. An estimate of US$398 per disability-adjusted life year was made for the cost of delivering all levels of treatment to all low- and middle-income nations (Table 1.3).

Table 1.3. *Length of Hospital Stay, Costs, and 30-Day Readmission Rates Among Older Adults Hospitalized for Targeted Conditions*

Hospitalization Metric	Overall Sample	CAP	DM	MI	Stroke	*p*-Value
LOS (days)	5.5 ± 4.7	5.2 ± 3.8	4.6 ± 3.8	4.3 ± 3.6	5.6 ± 5.5	-
LOS (Median)	4	4	3	3	4	<0.0001
Total charges	$51,612 ± 52,478	$35,480 ± 36,149	$35,341 ± 38,580	$72,077 ± 60,105	$46,785 ± 44,219	-
Total charges (Median)	$33,637	$24,309	$23,222	$56,016	$32,458	<0.0001
Total Cost	$13,425 ± 12,366	$9686 ± 8340	$9057 ± 9246	$18,148 ± 13,088	$12,188 ± 10,283	-
Total Cost (Median)	$9317	$7282	$6217	$14,802	$8772	<0.0001
Total summed costs (Millions)	$3312	$1130	$304	$1059	$819	<0.0001
30-day readmission rates	15.7%	17.0%	20.3%	15.0%	11.5%	<0.0001

Abbreviation: LOS = Length of stay.

Source: Olasupo O, Xiao H, Brown JD. Relative Clinical and Cost Burden of Community-Acquired Pneumonia Hospitalizations in Older Adults in the United States—A Cross-Sectional Analysis. Vaccines. 2018; 6(3):59. https://doi.org/10.3390/vaccines6030059.

The relative cost-effectiveness rankings for the strategies were the same across all regions, and regional variations in the CER for each case-management category were solely caused by variations in the intervention costs because we assumed that effectiveness rates would remain constant. Regional differences in the ratios of urban to rural populations also contributed to variation in the CERs for delivering all categories of care. 80% of nonseverely ill patients in rural areas receive treatment at the community level, and the remaining patients seek treatment at the facility level. This is based on our assumption that all patients in urban areas seek treatment at the facility level or higher.

1.2.4. Implementation of ARI Control Strategies: Lessons of Experience

The lessons of ARI prevention and control strategies that have been implemented by national programs include the vaccination and case-management strategies discussed below.

1.2.4.1. Vaccine Strategies

In Western Europe and North America, the Hib vaccine was added to the infant immunization schedule in the early 1990s. Though there are still significant obstacles, efforts to introduce vaccination in developing nations are progressing thanks to the creation of the Vaccine Fund and the Global Alliance for Vaccines and Immunization (GAVI). Only 84 of the 193 WHO member countries had made the Hib vaccine available by 2002. Since then, GAVI has approved support for five countries to help introduce the Hib vaccine in 2004–2005. In 2000, the US expanded its infant immunization program to include 7-PCV. While some developed nations advise using the vaccine only in certain high-risk groups, others intend to incorporate it into their national immunization programs in 2005. A significant percentage of all infants are included in the definition of "high risk" in some of these final countries, which is fairly expansive. Although some serotypes that are crucial in developing nations are absent from the currently licensed 7-PCV, the 9-PCV and 11-PCV would cover nearly 80% of the serotypes that cause serious disease globally.

Uptake in developing nations has been sluggish despite the Hib vaccine's success in developed nations and the widely acknowledged significance of LRIs as a cause of childhood mortality due to several interrelated factors. In certain of the nations where the vaccine has been introduced, its continued use is in jeopardy. Initially, the extent of the illness and fatalities brought on by Hib is not acknowledged in these nations, in part due to the underutilization of bacteriological diagnosis (caused by a lack of facilities and resources). Second, increasing the number of vaccines has not been prioritized since many countries still have low vaccination rates despite the implementation of the traditional Expanded Program on Immunization. Third, it took several years for industrialized countries to license and routinely use the vaccine before developing nations started to investigate the vaccine's usefulness. As a result, the Hib vaccination has been seen as a wealthy nation's intervention. Despite the availability of support through GAVI and the Vaccine Fund, there has been little actual demand for the vaccine due to all these factors.

A Hib task force was established in 2004 by the GAVI board to investigate the best ways to assist national initiatives aimed at making evidence-based decisions regarding the introduction of the Hib vaccine. The Hib Initiative was approved by the GAVI board based on the task force's recommendations. This initiative aims to assist countries that want to continue vaccinating against the Hib virus or investigate whether introducing the vaccine should be a top priority for their health systems. To spearhead this effort is a consortium made up of the WHO, the London School of Hygiene and Tropical Medicine, the Johns Hopkins Bloomberg School of Public Health, and the Centers for Disease Control and Prevention.

1.2.4.2. Case-Management Strategies

The ARI case-management strategy's effects on mortality were evaluated in 10 studies, seven of which included a concurrent control group, as part of a meta-analysis of community-based trials. Within neonates, infants, and children aged one to four, the meta-analysis revealed a reduction in all-cause mortality of 27%, 20%, and 24%, respectively. 42, 36, and 36%, respectively, less people died in LRIs. The aforementioned data unambiguously demonstrate that ARI case management, which is comparatively straightforward but standardized, can significantly reduce mortality in children under four years old, encompassing not only pneumonia mortality but also related causes. Right now, the IMCI strategy—which is being used in more than 80 countries—incorporates the ARI case-management approach. The promise of simplified case management has not been effectively realized worldwide, despite the significant number of people who succumb to pneumonia every year. When ARIs kill a lot of children, one major contributing factor is the underutilization of medical facilities in those nations or communities. 92% of sick children in Bangladesh, for instance, are not sent to the proper hospitals. Of the children who passed away in Bolivia, 62% had not been taken to a doctor when they were sick. Of the sick children in Guinea who passed away, 61% had not been seen by a doctor. A study conducted in Tanzania reveals that only 41% of sick children are admitted to a medical facility and that children from lower-income families are less likely than those from higher-income families to receive antibiotics for pneumonia. Research has thus repeatedly shown that ill children do not visit hospitals, particularly those from low-income families.

Some countries have established large-scale, sustainable programs for treatment at the community level:

- The Gambia has a national program for community-level management of pneumonia.
- In the Siaya district of Kenya, a nongovernmental organization efficiently provides treatment by community health workers for pneumonia and other childhood diseases.
- In Honduras, ARI management has been incorporated into the National Integrated Community Child Care Program, whereby community volunteers conduct growth monitoring, provide health education, and treat pneumonia and diarrhea in more than 1,800 communities.
- In Bangladesh, the Bangladesh Rural Advancement Committee and the government introduced an ARI control program covering 10 subdistricts, using volunteer community health workers. Each worker is responsible for treating childhood pneumonia in some 100 to 120 households after a three-day training program.
- In Nepal during 1986–89, a community-based program for the management of ARIs and diarrheal disease was tested in two districts and showed substantial reductions in LRI mortality. As a result, the program was integrated into Nepal's health services and is being implemented in 17 of the country's 75 districts by female community health volunteers trained to detect and treat pneumonia.
- In Pakistan, the Lady Health Worker Program employs approximately 70,000 women, who work in communities providing education and management of childhood pneumonia to more than 30 million people (Hargreave and Nair, 2009; Bush and Fleming, 2015; Asthma Guidelines Briefing Document, 2017; GINA, 2017).

1.2.5. Research and Development Agenda

The research and development agenda outlined below summarizes the priorities that have been established by advisory groups to the Initiative for Vaccine Research (vaccine intervention strategies) and the WHO Division of the Child and Adolescent Health (case-management strategies).

1.2.5.1. Vaccine Intervention Strategies

Many recommendations, which differ based

on the nation, were made by the GAVI task force on Hib vaccination. To guarantee ongoing support for such vaccination programs, nations that have implemented the Hib vaccine should concentrate on recording its effects and utilize the information to advise national authorities, development partners, and other public health organizations. A lack of local data and a lack of knowledge about regional data frequently impede GAVI-eligible nations from introducing Hib vaccinations. Subregional meetings are one way they can address these issues, as country experts can review and pool information from other countries. Furthermore, economic analyses based on standardized instruments are required in the majority of countries. To determine the incidence of Hib meningitis at particular sites, laboratory facilities must be developed in all countries with a high burden of Hib disease. Using protocols based on surveillance for meningitis invasive disease, countries, where the disease burden is still unknown, may not be able to record the incidence of Hib disease. They must investigate the potential for utilizing different approaches, such as vaccine-probe studies, to gauge the burden of disease.

Preemptively, GAVI launched an initiative in 2003 to implement an accelerated development and introduction program for pneumococcal vaccines, based at the Johns Hopkins School of Public Health in Baltimore, drawing on lessons learned from the introduction of the Hib and hepatitis B vaccines. The goal of the program is to promote the distribution of pneumococcal vaccinations and to establish and convey their importance. Producing local data regarding the prevalence of disease and the possible impact of vaccines on public health is necessary to determine the vaccine's value. In a few chosen leading countries, this endeavor can be achieved through relevant clinical trials and improved disease surveillance. As soon as the evidence base is established, it will be shared with influential opinion leaders and decision-makers to guarantee that decisions are based on facts. Once routine vaccination has been shown to be cost-effective, countries will need financial support to integrate the vaccines into their immunization programs and establish delivery systems. To inform capacity planning, product availability, and pricing, these activities are being started before the launch of vaccine formulations intended for use in developing nations.

1.2.5.2. Case-Management Strategies

In 2003, WHO's Division of Child and Adolescent Health convened a meeting to review data and evidence from recent ARI case-management studies and to suggest the following revisions to case-management guidelines and future research priorities:

- Nonsevere pneumonia
  - Improve the specificity of clinical diagnostic criteria.
  - Reassess WHO's current recommended criteria for detecting and managing treatment failure, given the high rates of therapy failure.
  - Reanalyze data from short-course therapy studies to better identify determinants of treatment failure.
  - Carry out placebo-controlled trials among children presenting with wheezing and pneumonia in selected settings that have a high prevalence of wheezing to determine whether such children need antibiotics.
- **Severe pneumonia**: In a randomized clinical trial in a controlled environment, oral amoxicillin is as effective as

parenteral penicillin or ampicillin; however, the following actions need to be undertaken before it can be recommended on a general basis:

- Analyze data on exclusions from the trial.
- Identify predictors that may help distinguish children who require hospitalization and who subsequently deteriorate.
- Reassess WHO's current recommended treatment failure criteria for severe pneumonia, given the overall high rates of therapy failure.
- Conduct descriptive studies in a public health setting in several centers worldwide, to evaluate the clinical outcomes of oral amoxicillin in children aged 2 to 59 months who present with lower chest wall indrawing.
- Document the effectiveness of WHO's treatment guidelines for managing children with pneumonia and HIV infection.

• LRI deaths
  - To help develop more effective interventions to reduce LRI mortality, study the epidemiology of LRI deaths in various regions in detail, using routine and advanced laboratory techniques.
  - Oxygen therapy:
  - Carry out studies to show the effectiveness of oxygen for managing severe respiratory infections.
  - Collect baseline information about the availability and delivery of oxygen and its use in hospital settings in low-income countries.
  - Explore the utility of pulse oximetry for optimizing oxygen therapy in various clinical settings.
  - Undertake studies to improve the specificity of clinical signs in the overlapping signs and symptoms of malaria and pneumonia.
  - Study rapid diagnostic tests for malaria to assess their effectiveness in differentiating between malaria and pneumonia.
  - Examine the effect of widespread use of co-trimoxazole on sulfadoxine-pyrimethamine resistance to *Plasmodium falciparum*.

Etiology: Data on the etiology of pneumonia in children are somewhat out of date, and new etiological studies are needed that use modern technology to identify pathogens.

1.3. Asthma Management in Pediatric Patients

Children with asthma, a chronic inflammatory disease of the airways, can benefit from a comprehensive approach to asthma management that aims to control symptoms, prevent exacerbations, optimize lung function, and promote overall well-being. Accurately diagnosing and classifying the severity and control of asthma is essential to managing the condition because it informs treatment choices and monitoring tactics. To confirm reversible airflow obstruction and gauge the severity of the disease, the diagnosis usually entails a clinical assessment that includes a thorough medical history, physical examination, and pulmonary function testing, such as spirometry and bronchodilator responsiveness testing. Evidence-based guidelines, like those offered by the National Asthma Education and Prevention Program (NAEPP) and the Global Initiative for Asthma (GINA), serve as a guide for treatment strategies in the management of pediatric asthma. These guidelines are customized to the unique needs, symptoms, and severity of each child's asthma. The foundation of managing asthma is pharmacotherapy, which involves using controller drugs like immunomodulators, leukotriene receptor antagonists (LTRAs), long-acting beta-agonists (LABAs), and inhaled corticosteroids (ICS) to decrease airway inflammation and avoid symptoms. During acute exacerbations, rescue drugs like short-acting beta-agonists (SABAs) are used to quickly relieve symptoms.

Non-pharmacological therapies, such as asthma action plans, environmental control strategies, and patient education, are equally important in managing pediatric asthma in addition to medication. To empower kids and families to identify early warning signs, follow treatment plans, and effectively manage asthma triggers and exacerbations, patient, and caregiver education is a crucial part of asthma management. Environmental control strategies help limit exposure to asthma triggers and disease exacerbations. Examples include avoiding allergens, quitting smoking, and improving indoor air quality. Personalized treatment strategies based on asthma severity and control are outlined in asthma action plans, which are created in partnership with healthcare providers. These strategies include medication dosages, step-up or step-down therapy, instructions for symptom management, and guidance on when to seek medical attention. These action plans increase treatment adherence, decrease ER visits, and improve overall asthma outcomes by empowering kids and families to effectively self-manage their asthma. Pediatric asthma care requires regular monitoring and follow-up, which enables medical professionals to evaluate the effectiveness of treatment, modify therapy as necessary, and offer children and families continuing support and education. Assessment of symptoms, lung function testing, medication adherence tracking, assessment of asthma control, frequency of exacerbations, and quality of life are a few examples of monitoring techniques.

A varied chronic airway disease that is very common in children, asthma is characterized by a variety of respiratory symptoms, such as coughing, wheezing, chest tightness, and breathlessness, along with varying obstruction of expiratory airflow. Concerns regarding asthmatic patients' ability to control their symptoms and the possibility of unfavorable outcomes in clinical practice are common. It follows that the availability of multiple guidelines to assist medical professionals in managing asthma in both adults and children is not surprising. Two widely recognized documents, published in the USA and Europe, respectively, are the Global Strategy for Asthma Management and Prevention (GINA) and the British Thoracic Society (BTS)/Scottish Intercollegiate Guideline Network (SIGN). The GINA Science Committee was founded in 2002 to review published studies on asthma. Leading authorities on asthma research in adults and children convene frequently to critically evaluate asthma-related scientific literature at international conferences of the European Respiratory Society (ERS) and the American Thoracic Society (ATS). In 2017, the GINA underwent a significant revision that included updated recommendations regarding the diagnosis and management of asthma.

The first BTS guideline was published in 1990, and the SIGN guidelines were published in 1996. However, in 1999, the two societies worked together to create a new asthma guideline that was published on websites and updated yearly until 2016. Both guidelines are widely used and offer current recommendations for managing and preventing asthma, but they offer contradictory advice and reach different conclusions about what constitutes and how to treat asthma. The National Institute for Health and Care Excellence (NICE) of the United Kingdom (UK) also published a consultation document in 2015 regarding asthma diagnosis and monitoring. Later, in December 2016, NICE released additional information regarding the management of chronic asthma, including cost-benefit analyses that were not taken into account in the BTS/SIGN guidelines. A working committee comprising experts in the field conducted an International Consensus on Pediatric Asthma in 2012, examining in detail the disparities between the current international guidelines mentioned above as well as other reports such as the Japanese Guideline for Childhood Asthma and the Australian Asthma Management document. It is important to try non-pharmacological treatments, especially for young patients, as they may enhance quality of life and lessen symptoms in asthmatic individuals. These include avoiding food or drug triggers in individuals who are susceptible to them, avoiding indoor and/or outdoor pollutants and irritants, and avoiding exposure to tobacco smoke in the environment or quitting smoking among teenagers. Patients who are overweight should be encouraged to lose weight; breathing exercise regimens and physiotherapy techniques should also be promoted.

Nonetheless, the cornerstone of treating asthma in both adults and children is pharmacotherapy. The global reports outline the fundamentals of managing pharmacological asthma and provide age-appropriate treatments in a stepwise manner based on clinical severity and the degree of disease control, which is dictated by the interplay of the patient's genetic background, current course of treatment, surroundings, and psychological variables. The amount of treatment needed to control symptoms and exacerbations of asthma is used to retrospectively determine the severity of the condition, which can vary over months. Personalized phenotype-guided asthma treatments are being investigated, taking into account the patient's therapy adherence issues. Asthma phenotypes have been defined based on specific pathologic features, demographic, and clinical patterns or therapy responses. Based on the most recent recommendations from international guidelines, this review highlights the important features and variations of these documents while providing a practical viewpoint on the most widely used medications and the fundamental steps in managing asthma in children and adolescents (Hargreave and Nair, 2009; Bush and Fleming, 2015; Asthma Guidelines Briefing Document, 2017; GINA, 2017).

1.3.1. Categories of Asthma Medications and Step-Wise Strategies of Treatment

According to their intended use, the pharmacological options for treating asthma include: reliever medications, which are drugs that, when used in conjunction with high-dosage controller medications, allow patients to experience relief from symptoms within a few minutes during worsening asthma or exacerbations. They are also used to prevent exercise-induced bronchoconstriction. Add-on therapies are recommended for patients who continue to experience severe persistent asthma symptoms and exacerbations despite receiving high-dose controller medications. The three drug classes most commonly used to treat asthma are corticosteroids, leukotriene modifiers (usually montelukast), and beta-2 adrenergic agonists. For the treatment of asthmatic patients with medication, a step-by-step method has been suggested (Table 1.4). Starting treatment at the step where asthma is most appropriate for its initial severity is best. Once good asthma control and the patient's lowest effective level of treatment have been found and maintained for about three months, treatment step-down may be attempted. If control is not achieved within three months, stepping-up should be tried after reevaluating adherence to therapy, environmental factors, and associated co-morbidities. Every recommendation in all guidelines has been evaluated for adults, adolescents (over 12), and children (ages 5 to 12 and younger than 5).

Table 1.4. *Characteristics and Main Findings of the Studies Applying Pharmaco-Metabolomics in Pediatric Asthma*

Study Design and Number of Subjects Included	Main Result	Biofluid Analyzed	Analytical Platform	Main Metabolites Involved	Putative Biochemical Pathways
multicenter, randomized, double-masked, clinical trial, 565 children (8.8 years followed up for 16 years)	Specific metabolites may modify the estimated effect of age on bronchodilator response	Blood	LC-MS	Metabolites directly associated with the decline in bronchodilator response: 2-hydroxyglutarate; metabolites inversely associated with the decline in bronchodilator response: cholesterol esters, GABA, and robothymidine	Lipid metabolism, amino acid metabolism
multicenter prospective study, 52 children (mean age 12 years)	Children with severe asthma responding to omalizumab showed a different metabolomic urinary profile at baseline compared to non-responders	Urine	LC-MS	Biomarkers increased in responders were dipeptides and amino acids (the better characterized: histamine precursor L-Histidine); biomarker increased in non-responders is uric acid	Histamine pathway, protein metabolism, urea, and nitrogen metabolism

Study Design and Number of Subjects Included	Main Result	Biofluid Analyzed	Analytical Platform	Main Metabolites Involved	Putative Biochemical Pathways
case-control design, 26 asthmatic children (median age 9.1 years) and 16 healthy children (median age 10.2)	Asthmatic children treated with a three-week course of inhaled beclomethasone dipropionate showed no significant differences in the EBC metabolic arrangement and urinary steroid profile	EBC and urine	LC-MS	After beclomethasone dipropionate treatment, there were no changes in EBC metabolomic profile nor in urinary endogenous steroid profile	None
cohort study, 14,000 individuals in four cohorts (adults and adolescents)	The largest reduction in steroid levels was associated with inhaled corticosteroid (ICS) use	Blood	LC-MS	34 corticosteroid, androgenic, and pregnenolone steroid metabolites	Steroid metabolism

Abbreviations: LC-MS = Liquid Chromatography–Mass Spectrometry; EBC = Exhaled Breath Condensate.

Source: *Ferraro VA, Zanconato S, Carraro S. Metabolomics Applied to Pediatric Asthma: What Have We Learnt in the Past 10 Years? Children. 2023; 10(9):1452. https://doi.org/10.3390/children10091452.*

1.3.2. Medications Used for Rapid Relief of Symptoms

As of right now, the only treatment for Step 1 is inhaled short-acting beta2-agonists (SABAs), most commonly salbutamol, as needed. SABAs are primarily used in patients with normal lung function but sporadic daytime symptoms to provide acute relief from asthma symptoms. Second-line treatments include inhaled anticholinergic drugs, such as ipratropium. While they are less effective than SABA, they may work in concert with SABA to reduce hospitalization rates in patients experiencing severe exacerbations. Although they have a slower onset of action than inhaled SABA and a higher risk of side effects, oral SABA or short-acting theophylline are viable alternatives to SABA in adults. It is not advised to use these medications on children (Hargreave and Nair, 2009; Bush and Fleming, 2015; Asthma Guidelines Briefing Document, 2017; GINA, 2017).

1.3.3. Medications Used for Long-Term Asthma Symptoms Control

1.3.3.1. Inhaled corticosteroids (ICS)

Indicators of the need for routine controller treatment include more frequent symptoms or the existence of any exacerbation risk factors. Long-term asthma control in children may benefit from a maintenance regimen that includes SABA when needed along with therapeutic doses of ICS.

Asthma symptoms and lung function are improved with regular low dose ICS, which also reduces the need for extra medication and hospital stays. The drug combination in question is the initial treatment option included in Step 2 according to international reports. While there may be some variations in the effects of beclomethasone dipropionate (BDP) and budesonide when using different delivery devices, the potencies and bioavailability of ICS vary. The clinical activity of mometasone and fluticasone propionate seems to be equivalent to that of budesonide and BDP at a dosage of half. Based on the severity of the disease, the initial dose of ICS should be administered (Table 1.5). The recommended initial twice-daily dose of ICS for children and adolescents is typically 200 micrograms BDP or less. (except ciclesonide proposed once daily). Over 400 µg would be regarded as a pediatric high dose and over 200–400 µg BDP or equivalent as a pediatric moderate dosage. Subsequently, the ICS dosage ought to be gradually increased to the minimum level that effectively manages asthma. Growing data indicates that ICS are safe and beneficial for young children with asthma when taken at recommended dosages.

Table 1.5. *Daily Total Dose of ICS Recommended to Adolescents Aged ≥12 for Asthma Treatment Based On GINA 2022* (Keeley and Baxter, 2018)

Adolescents ≥12 Years Old			
ICS Type	Daily Total Dose of ICS (mcg)		
	Low	Medium	High
Beclomethasone dipropionate (pMDI, standard particles, HFA)	200–500	>500–1000	>1000
Beclomethasone dipropionate (DPI or pMDI, extra fine particles, HFA)	100–200	>200–400	>400
Budesonide (DPI or pMDI, standard particles, HFA)	200–400	>400–800	>800
Ciclesonide (pMDI, extra fine particles, HFA)	800–160	>160–320	>320
Fluticasone furoate (DPI)	100		200
Fluticasone propionate (DPI)	100–250	>250–500	>500
Fluticasone proprionate (pMDI, standard particles, HFA)	100–250	>250–500	>500
Mometasone furoate (DPI)	It depends on the used device—see product information		
Mometasone furoate (pMDI, standard particles, HFA)	200–400		>400

Abbreviations: DPI: dry powder inhaler; HFA: hydrofluoroalkane propellant; ICS: inhaler corticosteroid; pMID: pressurized inhaler with fixed dose.

Source: *Ioniuc I, Miron I, Lupu VV, Starcea IM, Azoicai A, Alexoae M, Adam Raileanu A, Dragan F, Lupu A. Challenges in the Pharmacotherapeutic Management of Pediatric Asthma. Pharmaceuticals. 2022; 15(12):1581. https://doi.org/10.3390/ph15121581.*

Long-term follow-up studies have, however, shown that chronic use of intermediate-high doses of ICS can have some effects, such as growth retardation in prepubescent children during the first years of treatment and a reduction in adult final height. Individuals with uncontrolled asthma may experience growth disturbances. Consequently, ICS medication should be gradually tapered to the lowest effective dose once symptom control has been attained. A few kids who received ICS treatment have also been reported to have clinical adrenal suppression. It is unknown how long ICS treatment could expose a child at risk of developing clinical adrenal insufficiency, but it is likely to happen at high daily doses (≥800 µg BDP or equivalent). It is unclear how often tests of adrenal function, such as the low-dose adrenocorticotrophic hormone (ACTH) test, would need to be repeated in children to predict clinically relevant adrenal insufficiency in a child receiving high-dose ICS. Additionally, comparing extra-fine (diameter <2 µm) vs. In a meta-analysis of observational studies, fine particle BDP given as monotherapy or in conjunction with LABA, has demonstrated a reduction in exacerbation rates in patients with severe asthma. Another particular problem being researched is corticosteroid insensitivity; various molecular mechanisms, such as modification of the glucocorticoid receptor, have been suggested. A step up may be necessary for patients who continue to experience symptoms or recurrent exacerbations even after using low-dose ICS. This is after comorbidities like obesity, obstructive sleep apnea, reflux disease, and rhinosinusitis have been evaluated, as well as medication adherence, inhaler technique, and continuous allergen exposure.

1.3.3.2. Long-Acting Beta-2 Adrenergic Agonists (LABA)

Asthma outcomes in adolescents and adults should combine ICS and LABA, such as salmeterol and formoterol, rather than using higher doses of ICS. This combination should be taken into account before increasing the daily dose of 400 µg BDP or its equivalent, and definitely before using 800 µg of BDP. For asthma, a LABA should only be used in fixed-dose combination devices that also include an ICS rather than as monotherapy. According to recent research, patients with asthma who take LABA in addition to steroids have an equivalent risk of experiencing side effects from using corticosteroids alone. When compared to ICS alone, it is more costly and does not lower the chance of future exacerbations. Furthermore, an international trial that tracked 6208 children aged 4–11 years with asthma and an exacerbation in the previous year found that adding salmeterol to fixed fluticasone doses is effective and does not increase the risk of serious asthma-related adverse outcomes compared to using ICS alone. These findings complement studies that provide reassurance regarding the use of LABA in adolescents and adults.

1.3.3.3. Leukotriene Receptor Antagonists (LTRAs)

Leukotrienes, which are released during an asthmatic reaction by cells involved in the pathophysiology of asthma, mediate certain inflammatory responses that LTRAs block, including the tightening of airway muscles and the secretion of mucus. International guidelines recommend LTRA as the second choice for monotherapy as the first line of treatment for chronic asthma, after low-dose ICS. As we move on to the next steps, they are also regarded as additional medications, typically used in conjunction with ICS to improve pulmonary function and symptoms through increased antiinflammatory activity. They work particularly well in treating exercise-induced asthma, and they may be particularly worth considering for patients who have had adverse effects from ICS or for younger patients. Treatment options at

Step 3 vary based on the age group. For young children, the best course of action is to combine a medium dose of ICS with as-needed SABA. However, for adults and adolescents, low-dose ICS/LABA (BDP/formoterol or budesonide/formoterol) as a maintenance treatment and as-needed SABA as a reliever, or low-dose ICS/LABA (BDP/formoterol) as both maintenance and reliever treatment, may be taken into consideration. When combined with a lower dose of ICS and SABA as needed, adding LABA to the same low dose of ICS appears to improve lung function and symptoms in this age group while lowering the risk of exacerbations. If adults' and teenagers' asthma control is still subpar, they have the option of increasing their ICS dosage to a medium level, though this is less efficient than adding a LABA. Other less effective options include low-dose sustained-release theophylline or low-dose ICS combined with either LTRA or LTRA plus.

Step 4 suggests low-dose maintenance and reliever ICS/LABA with as-needed SABA for both adult and adolescent patients; if necessary, medium-dose ICS may be considered for patients whose symptoms are not completely controlled. If the child's asthma cannot be controlled with ICS at a moderate dosage for children under 12 years old, a referral for an expert assessment is advised. Only in cases where good asthma control cannot be obtained with ICS at a medium dose in addition to LABA and/or a third controller, like LTRA, is a high dose advised. On the other hand, there is a higher chance of side effects and typically little extra benefit from increasing the ICS dosage. Conflicting recommendations regarding important aspects of managing asthma in primary care are included in the NICE publication. The use of LTRA as the first-choice adjunct therapy for patients whose asthma is not well controlled with low dose ICS is one contentious distinction. According to NICE's analysis, LABA is marginally more effective than LTRA, which helps to justify the higher cost. The Primary Care Respiratory Society UK has recommended a preliminary trial of LTRA as a supplement to low-dose ICS, but emphasizes that patients who are already responding well to a LABA regimen should not have their treatment altered. Various pharmacological options can be considered at Step 5 when patients continue to experience symptoms or exacerbations even after receiving high-dose ICS or ICS/LABA, or other Step 4 treatment options.

1.3.3.4. Oral Corticosteroids

Oral corticosteroids at low doses (≤7.5 mg/day equivalent to prednisone) may be added, but they carry some risk of side effects, particularly when used for extended periods of time. When it comes to treating patients with chronic asthma, prednisolone is the most often used steroid. It is important to routinely check blood pressure, blood sugar or urine, cholesterol, bone mineral density, growth (weight and height centiles), and cataracts in patients taking steroid pills.

1.3.3.5. Omalizumab

Another treatment option for patients over the age of 12 who have severe allergic asthma, reduced lung function, and established IgE-mediated sensitivity to inhaled allergens is anti-immunoglobulin E (anti-IgE) medication. Omalizumab is a humanized monoclonal antibody that lowers serum IgE levels and prevents IgE from binding to receptors, thus disrupting the inflammatory cascade. Subcutaneous injections are administered every two or four weeks, based on the patient's weight and total serum IgE levels. It shows a good clinical result in terms of lowering exacerbations and enhancing asthma management. In long-term trials, school-age children and adolescents with moderate-to-severe asthma who received omalizumab treatment experienced a significant reduction in the frequency of exacerbation attacks, an improvement in their quality of life, and a decrease in the need for additional standard asthma medications. Although omalizumab is well tolerated and safe, its subcutaneous delivery method and high cost are drawbacks.

1.3.3.6. Immunotherapy

Research has shown that in children who do not fully respond to other preventative measures, such as inhaled cortical steroids (ICS), subcutaneous, and sublingual allergen immunotherapy (SCIT and SLIT) is beneficial in lowering bronchial hyperreactivity and asthma symptoms. It appears that SLIT has a higher safety profile than SCIT. To be precise, it is difficult to determine where immunotherapy fits into the step-by-step management of asthma because there aren't many studies combining it with ICS.

1.3.3.7. Mepolizumab

It is controversial to use eosinophilia (>3%) in induced sputum as a biomarker for specific anti-IL5 monoclonal antibody treatment (mepolizumab) to identify responsive patients. According to certain trials, an anti-eosinophil biologic medication may help treat severe systemic corticosteroid-dependent asthma in patients with an "eosinophilic" endotype, whose illness is primarily caused by eosinophil pathophysiology. The medication works by improving airway remodeling (Hargreave and Nair, 2009; Bush and Fleming, 2015; Asthma Guidelines Briefing Document, 2017; GINA, 2017).

1.3.4. Other Pharmacological Options

1.3.4.1. Theophylline and Chromones

Theophylline, the most commonly used methylxanthine, is another medication that is not advised for regular use. It has a suitable safety profile but is not very effective in treating asthma bronchoconstriction. It also has common side effects, especially when taken in higher doses. Chromones, such as sodium cromoglycate and nedocromil sodium, are used as mast cell stabilizers and have low efficacy. As second-line medications in the first stages of treatment and for preventing exercise-induced asthma, they are listed in the guidelines.

1.3.4.2. Intramuscular Triamcinolone

Triamcinolone injections (intramuscular) have been used to treat severe asthma. Studies on children with severe asthma indicate that it may influence eosinophilic inflammation, enhance airway obstruction, and prevent exacerbation attacks; however, using it has more side effects than when using oral corticosteroids.

1.3.4.3. Anticholinergic Agents

Patients with severe persistent asthma in adults have shown improved lung function and improved control of asthma symptoms when tiotropium bromide, a long-acting inhaled anticholinergic agent, is added to ICS plus LABA. Studies on tiotropium use in children with asthma have not been conducted.

1.3.4.4. Metotrexate, Antifungal Agents, Macrolides

Metotrexate's effectiveness in treating childhood asthma is not well-established. Despite a high recurrence of adverse effects, a meta-analysis examining the steroid-sparing effect of oral methotrexate in asthmatics revealed a slight benefit. When an asthmatic patient does not have allergic bronchopulmonary aspergillosis, antifungal medications are not advised. Vicencio et al. have reported that a significant proportion of kids suffering from refractory asthma exhibited fungal sensitization, which was associated with the intensity of their condition. After removing mold from the environment, the authors propose that antifungal therapy may be a potentially effective treatment for some patients exhibiting signs of fungal sensitization, based on a case report of a child with severe asthma who responded favorably to itraconazole treatment. Because of their anti-inflammatory and antimicrobial properties, macrolides have also been suggested as a combination for the treatment of childhood asthma to reduce the patient's daily corticosteroid dosage. A 3-week course of clarithromycin given as add-on therapy to regular treatment was linked to improved symptom control and a reduction in the length of asthma exacerbations, according to a recent study involving 40 school-aged asthmatic children. Given the relative safety of this antibiotic when compared to other drugs, it might be recommended for severe asthmatic patients who exhibit resistance to other forms of therapy and primarily exhibit neutrophilic airway inflammation. However, the development of macrolide resistance among respiratory pathogens should be taken into account in long-term treatment (Hargreave and Nair, 2009; Bush and Fleming, 2015; Asthma Guidelines Briefing Document, 2017; GINA, 2017).

1.3.5. Asthma Severity Assessment

Asthma severity can be assessed when the patient is in regular control of symptoms with continuous treatment:

- Asthma that responds well to Step 1 or Step 2 treatment is considered mild: either with low-dosage controller treatment such as low-dose ICS, LTRA, or chromones, or with as-needed reliever medication alone.
- Moderate asthma is asthma that is well controlled with Step 3 treatment e.g., low-dose ICS/LABA.
- Asthma that necessitates Step 4 or Step 5 treatment is considered severe: high-dose ICS/LABA to keep asthma from getting "uncontrolled," or asthma that doesn't get better with treatment. International guidelines offering definitions and guidance regarding the management of patients with uncontrolled asthma have been published by the ERS/ATS Task Force on Severe Asthma (Hargreave and Nair, 2009; Bush and Fleming, 2015; Asthma Guidelines Briefing Document, 2017; GINA, 2017).

A Closer Look

Cystic Fibrosis Care in Pediatric Patients

Cystic fibrosis (CF) care in pediatric patients involves a multifaceted approach aimed at managing the complex manifestations of this genetic disorder, optimizing lung function, and improving overall quality of life. CF is characterized by abnormal mucous secretion, leading to obstructive lung disease, pancreatic insufficiency, and other multi-system complications. The management of CF in children requires a comprehensive understanding of the underlying pathophysiology, early diagnosis, and proactive treatment strategies to address both respiratory and non-respiratory aspects of the disease.

One of the primary goals of CF care is to maintain pulmonary health and prevent disease progression by managing airway obstruction, reducing inflammation, and preventing pulmonary infections. This often involves a combination of airway clearance techniques, such as chest physiotherapy, percussion, and vibration, to mobilize and remove thickened mucous secretions from the airways. Inhaled medications, including bronchodilators, mucolytics, hypertonic saline, and dornase alfa (recombinant human DNase), are also commonly used to improve airway clearance, reduce mucous viscosity, and enhance mucociliary clearance.

Additionally, aggressive treatment of pulmonary infections is essential in CF management to prevent exacerbations and preserve lung function. Antibiotics, both oral and inhaled, are used for the treatment of acute exacerbations and chronic infection control, targeting bacterial pathogens commonly found in CF airways, such as *Pseudomonas aeruginosa* and *Staphylococcus aureus*. Long-term antibiotic therapies, such as azithromycin, may also be prescribed for their anti-inflammatory and immunomodulatory effects in CF.

Nutritional support is another cornerstone of CF care in pediatric patients, addressing malnutrition, pancreatic insufficiency, and poor weight gain commonly seen in CF. Pancreatic enzyme replacement therapy (PERT) is prescribed to facilitate digestion and absorption of nutrients, while high-calorie, high-protein diets and nutritional supplements are recommended to meet increased energy requirements and promote growth and development. Regular monitoring of nutritional status, including weight, height, and body mass index (BMI), is essential to ensure adequate nutritional intake and optimize growth outcomes.

Furthermore, CF care involves the management of extra-pulmonary manifestations and comorbidities associated with CF, including gastrointestinal complications, liver disease, bone health, and reproductive issues. Multidisciplinary care teams, consisting of pediatric pulmonologists, gastroenterologists, nutritionists, respiratory therapists, nurses, and social workers, collaborate to provide comprehensive care, address individual needs, and optimize outcomes for pediatric patients with CF. Advancements in CF research and therapy, including the development of CFTR modulator therapies targeting specific gene mutations underlying CF, have revolutionized the management of CF in recent years, offering promising treatment options to improve lung function, reduce exacerbations, and extend survival in pediatric patients. However, ongoing monitoring, adherence to treatment regimens, and proactive management remain crucial components of CF care to optimize long-term outcomes and enhance the quality of life for children living with CF.

Summary

- Pediatric pulmonology is a specialized field of medicine focused on the diagnosis, treatment, and management of respiratory disorders in infants, children, and adolescents.
- Pulmonary infections remain a major cause of infant and child mortality worldwide and are responsible for a substantial burden of morbidity.
- Bacterial pathogens were identified in a minority of cases, with viruses, particularly respiratory syncytial virus (RSV) in the younger subjects and rhinovirus in older children, being identified in the majority.
- Acute respiratory infections (ARIs) are classified as upper respiratory tract infections (URIs) or lower respiratory tract infections (LRIs). The upper respiratory tract consists of the airways from the nostrils to the vocal cords in the larynx, including the paranasal sinuses and the middle ear.
- Acute pharyngitis is caused by viruses in more than 70% of cases in young children. Mild pharyngeal redness and swelling and tonsil enlargement are typical. Streptococcal infection is rare in children under five and more common in older children.
- Bronchiolitis occurs predominantly in the first year of life and with decreasing frequency in the second and third years. The clinical features are rapid breathing and lower chest wall indrawing, fever in one-third of cases, and wheezing.
- Interventions to control ARIs can be divided into four basic categories: immunization against specific pathogens, early diagnosis and treatment of disease, improvements in nutrition, and safer environments.
- The simplification and systematization of case management for early diagnosis and treatment of ARIs have enabled significant reductions in mortality in developing countries, where access to pediatricians is limited.
- The choice of an antimicrobial drug for treatment is based on the well-established finding that most childhood bacterial cases of pneumonia are caused by *S. pneumoniae* or *H. influenzae*.

References

1. Addo-Yobo, E., Chisaka, N., Hassan, M., Hibberd, P., Lozano, J. M., Jeena, P., et al. (2004). Oral amoxicillin versus injectable penicillin for severe pneumonia in children aged 3 to 59 months: A randomized multicenter equivalency study. *The Lancet, 364*(9440), 1141–1148.
2. Adegbola, R. A., Falade, A. G., Sam, B. E., Aidoo, M., Baldeh, I., Hazlett, D., et al. (1994). The etiology of pneumonia in malnourished and well-nourished Gambian children. *Pediatric Infectious Disease Journal, 13*(11), 975–982
3. Adegbola, R. A., Usen, S. O., Weber, M., Lloyd-Evans, N., Jobe, K., Mulholland, K., et al. (1999). Haemophilus influenzae type b meningitis in The Gambia after introduction of a conjugate vaccine. *The Lancet, 354*(9184), 1091–1092.
4. Aguilar, A. M., Alvarado, R., Cordero, D., Kelly, P., Zamora, A., & Salgado, R. (1998). *Mortality Survey in Bolivia: The Final Report—Investigating and Identifying the Causes of Death for Children Under Five.* Basic Support for Institutionalizing Child Survival Project.

5. Berman, S. (1995). Otitis media in children. *New England Journal of Medicine, 332*(23), 1560–1565.

6. Bhattacharyya, K., Winch, P., LeBan, K., & Tien, M. (2001). *Community Health Worker Incentives and Disincentives: How They Affect Motivation, Retention, and Sustainability*. Basic Support for Institutionalizing Child Survival Project for the U.S. Agency for International Development.

7. Black, R. E., Morris, S. S., & Bryce, J. (2003). Where and why are 10 million children dying every year? *The Lancet, 361*(9376), 2226–2234.

8. Black, S. B., Shinefield, H. R., Fireman, B., & Hiatt, R. (1992). Safety, immunogenicity, and efficacy in infancy of oligosaccharide conjugate Haemophilus influenzae type b vaccine in a United States population: Possible implications for optimal use. *Journal of Infectious Diseases, 165*(Suppl. 43), S139–S143.

9. Black, S. B., Shinefield, H. R., Fireman, B., Lewis, E., Ray, P., & Hansen, J. R. (2000). Efficacy, safety, and immunogenicity of heptavalent pneumococcal conjugate vaccine in children. *Pediatric Infectious Disease Journal, 19*(3), 187–195.

10. Black, S. B., Shinefield, H. R., Hansen, J., Elvin, L., Laufer, D., & Malinoski, F. (2001). Postlicensure evaluation of the effectiveness of seven-valent pneumococcal conjugate vaccine. *Pediatric Infectious Disease Journal, 20*(12), 1105–1107.

11. Bush, A., & Fleming, L. (2015). Diagnosis and management of asthma in children. *BMJ, 350*, h996. https://doi.org/10.1136/bmj.h996.

12. Global Initiative for Asthma. (2017). *GINA Report: Global Strategy for Asthma Management and Prevention*. https://ginasthma.org/gina-reports/ (accessed on 22 October 2024).

13. Hargreave, F. E., & Nair, P. (2009). The definition and diagnosis of asthma. *Clinical & Experimental Allergy, 39*(12), 1652–1658. https://doi.org/10.1111/j.1365-2222.2009.03321.x.

14. Keeley, D., & Baxter, N. (2018). Conflicting asthma guidelines cause confusion in primary care. *BMJ, 360*, k29. https://doi.org/10.1136/bmj.k29.

15. Primary Care Respiratory Society UK. (2017). *Asthma Guidelines Briefing Document*. https://pcrs-uk.org/briefing-asthma-guidelines (accessed on 22 October 2024).

Chapter

ALLERGIC CONDITIONS

2

Contents

Introduction

The diagnosis, treatment, and management of a variety of childhood respiratory disorders, including allergic disorders, fall under the purview of pediatric pulmonology. In pediatric pulmonology, allergic conditions cover a broad spectrum of illnesses, from moderate allergic rhinitis to severe exacerbations of asthma brought on by allergens. These illnesses can have a serious negative influence on a child's quality of life and may necessitate extensive management techniques to successfully manage symptoms. Allergy rhinitis, or hay fever, is one of the most common allergic conditions seen in pediatric pulmonology. It appears as watery eyes, itching, congestion in the nose, and sneezing in reaction to allergens like dust mites, pollen, or pet dander. Even though allergic rhinitis is usually not fatal, if treatment is not received, it can seriously affect a child's everyday activities, sleep habits, and academic achievement.

Asthma is another common allergy condition seen in pediatric pulmonology. It is a long-term inflammatory respiratory disease. Recurrent episodes of wheezing, coughing, tightness in the chest, and dyspnea caused by allergens like mold, pollen, or animal dander are the hallmarks of allergic asthma. Exposure to these allergens can cause inflammation and constriction of the airways in susceptible individuals, resulting in mild to severe symptoms of asthma.

In pediatric pulmonology, pharmacological interventions are essential for managing allergic conditions. Depending on the particular symptoms and severity of the condition, this may involve the use of leukotriene receptor antagonists, short- or long-acting bronchodilators, antihistamines, and intranasal corticosteroids. To attain the best possible control in more severe cases of allergic asthma, controller drugs like biological agents or inhaled corticosteroids might be required.

If pharmacological treatments and allergen avoidance are insufficient for children with asthma or allergic rhinitis, immunotherapy—also referred to as allergy shots—may be suggested. In immunotherapy, allergens are progressively added to larger doses to gradually desensitize the immune system and lessen allergic reactions. It may be a useful long-term therapy choice for kids who have persistent allergy symptoms. In pediatric pulmonology, allergic conditions are frequently encountered and can significantly affect a child's respiratory health and overall quality of life. Healthcare professionals can effectively manage allergic conditions in children and improve outcomes by using a comprehensive approach that includes allergen avoidance, pharmacological interventions, and immunotherapy when appropriate.

Orientation and Directional Terms

Term	Definition	Illustration
Diagnosis	Diagnosis is the identification of the nature and cause of a certain phenomenon.	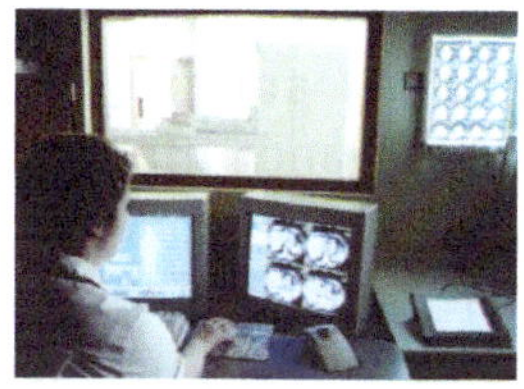
Pulmonology	Pulmonology is a medical specialty that deals with diseases involving the respiratory tract.	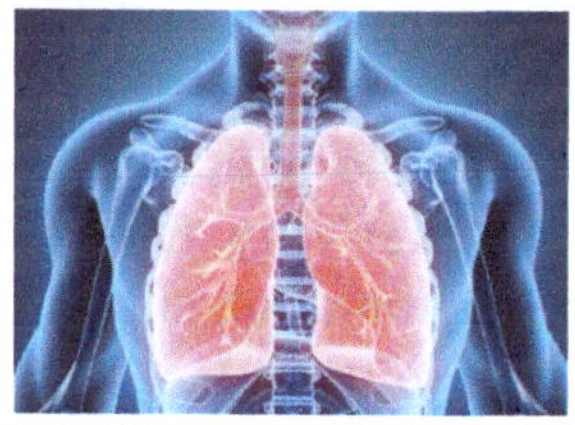
Asthma	Asthma is a condition in which your airways narrow and swell and may produce extra mucus.	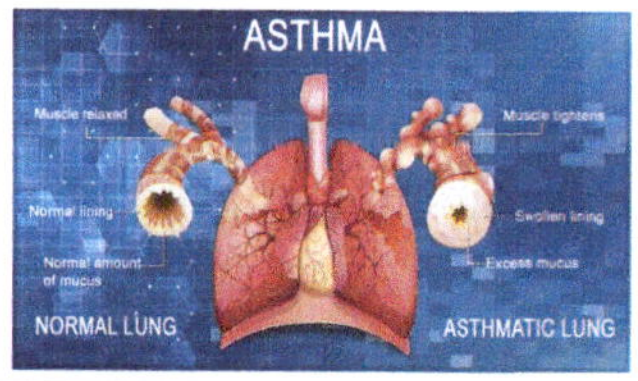
Mucoid impaction	A mucoid impaction is generally the result of the inspissation of copious mucus and other secretions in the tracheobronchial tree.	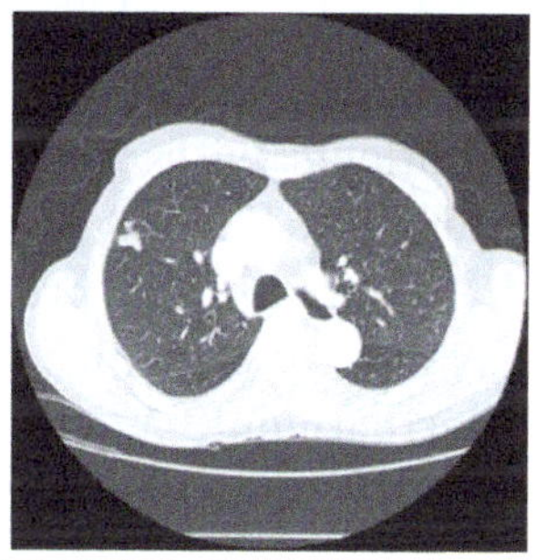
Aspergillus fumigatus	*Aspergillus* fumigatus is a species of fungus in the genus *Aspergillus* and is one of the most common *Aspergillus* species to cause disease in individuals with an immunodeficiency.	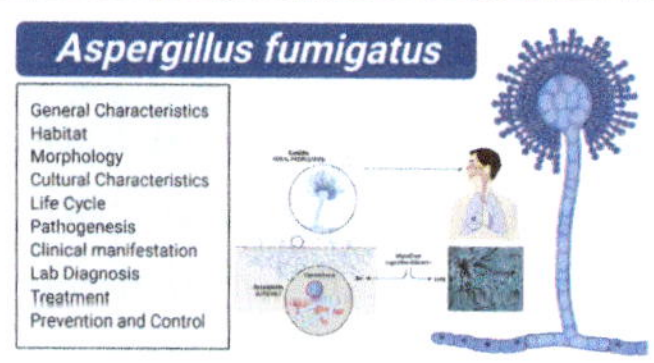

2.1. Bronchopulmonary Aspergillosis

A group of illnesses known as bronchopulmonary aspergillosis (BPA) are brought on by the *Aspergillus* fungus and affect the lungs and airways. It includes a spectrum of clinical manifestations with variable severity and immune response, ranging from invasive pulmonary aspergillosis (IPA) to allergic bronchopulmonary aspergillosis (ABPA). BPA mainly affects people with weakened immune systems and underlying lung diseases like cystic fibrosis, asthma, or chronic obstructive pulmonary disease (COPD).

Aspergillus antigens colonizing the airways can cause hypersensitivity reactions, such as allergic bronchopulmonary aspergillosis (ABPA). It is characterized by recurrent episodes of wheezing, coughing, and worsening asthma symptoms; peripheral eosinophilia and elevated serum IgE levels are frequently present as well. Usually, patients with cystic fibrosis or asthma experience it. If ABPA is not treated, it can result in fibrosis and bronchiectasis, which emphasizes the significance of early detection and treatment. A combination of clinical, radiological, and laboratory findings are used to diagnose ABPA. Radiology reports can show transient pulmonary infiltrates, mucoid impaction, and central bronchiectasis; eosinophilia and elevated serum IgE levels are frequently found in laboratory tests. The diagnosis is further supported by precipitating antibodies to *Aspergillus* antigens. Accurate diagnosis and management require a high degree of clinical suspicion and a multidisciplinary approach involving allergists, radiologists, and pulmonologists.

The goals of ABPA treatment are to lessen airway inflammation, manage symptoms, and stop the disease from getting worse. This usually entails a combination of antifungal medications like voriconazole or itraconazole to eradicate *Aspergillus* colonization, bronchodilators to relieve airflow obstruction, and systemic corticosteroids to suppress the immune response. Maintenance corticosteroid therapy and vigilant monitoring for disease recurrence or exacerbations may be necessary for long-term management. On the other hand, *Aspergillus* hyphae invasion of the lung parenchyma, blood vessels, or airways causes invasive pulmonary aspergillosis (IPA), a serious and frequently fatal infection. Immunocompromised people are the main victims, such as those receiving long-term corticosteroid therapy, organ transplants, or chemotherapy. If not identified and treated right away, influenza-like pneumonia (IPA) can quickly progress to respiratory failure. IPA symptoms include fever, cough, dyspnea, and hemoptysis.

A high index of suspicion is necessary for the diagnosis of IPA, which is made up of clinical, radiological, and microbiological findings. Nodules, cavitation, and the halo sign on chest imaging are examples of radiographic features. *Aspergillus* species isolation from respiratory specimens or lung tissue histological analysis are methods used for microbiological confirmation. For patients with IPA, early initiation of antifungal therapy with medications like voriconazole or isavuconazole is essential to improving outcomes.

Apart from *Aspergillus* bronchitis and *Aspergillus* bronchial mycosis, there are other types of bronchopulmonary aspergillosis such as chronic necrotizing pulmonary aspergillosis (CNPA) and ABPA. These conditions exhibit unique radiological and clinical characteristics. While bronchial mycosis and *Aspergillus* bronchitis mainly affect immunocompetent people and are linked to chronic coughing and sputum production, community-onset pneumonia (CNPA) usually affects patients who already have a lung condition and presents as a slowly progressing pneumonia with cavitary lesions.

The term "bronchopulmonary aspergillosis" refers to a group of illnesses affecting the lungs and airways that are brought on by *Aspergillus*. For patients suffering from pulmonary involvement, including invasive pulmonary aspergillosis (IPA) and allergic bronchopulmonary aspergillosis (ABPA), early identification, precise diagnosis, and timely initiation of suitable treatment are critical to improving outcomes. This is especially true for patients with weakened immune systems or underlying lung conditions.

2.1.1. Allergic Bronchopulmonary Aspergillosis/Mycosis: An Underdiagnosed Disease

After *Aspergillus* fumigatus has colonized the airways, a hypersensitive reaction to its antigens causes allergic bronchopulmonary aspergillosis (ABPA), an immune-allergic lung disease. Patients with cystic fibrosis (CF) and bronchial asthma are the most common populations affected. Even after being identified as a separate condition almost 70 years ago, this illness is still underdiagnosed. This could be because of the diagnostic criteria used, the diagnostic procedures used, or the absence of standardized testing. The primary therapy for ABPA is systemic steroid therapy. As a preferred method for sparing corticosteroids, azole antifungal drugs offer an alternative for treating exacerbations. Based on their mechanisms of type 2 inflammation inhibition, eosinophil, and IgE regulation, and inflammatory cytokine modulation, biologic drugs are anticipated to be important in the treatment of ABPA. Dr. K. first recognized allergic bronchopulmonary aspergillosis (ABPA) in 1952. F. W. Hinson, who detailed eight instances with typical clinical features such as eosinophilia, bronchiectasis, and/or mucus plugs, bronchitis/asthma, and *Aspergillus* fumigatus isolation in lung tissue. Although our department at Federal University of Rio de Janeiro in Brazil reported the first case of ABPA six years after it was first reported in the United States in 1968, the condition is still underdiagnosed globally and in Brazil in particular.

An exaggerated hypersensitivity reaction to the *Aspergillus* fumigatus species causes ABPA, a complex pulmonary disorder that manifests as bronchiectasis, mucus plugging, and airway inflammation. People who have cystic fibrosis (CF) or asthma are most at risk of developing ABPA. It is imperative to develop screening protocols for ABPA in these patients due to the disease's tendency to cause irreversible complications. A better prognosis depends on early disease detection.

2.1.2. Epidemiology

The frequency of ABPA is still unknown and is probably varies by region. Subject to variations within the studied population, ABPA affects 2.5–15% of patients with asthma and 7–9% of patients with CF. Asthmatic adults who were sensitized to A had a pooled prevalence of ABPA of 11.3%, according to a systematic literature review fumigatus (Af) accounted for 37%. The combined prevalence of ABPA in children who had asthma was 9.9%. Research carried out at our facility showed that children with CF had a prevalence of 12.5% for ABPA and 19% for asthmatics sensitized to Af. Over 4 million individuals globally are impacted by ABPA.

Furthermore, in vulnerable people, genetic predispositions like particular HLA-DR alleles may play a role in the development of ABPA. The incidence of ABPA is not age- or gender-specific, though it is less common in people without CF or asthma. Because of the diagnostic criteria used, lack of standardized tests, diagnostic methods used, and populations studied, it is challenging to determine the true prevalence of ABPA.

2.1.3. Pathogenesis

Aspergillus is a saprophytic fungus that grows on decomposing vegetation, spreads through the air, and is commonly found in soil. Because its spores are tiny (2–3 µm), they can be more easily deposited in the airways. When inhaled, *Aspergillus* spores can colonize and germinate in the respiratory tracts of susceptible individuals, such as those with cystic fibrosis (CF) or asthma. *Aspergillus* spores may germinate into mycelial filaments and remain in the lower respiratory tracts. This germination results in metabolite secretion, triggering an innate immune response in the mucosa and exposing *Aspergillus*. Due to impaired mucociliary clearance and heightened local immune response, *Aspergillus* hyphae are able to persist in the airways of these individuals.

The hallmark of allergic bronchopulmonary aspergillosis (ABPA) is a combination of type I (immediate) and type III (immune complex-mediated) hypersensitivity reactions. In type I hypersensitivity, *Aspergillus* antigens attach to immunoglobulin E (IgE) on mast cell and basophil surfaces, releasing inflammatory mediators like prostaglandins, histamine, and leukotrienes that result in mucus production, bronchoconstriction, and increased vascular permeability. In type III hypersensitivity, immunoglobulin G (IgG) and *Aspergillus* antigens form immune complexes that accumulate in lung tissue, activating complement and attracting inflammatory cells, which causes tissue damage and eosinophilic inflammation. Eosinophils are essential to ABPA pathophysiology, promoting mucus production, airway inflammation, and bronchial hyperresponsiveness.

In ABPA, significant type-2 (T2) inflammation occurs, marked by high levels of polyclonal IgE and substantial eosinophil infiltration of the airways. Cytokines produced by Th2 cells, including interleukins IL-4, IL-5, and IL-13, promote eosinophil recruitment, activation, and survival. Furthermore, IL-4 and IL-13 induce goblet cell hyperplasia, increasing mucus secretion and encouraging B cells to produce IgE. This airway inflammation results in the production of thick eosinophil mucus containing Charcot–Leyden crystals, which obstructs the airways. The potential involvement of CF transmembrane conductance regulator (CFTR) mutation in ABPA, even in the absence of CF, remains uncertain.

2.1.4. Clinical Manifestation

There is a wide range in the clinical presentation of ABPA, from mild to severe respiratory symptoms. The main clinical signs of ABPA are respiratory symptoms, which can be difficult to distinguish from those of asthma or cystic fibrosis because they frequently resemble each other. Chest tightness, dyspnea, wheezing, and paroxysmal coughing episodes are common respiratory symptoms of ABPA. Additionally, pulmonary exacerbations—which are marked by worsening respiratory symptoms and increased production of sputum—may occur frequently in patients with ABPA.

The expectoration of brownish-black mucus plugs containing eosinophilic material and fungal hyphae is a characteristic feature of ABPA. These mucus plugs can impede mucociliary clearance and cause airway obstruction, which can exacerbate bronchiectasis and recurrent infections. In ABPA, systemic symptoms like fever, malaise, and weight loss are possible, especially during exacerbations. It is believed that the immune system's reaction to *Aspergillus* antigens and the release of inflammatory mediators are connected to these symptoms. Exacerbations of ABPA, which are defined by the beginning or worsening of the disease's clinical manifestations and are frequently linked to radiological anomalies, elevated eosinophil counts, and elevated total IgE, are indicative of evolution (Oliveira Rodrigues et al, 2023).

2.1.5. Diagnostic Criteria

The majority of people with ABPA have been diagnosed with CF or asthma. The diagnosis is made using a combination of immunological, radiological, and clinical characteristics. A careful review of the literature in the field emphasizes how crucial it is to identify ABPA early and treat it appropriately to stop the disease from getting worse and developing complications.

Over the years, the diagnostic criteria and approaches for ABPA have evolved significantly (Table 2.1).

Table 2.1. *Diagnostic Criteria for ABPA*

Rosenberg-Patterson 1977 Criteria for Diagnosis of ABPA	
Primary criteria (1–6 suggestive, +7 definite)	
1.	Episodic bronchial obstruction
2.	Peripheral eosinophilia
3.	Positive immediate skin test to *Aspergillus*
4.	Positive preciptin test to *Aspergillus*
5.	Increased total serum IgE
6.	History of transient or fixed lung infiltrates
7.	Proximal bronchiectasis
Secondary (supportive) criteria	
1.	Brown plugs/flecks in sputum
2.	Positive late (6–12 h/Arthus) skin test to *Aspergillus*
Modified ISHAM working group 2013 criteria for diagnosis of ABPA	
1.	Predisposing asthma or CF
2.	Obligatory criteria
a.	IgE > 1000 IU/mL and
b.	Positive immediate skin test or increased IgE antibody to *Aspergillus*
3.	Supportive (≥2) criteria
a.	Eosinophila > 500
b.	Precipitins or increased IgG antibody to *Aspergillus*
c.	Consistent radiographic opacities

Source: Tracy MC, Okorie CUA, Foley EA, Moss RB. Allergic Bronchopulmonary Aspergillosis. Journal of Fungi. 2016; 2(2):17. https://doi.org/10.3390/jof2020017.

The initial ABPA diagnostic criteria were mainly based on radiological findings, blood eosinophilia, and clinical features. Following the identification of the IgE antibody isotype in the 1970s, serology began to play a major role in the diagnosis of ABPA. Two sets of criteria were put forth by Rosenberg and Patterson to enhance diagnosis. Since then, the most common criteria for diagnosing ABPA have been these seven primary and three secondary criteria.

These criteria, however, lacked specificity and sensitivity, which resulted in an incorrect or underdiagnosed diagnosis. To provide standardized guidelines for ABPA diagnosis, the International Society for Human and Animal Mycology (ABPA-ISHAM). Working Group on ABPA proposed new diagnostic criteria in 2013. Thereafter, more information regarding the "sensibility and specificity" of the ISHAM criteria became available. This evidence was discovered during a study that examined how well several new and established diagnostic criteria performed using a latent class analysis. It has been shown that IgE-specific tests are more sensitive than skin tests to detect *Aspergillus* sensitization and that the sensitivity and specificity are enhanced when a threshold for total IgE of 500 kIU/l is used. Furthermore, a cut-off for particular IgG to *Aspergillus* was suggested. The ISHAM changed the diagnostic standards in response to this evidence. These changes were released in 2021 and provided better diagnostic performance. The ISHAM criteria were validated, however it was found that the sensitivity was low for cases of non-ABPM (*Aspergillus* Allergic Bronchopulmonary Mycosis). Asano et al. proposed and validated new diagnostic criteria that showed improved sensitivity and specificity compared to previous criteria of Rosenberg-Paterson and ISHAM, even in atypical cases without asthma or non-*Aspergillus* ABPM (Table 2.1).

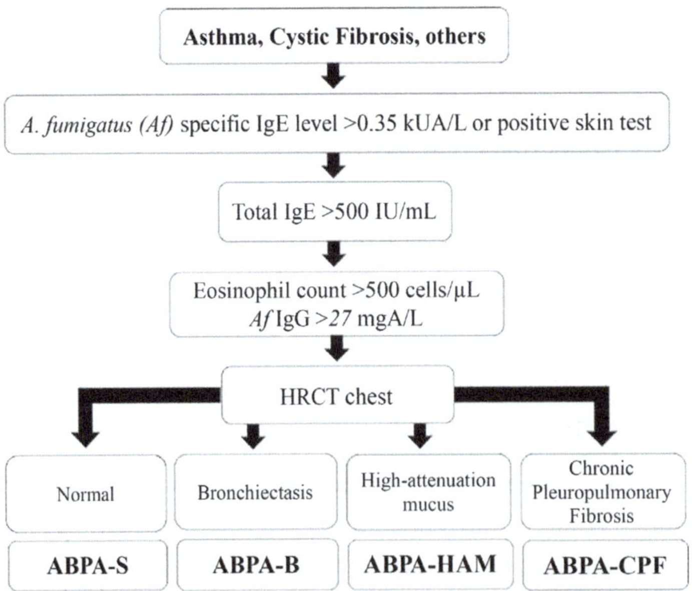

Figure 2.1. *Algorithm to diagnosis and radiographic classification of ABPA. Af: Aspergillus fumigatus; HCTR: High-resolution computed tomography; ABPA-S: Serologic ABPA; ABPA-B: ABPA with bronchiectasis; ABPA-HAM: ABPA with high-attenuation mucus; ABPA-CPF: ABPA with chronic pleuropulmonary fibrosis.*

Source: Oliveira Rodrigues Valle, S, Sarquis Serpa, A, & Sarquis Serpa, F. (2023). Allergic Bronchopulmonary Aspergillosis/Mycosis: An Underdiagnosed Disease. IntechOpen. doi: 10.5772/intechopen.112166.

The diagnostic of ABPA often follows an algorithm that integrates multiple pieces of clinical, immunological, and radiological information. The starting point is a clinical assessment, looking for key symptoms and risk factors, especially asthma or CF and then elevated specific IgE to *Af*. Total serum IgE levels are also evaluated, which typically exceed 500 IU/mL, while peripheral eosinophils >500 cels/μL and specific IgG-*Af*> 27 mg_A/l provide further evidence of a patient's immunological response to the fungus. Chest high-resolution computed tomography (HRCT) is another essential component of the algorithm because it provides a classification of ABPA based on the features observed (Figure 2.1).

Even with the recent improvements to the diagnostic criteria, diagnosing ABPA in clinical practice is still difficult. It is crucial to remember that the diagnostic algorithm may change slightly in response to particular recommendations and advancements in diagnostic technology. For instance, there is disagreement over which IgE levels are indicative of ABPA. Patterson along with others. had previously reported in 1983 that patients with ABPA had twice as much specific IgE and IgG for Af than patients with Af-sensitive asthma. An overdiagnosis of ABPA may occur if a cutoff of 0.35 kUA/L is used for Af-IgE. Additionally, the ImmunoCAP® method was used to determine the cutoff to IgG-Af proposed in the ISHMA criteria in an Asian population. The results were significantly lower than those reported by other European studies in patients with ABPA.

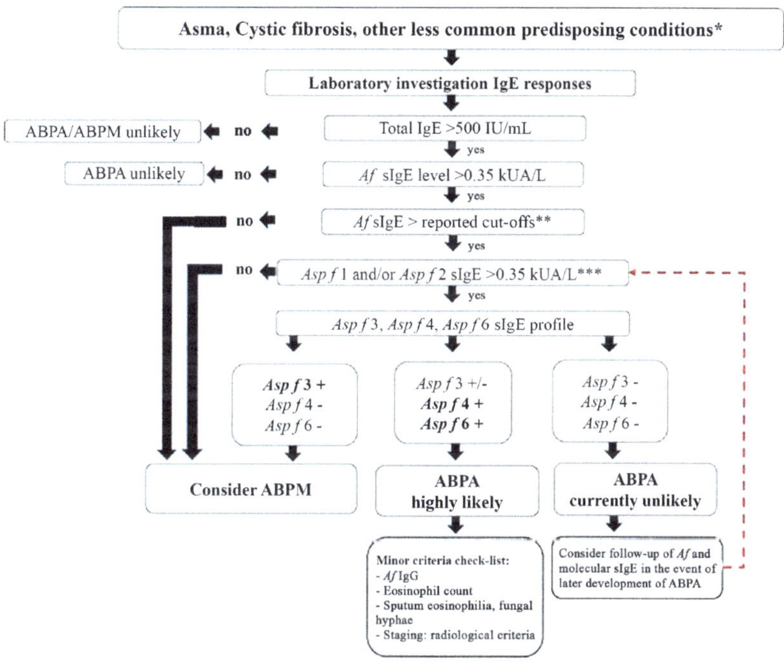

Figure 2.2. *Laboratory investigation of recombinant Aspergillus antigen-based algorithm for diagnosing ABPA. Chronic obstructive pulmonary disease, altered bronchopulmonary structure; consider the establishment of locally validated cut-offs; consider the ratio of sIgE to molecular allergens vs. Af sIgE.*

Source: Oliveira Rodrigues Valle, S, Sarquis Serpa, A, & Sarquis Serpa, F. (2023). Allergic Bronchopulmonary Aspergillosis/Mycosis: An Underdiagnosed Disease. IntechOpen. doi: 10.5772/intechopen.112166.

It has been suggested recently to use molecular allergology. These tests assess IgE directed against allergen components of Af (rAsp) to enhance diagnosis, considering that IgE specific to Af is unable to differentiate between Af allergy and sensitization. Since it is well known that certain Af proteins may be important in ABPA, this method can be used to identify them. **Table 2.2.** *Radiographic Features Described in ABPA*

Chest Radiography Findings	
Transitory	• Peripheral infiltrate • Air-fluid levels • Consolidations • Toothpaste image • Train line image • Lobe or segmental collapse
Permanent	• Bronchiectasis • Parallel line image • Ring shadow • Pulmonary fibrosis
High-Resolution Chest Tomography Findings	
Bronchi	• Bronchiectasis • Mucus plug with high attenuation • Dilated bronchi • Occluded bronchi • Bronchial thickening
Parenchyma	• Cavitation • Bullous emphysema • Pleural involvement • Pneumothorax • Pleural fibrosis

Source: Oliveira Rodrigues Valle, S, Sarquis Serpa, A, & Sarquis Serpa, F. (2023). Allergic Bronchopulmonary Aspergillosis/Mycosis: An Underdiagnosed Disease. IntechOpen. doi: 10.5772/intechopen.112166.

When diagnosing ABPA in patients with asthma and cystic fibrosis (CF), the presence of either rAsp f1 or rAsp f3 showed high sensitivity and rAsp f4 or rAsp f6 showed high specificity. Based on the proposal of a diagnostic algorithm that includes r*Asp* to improve the accuracy of diagnosis, the EAACI ABPA Task Force proposed changes to the algorithm and reinforced the need for adequate recommendations for countries with limited resources (Figure 2.2).

The diagnosis and treatment of ABPA depend heavily on chest radiography, which can show characteristics ranging from normal to pulmonary fibrosis manifestations (Table 2.2). This range of symptoms is indicative of both the disease's possible course and each person's unique reaction to *Aspergillus*. These radiographic features have been the subject of several studies. It has been shown that HRCT is the gold standard for locating the distribution of bronchiectasis and spotting minute radiographic abnormalities like tree-in-bud opacities, which could be signs of small airway involvement in ABPA.

Transient pulmonary infiltrates, which usually appear as patchy opacities or consolidation, may be seen in the acute stage of ABPA. These infiltrates may go away on their own or get better with medicine. More pronounced, long-lasting alterations in HRCT can be seen as ABPA advances. Among them is central bronchiectasis, which primarily affects the upper lobes. Another crucial characteristic is the presence of high-attenuation mucus (HAM) in the bronchi, which is frequently linked to bronchial dilatation that resembles the "finger-in-glove" sign. When the density of mucus is noticeably higher than that of the paraspinal muscle, it is said to be associated with hypertrophic mucus, calcium salts, metal ions (iron or manganese), and/or desiccated mucus. Indicators of the chronic stage also include thickening of the bronchial wall and parenchymal scarring, which are indicative of chronic inflammation and damage. ABPA patients frequently have centrilobular nodules with a "tree-in-bud" pattern, which is suggestive of small airway inflammation and frequently linked to chronic inflammation. Fibrosis and architectural distortion, primarily affecting the upper lobes, are indicative of the fibrotic end stage of the disease. Traction bronchiectasis, honeycombing, and volume loss on HRCT are some of the symptoms of pulmonary fibrosis.

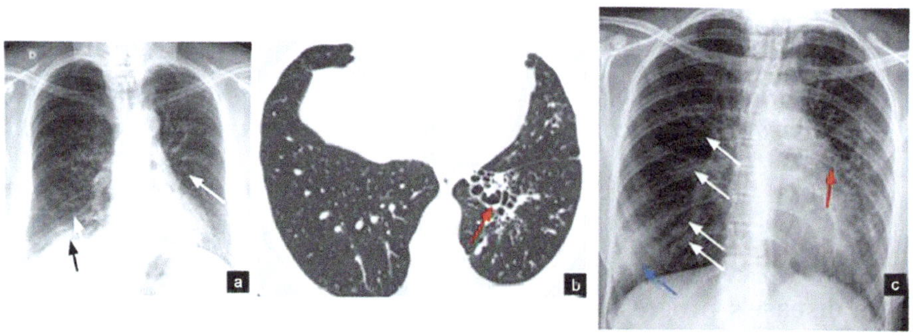

Figure 2.3. *(a) A 64-year-old female. Radiograph with consolidation in the right lower lobe (black arrow), in addition to some bilateral bronchiectasis with parietal thickening (white arrows). (b) Chest CT of the same patient demonstrates multiple central bronchiectasis in the left lower lobe with thickening and interspersed hyperdense content, a finding highly specific for ABPA (allergic bronchopulmonary aspergillosis). (c) a 16-year-old female. The radiograph shows consolidations in the peripheral region of the left lung (red arrow) and in the right lower lobe (blue arrow), in addition to bronchiectasis with thickened walls, and the tram-track sign (white arrows).*

Source: *Oliveira Rodrigues Valle, S, Sarquis Serpa, A, & Sarquis Serpa, F. (2023). Allergic*

Bronchopulmonary Aspergillosis/Mycosis: An Underdiagnosed Disease. IntechOpen. doi: 10.5772/intechopen.112166.

HRCT plays a crucial role in the image-based classification of ABPA because it provides detailed insights into the nature and extent of the disease. ABPA can be divided into four types, or phenotypes, using HRCT. Individuals with serologic ABPA are those who have no abnormalities on a chest scan (ABPA-S). On the other hand, people with central bronchiectasis are diagnosed with ABPA Central Bronchiectasis (ABPA-CB). The illness is classified as ABPA-High Attenuation Mucus (ABPA-HAM) due to the presence of HAM.

Lastly, if at least two radiological features suggestive of fibrosis (fibrocavitary lesions, pulmonary fibrosis, and pleural thickening) are observed in the absence of mucoid impaction (or HAM), the disease is classified as ABPA-Chronic Pleuropulmonary Fibrosis (ABPA-CPF) (Figures 2.1, 2.3, and 2.4). Timely recognition and appropriate monitoring of radiographic changes are essential for optimizing patient care and outcomes in ABPA.

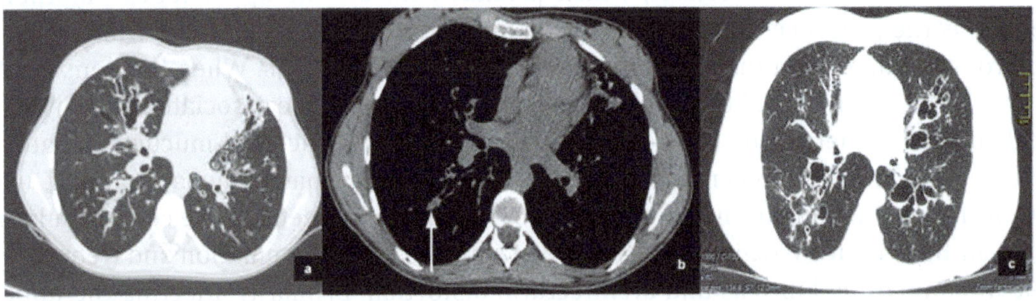

Figure 2.4. *CT imaging of patients diagnosed with ABPA: (a) multiple bilateral bronchiectasis with parietal thickening and mucoid impactation; (b) mucoid impactation in mediastinal window of the same patient (white arrow); (c) central bronchiectasis in a corticosteroid-dependent patient who has experienced multiple exacerbations.*

Source: Oliveira Rodrigues Valle, S, Sarquis Serpa, A, & Sarquis Serpa, F. (2023). Allergic Bronchopulmonary Aspergillosis/Mycosis: An Underdiagnosed Disease. IntechOpen. doi: 10.5772/intechopen.112166.

2.1.6. Staging of ABPA

Understanding the disease's progression and diagnosing ABPA all depend on the staging of the condition. The first suggested these stages and are frequently employed. Agarwal et al. have reviewed and updated the staging. , who put forth a more thorough six-stage system that further divides some stages according to radiological results (Table 2.3).

Table 2.3. *Staging of ABPA*

Stage	Clinical, Radiographic, and Laboratorial Features
0 – Asymptomatic	• No previous diagnosis of ABPA • Controlled asthma • Fulfilling the diagnostic criteria of ABPA
1 – Acute	• No previous diagnosis of ABPA • Uncontrolled asthma/symptoms consistent with ABPA • Satisfying the diagnostic criteria of ABPA
1a – With mucoid impaction	• Mucoid impaction observed on thoracic imaging
1b – Without mucoid impaction	• Absence of mucoid impaction on thoracic imaging
2 – Remission	• Clinical and/or radiological improvement and • Decline in serum total IgE by ≥25% of baseline at 8 weeks
3 – Exacerbation	• Clinical and/or radiological worsening and • Increase in serum total IgE by at least 50% from the new baseline established during response/remission
4 – Remission	• Sustained clinical and radiological improvement and • Serum total IgE levels persisting at or below baseline (or increase by <50%) for ≥6 months off treatment
5a – Treatment-dependent ABPA	• Two or more exacerbations within 6 months of stopping therapy OR • Clinical and/or radiological worsening, along with increase in serum total IgE levels, on tapering oral steroids/azoles
5b – Steroid dependent asthma	• Systemic corticosteroids required for control of asthma while the ABPA activity is controlled (as indicated by serum total IgE and thoracic imaging)
6 – Advanced ABPA	• Extensive bronchiectasis due to ABPA on chest imaging AND • Complications (cor pulmonale and/or chronic Type II respiratory failure

Source: Oliveira Rodrigues Valle, S, Sarquis Serpa, A, & Sarquis Serpa, F. (2023). Allergic Bronchopulmonary Aspergillosis/Mycosis: An Underdiagnosed Disease. IntechOpen. doi: 10.5772/intechopen.112166.

2.1.7. Differential Diagnosis

Several pulmonary conditions, including asthma with Af sensitization, tuberculosis, nontuberculous mycobacterial infections, eosinophilic granulomatosis with polyangiitis, and idiopathic chronic eosinophilic pneumonia, are included in the differential diagnosis of ABPA. These conditions also share radiological and clinical features with ABPA. A comprehensive clinical assessment, including the identification of risk factors, is necessary to differentiate ABPA from these conditions. Appropriate testing should also be performed to confirm or rule out these conditions.

2.1.7.1. Treatment

In individuals with bronchiectasis, ABPA is acknowledged as a treatable characteristic. Treatment is expected to prevent lung damage and improve quality of life. Depending on the disease's stage, the management of ABPA entails a combination of systemic corticosteroid, antifungal therapy, immunobiological agents, and airway clearance techniques catered to the specific needs of each patient to accomplish these goals (Table 2.4).

Table 2.4. *Drugs Used in the Management of ABPA*

Drugs		Indication
Oral corticosteroids	Prednisolone (or equivalent), 0.5 mg/kg over a period of 14 days, followed by 0.5 mg/kg/day on alternate days for 8 weeks, then reduce 5 mg every 2 weeks. Total duration of 3–5 months or Prednisolone (or equivalent), 0.75 mg/kg/day for 6 weeks, then reduce 5 mg every 6 weeks. Total duration: 6–12 months	• Acute stage • Exacerbation stage
Intravenous corticosteroid	• Methylprednisolone, 15 mg/day (note exceeding 1 g) intravenous for 3 consecutive days	• To minimize the side effects of daily corticosteroid therapy • Refractory ABPA exacerbations
Antifungal	Oral antifungal therapy: Itraconazol 200 mg twice a day for 16 weeks OR Voriconazole 200 mg twice a day, for at least 24 weeks Nebulized antifungal therapy: Amphotericin B	• Acute stage • Exacerbation stage
Immunobiological	Omalizumab 150 mg: approved for ages ≥6 years, SC injection. Dose and frequency depend on the patient's weight and the serum IgE level at the start of treatment. Highest permitted serum total IgE is 1500 IU/mL OR Mepolizumab 40 mg or 100 mg: approved for ages ≥6 years. For children 6–11 years, 40 mg SC injection every 4 weeks. For ≥12 years, 100 mg SC injection every 4 weeks OR Benralizumab 30 mg: approved for ages ≥12 years, SC injection every 4 weeks for three doses then every 8 weeks OR Dupilumab 200 mg or 300 mg: approved for ages ≥6 years, SC injections every 2 weeks. For children 6–11 years, dose, and frequency depend on weight. For ages ≥12 years 300 mg for asthma corticosteroid-dependent severe asthma or concomitant moderate/severe atopic dermatitis OR • Tezepelumab 210 mg: approved for ages ≥12 years, SC injection every 4 weeks	• Refractory ABPA • Uncontrolled asthma • Adverse effects or • Contraindications to corticosteroids and azoles

Source: Oliveira Rodrigues Valle, S, Sarquis Serpa, A, & Sarquis Serpa, F. (2023). Allergic Bronchopulmonary Aspergillosis/Mycosis: An Underdiagnosed Disease. IntechOpen. doi: 10.5772/intechopen.112166.

2.1.7.1.1. Corticosteroids

The initial course of treatment for ABPA is oral corticosteroids. There exist multiple treatment regimens, each with different dosages and durations of use, but the optimal dosage and duration of treatment are still unknown. The most popular regimen starts with a daily dose of 0.5 mg/kg of prednisolone for 14 days. After that, it is tapered down to 0.5 mg/kg/day on alternate days for 8 weeks. This allows for a total steroid duration of 3–5 months.

Even though most patients who receive medium- to high-dose systemic corticosteroids achieve disease remission, relapse happens in a significant percentage of patients (13.5–45%), and these patients may develop a corticosteroid dependency. Oral administration of corticosteroids may be replaced with an intravenous pulse dose. Methylprednisolone has been used in children to treat refractory ABPA exacerbations and to reduce the side effects of daily corticosteroid therapy at a dose of 15 mg/day (note that this dose does not exceed 1 g).

2.1.7.1.2. Antifungal Therapy

Antifungal drugs reduce antigenic stimulus, the inflammatory response, the fungal burden in the airways, and they may also help lower systemic corticosteroid exposure. When treating ABPA, azole agents can be used either alone or in conjunction with corticosteroids. Itraconazole and other azoles are typically prescribed for 16 weeks at a dose of 200 mg twice a day. When comparing the one-year exacerbation rate, the combination of itraconazole and prednisolone was more effective than either medication alone.

However, the use may be restricted due to hepatotoxicity, drug interactions, and variable bioavailability. Treatment for ABPA has also shown promise with other azoles, including voriconazole and posaconazole, particularly in cases of itraconazole resistance or intolerance. Nebulized amphotericin B appears to have limited effectiveness in treating ABPA exacerbations. They might, however, be taken into account after all other options have been explored.

2.1.7.1.3. Immunobiological Drugs

Whether receiving oral corticosteroids, antifungal therapy, or both, posttreatment recurrences of ABPA are frequently observed, and prolonged treatment can have negative effects. Thus, it is evident that new, secure, and efficient treatment approaches are required. Because of the pathophysiology of ABPA, biologics that target type 2 inflammation and were first created to manage severe asthma are anticipated to be useful treatment options for ABPA. The advantages of targeting type 2 inflammation in the treatment of ABPA have been shown in recent case reports and case series, despite the lack of randomized controlled trials.

Omalizumab, an anti-IgE monoclonal antibody, has demonstrated promise in lowering the need for corticosteroids, enhancing lung function, and averting relapses. Every two to four weeks, omalizumabe is given subcutaneously. The dosage is established by taking the patient's weight and baseline serum total IgE levels into consideration. However, because of the high levels of IgE found in ABPA, the doses used may not have been ideal. Biologics that target the IL-5/eosinophil pathway include benralizumab, which has shown efficacy in treating resistant eosinophilic pulmonary disorders like ABPA, and monoclonal antibodies that target IL-5, such as mepolizumab and reslizumab, and those that target the IL-5 receptor-alpha chain (IL-5Rα). Anti-IL-5/IL-5Rα mAbs have demonstrated efficacy in decreasing the frequency of exacerbations, increasing the dosage of oral corticosteroids, and improving pulmonary function in patients suffering from asthma-complicated ABPA, including those who do not respond to omalizumab. Anti-IL-4Rα monoclonal antibody dupilumab has been demonstrated to have therapeutic effects on both pulmonary function and symptoms. Dupilumab treatment was effective for certain ABPA patients who were resistant to omalizumab or mepolizumab treatment. By restoring broad inflammatory pathways, ezepelumab, a human IgG2 monoclonal antibody that binds specifically to thymic stromal lymphopoietin (TSLP), has been shown to improve the management of severe asthma. A case study on a patient treated with mepolizumab was recently published, and it demonstrated improvements in symptom management as well as a decrease in pulmonary opacities and mucus plugs.

Patients with ABPA may benefit from airway clearance techniques like positive expiratory pressure devices and chest physiotherapy, especially if they also have coexisting CF. By using these methods, you can enhance lung function, get rid of mucus plugs, and lower your chance of getting infections again. The way that ABPA is treated for CF and asthma is not all that dissimilar. Treatment for CF patients is more complicated because they frequently have coexisting malabsorption. Oral medications, particularly itraconazole capsules, may not be absorbed well.

2.1.7.2. Monitoring of Treatment

Every eight weeks, measurements of the serum total IgE concentration, clinical parameters, and chest radiographs should be used to track the patient's response to treatment. Radiographic opacities should resolve, serum total IgE levels should drop by at least 25%, and the "new" baseline level needs to be established. A 50% increase in IgE levels combined with a worsening of clinical and/or radiological symptoms points to an exacerbation (Oliveira Rodrigues Valle et al., 2023).

2.2. Hypersensitivity Pneumonitis

Extrinsic allergic alveolitis (EAA), also known as hypersensitivity pneumonitis (HP), is a syndrome that develops in susceptible or sensitized individuals when they repeatedly inhale environmental antigens. Molds, bacteria, bird feces, dust from agriculture, bioaerosols, paint or plastic chemicals, and bird droppings are examples of common antigens. Individuals with this kind of lung inflammation (pneumonitis) are frequently exposed to the antigens through their jobs, interests, the outdoors, and animals. Inhaled antigens trigger a hypersensitivity immune response that inflames the lung's small airways, or bronchioles, and airspaces, or alveoli. Interstitial lung disease may eventually result from hypersensitive pneumonitis.

Extrinsic allergic alveolitis, or hypersensitivity pneumonitis (HP), is a complicated inflammatory lung disease brought on by inhaling different organic or inorganic antigens repeatedly. This causes an overabundance of immune response in the lung parenchyma. Depending on the duration and degree of antigen exposure as well as unique host factors, HP can present in a variety of clinical ways, from acute to subacute to chronic. An abnormal immune response to inhaled antigens is a pathogenesis of HP that leads to interstitial fibrosis, granuloma formation, and inflammation of the alveoli. When exposed to the offending antigen—such as mold spores, bird proteins, or dust from their jobs—their immune systems become activated, releasing pro-inflammatory cytokines, and drawing inflammatory cells into the interstitium of their lungs. Repeated exposure to the antigen over time causes fibrotic changes, tissue remodeling, and chronic inflammation in the lungs, which ultimately affects lung function and gas exchange. The length and degree of antigen exposure, in addition to host characteristics like age, genetic predisposition, and underlying lung disease, all affect how HP manifests clinically. Usually occurring hours to days after antigen exposure, acute HP presents as flu-like symptoms such as fever, chills, cough, dyspnea, and malaise that go away when the offending environment is removed. The subtle onset of progressive dyspnea, cough, exhaustion, and weight loss that characterize subacute and chronic forms of HP frequently resembles other interstitial lung diseases like sarcoidosis or idiopathic pulmonary fibrosis (IPF).

The diagnosis of HP involves a thorough assessment incorporating a detailed medical history, physical examination, imaging studies, pulmonary function tests, and serological testing for specific antibodies. High-resolution computed tomography (HRCT) of the chest typically shows characteristic findings like ground-glass opacities, centrilobular nodules, mosaic attenuation, and air trapping, which can be patchy or diffuse depending on the disease stage. Bronchoalveolar lavage (BAL) may reveal a predominance of lymphocytes, an elevated CD4/CD8 ratio, and increased levels of inflammatory markers like interleukin-8 (IL-8) or tumor necrosis factor-alpha (TNF-alpha). Histopathological examination of lung tissue obtained via biopsy may show lymphocytic bronchiolitis, non-necrotizing granulomas, or fibrosis consistent with HP.

The goal of managing HP is to find the offending antigen and eliminate it from the patient's surroundings to stop the disease from progressing and avoid additional exposure. This could mean making adjustments to the workspace or surroundings, like avoiding contaminated areas, putting dust control measures in place, or taking pets or birds inside the house. The primary goal of pharmacological treatment for acute or subacute forms of HP is to reduce inflammation and alter the immune response. Systemic corticosteroids are commonly used in this capacity. To lower disease activity and maintain lung function, immunosuppressive medications like azathioprine, mycophenolate mofetil, or rituximab may be considered for patients with chronic HP or those who do not respond well to corticosteroids.

The degree of lung involvement, the time it takes to remove antigens and start treatment, and the stage of the disease at presentation all affect the prognosis for HP. After being removed from the offending environment, acute HP typically has a good prognosis with full resolution of symptoms and radiographic abnormalities. If untreated, subacute, and chronic forms of HP can lead to irreversible fibrosis and respiratory failure, emphasizing the significance of early detection and treatment. Monitoring over an extended time is necessary to evaluate the state of the disease, track lung function, and identify any possible side effects like cor pulmonale or pulmonary hypertension.

Exaggerated immune response within the lung parenchyma results from repeated inhalation of different organic or inorganic antigens, which causes hypersensitivity pneumonitis, a complex inflammatory lung disease. Depending on the length and degree of antigen exposure, clinical presentation can vary. A thorough evaluation that includes imaging studies, serological testing, and medical history is necessary for diagnosis. To stop the disease from getting worse and maintain lung function, management strategies include avoiding antigens, taking medication, and doing long-term monitoring.

2.2.1. Signs and Symptoms

Hypersensitivity pneumonitis (HP) can be categorized as acute, subacute, and chronic based on the duration of the illness.

2.2.1.1. Acute

The dose of antigen exposure in the acute form of HP is typically very high, but it lasts only briefly. Four to six hours after intense exposure to the provoking antigen, symptoms may appear. Fever, chills, malaise, coughing, tightness in the chest, dyspnea, rash, swelling, and headache are among the symptoms. The symptoms go away after stopping the exposure in a matter of hours to days.

2.2.1.2. Subacute

Subacute HP patients experience pleurisy, anorexia, dyspnea, exhaustion, and a productive cough over time. While less severe and lasting longer, the symptoms are comparable to those of the acute form of the illness. Patients who have had recurrent acute episodes may exhibit findings.

2.2.1.3. Chronic

Chronic hypersensitivity pneumonitis typically involves low-volume doses of antigens over a long period of time. Patients may not have a history of acute episodes but instead experience a gradual onset of symptoms such as cough, dyspnea, fatigue, and weight loss. Symptoms can be partially or completely reversible with avoidance of further exposure to the allergen. Clubbing is seen in about half of patients, while tachypnea, respiratory distress, and crackles in the lower lung fields are common. Hypersensitivity pneumonitis can sometimes be mistaken for idiopathic pulmonary fibrosis due to the presence of pulmonary fibrosis and hypoxemia in many patients.

2.3. Eosinophilic Pneumonia

A rare but potentially dangerous respiratory disease known as eosinophilic pneumonia (EP) is characterized by an accumulation of eosinophils in the airways and lung parenchyma, which can cause tissue damage, inflammation, and poor gas exchange. Acute eosinophilic pneumonia (AEP), chronic eosinophilic pneumonia (CEP), and eosinophilic granulomatosis with polyangiitis (EGPA) are among the diseases that fall under the umbrella of EP. Each of these conditions has a unique clinical presentation, underlying cause, and mode of treatment.

The typical presentation of acute eosinophilic pneumonia (AEP) is a sudden onset of fever, cough, dyspnea, and hypoxemia. Chest imaging frequently shows diffuse pulmonary infiltrates in addition to these symptoms. Though the precise etiology of AEP is still unknown, it is frequently linked to the recent onset or exposure to medications, illegal drugs, or environmental triggers. Diffuse alveolar damage with prominent eosinophilic infiltration, pulmonary edema, and the formation of hyaline membranes are revealed by histopathological examination of lung tissue obtained through biopsy, all of which are consistent with an acute inflammatory response.

Chronic eosinophilic pneumonia (CEP) is a condition that usually begins slowly with symptoms such as a persistent cough, difficulty breathing, fatigue, and weight loss. It may take weeks to months before a diagnosis is made. Chest imaging typically shows areas of consolidation in the outer regions of the lungs, accompanied by an increase in eosinophils in the blood and higher than normal levels of IgE in the serum. The lung tissue of those with CEP often displays scattered areas of inflammation and eosinophil infiltration, along with changes resembling bronchiolitis obliterans organizing pneumonia (BOOP), indicating a long-lasting inflammatory process.

Formerly known as Churg-Strauss syndrome, Eosinophilic granulomatosis with polyangiitis (EGPA) is a systemic vasculitis characterized by asthma, eosinophilia, and small-to-medium vessel vasculitis affecting multiple organ systems, particularly the lungs. Common symptoms of EGPA include asthma exacerbations, sinusitis, neuropathy, and skin manifestations, along with pulmonary infiltrates and elevated eosinophils on lab tests. Histopathological features of EGPA include necrotizing vasculitis with eosinophilic infiltrates, granulomatous inflammation, and tissue eosinophilia.

A comprehensive assessment is necessary to diagnose eosinophilic pneumonia. This assessment should include a thorough medical history, physical examination, laboratory testing, imaging studies, and, in certain situations, a histopathological examination of lung tissue that was obtained through biopsy. In EP, peripheral blood eosinophilia is frequently observed, though it can also be absent in certain instances, especially in acute presentations. Bilateral pulmonary infiltrates with peripheral or basilar predominance are commonly seen on chest imaging, though the pattern may differ based on the specific EP subtype.

To control eosinophilic pneumonia, the underlying cause or inciting factor must be located, removed, and, if necessary, treated with medication to reduce inflammation and alleviate symptoms. To quickly decrease eosinophilic infiltration and avoid respiratory failure, acute eosinophilic pneumonia (AEP) frequently necessitates hospitalization and systemic corticosteroid treatment. Corticosteroid treatment for chronic eosinophilic pneumonia (CEP) may be effective, but relapses are frequent and long-term maintenance medication may be required to stop recurrence. To effectively manage asthma, vasculitis, and systemic manifestations of eosinophilic granulomatosis with polyangiitis (EGPA), pulmonologists, rheumatologists, and immunologists are needed. EGPA is often treated with a combination of corticosteroids, immunosuppressive agents, and biologic therapies.

A group of respiratory illnesses known as eosinophilic pneumonia is defined by the infiltration of eosinophils into the airways and lung parenchyma, which results in tissue damage, inflammation, and poor gas exchange. A thorough evaluation is necessary for diagnosis, and management entails locating and, if feasible, eliminating the underlying cause or inciting factor as well as starting the proper pharmacological therapy to reduce inflammation and ameliorate symptoms. To stop the disease progression and enhance the prognosis of eosinophilic pneumonia patients, early detection and treatment are crucial.

2.3.1. Classification of Eosinophilic Pneumonia

Depending on whether the cause of eosinophilic pneumonia can be identified or not, the condition is classified into various categories. Known causes include cancer, parasite infections, and specific drugs or environmental triggers. Eosinophilic granulomatosis with polyangiitis, a condition in which the immune system attacks the lungs, can also result in eosinophilic pneumonia. Idiopathic refers to eosinophilic pneumonia in cases where a cause is not identified. Acute and chronic forms of idiopathic eosinophilic pneumonia can also be distinguished based on the symptoms a patient is presenting with.

2.3.2. Signs and Symptoms

The signs and symptoms of the majority of eosinophilic pneumonia types are comparable. Cough, fever, dyspnea, and nocturnal sweats are common and almost universal indications and symptoms. The course of acute eosinophilic pneumonia usually proceeds quickly. It may take just one or two weeks for a fever and cough to appear before breathing problems worsen to the point where mechanical ventilation is necessary due to respiratory failure. The course of chronic eosinophilic pneumonia is typically slower. The illness progresses over several months and manifests as fever, coughing, dyspnea, wheezing, and weight loss. Before the right diagnosis of asthma is made, people with chronic eosinophilic pneumonia are frequently misdiagnosed as having asthma.

Similar to eosinophilic pneumonia brought on by drugs or environmental exposures, eosinophilic pneumonia develops following exposure to a recognized offending agent. Similar prodromes are present in eosinophilic pneumonia caused by parasite infections, along with a wide range of symptoms of the various underlying parasites. When cancer is present, eosinophilic pneumonia frequently occurs in the context of a confirmed diagnosis of lung cancer, cervical cancer, or another specific type of cancer.

2.3.3. Pathophysiology

The development of eosinophilic pneumonia can vary based on the underlying etiology of the illness. Eosinophils are essential for protecting the body from parasite infection. Excessive release of chemicals by eosinophils in response to environmental triggers is the cause of numerous diseases, including eczema and asthma e.g., cytokines as well as histamine. All causes of eosinophilic pneumonia have eosinophil overreaction or lung dysfunction as a common feature.

2.3.3.1. Medications and Environmental Exposures

Environmental exposures, drug abuse, and medication side effects can all cause eosinophil dysfunction. Drugs like nonsteroidal anti-inflammatory medications (e.g., nitrofurantoin, phenytoin, L-tryptophan, daptomycin, ampicillin, and painkillers like heroin and cocaine inhalation can cause an allergic reaction that leads to eosinophilic pneumonia. When inhaled, chemicals including sulfites, aluminum silicate, and cigarette smoke can result in eosinophilic pneumonia.

2.3.3.2. Parasitic Infections

Eosinophilic pneumonia is caused by parasites in three different ways. It is possible for parasites to enter the lungs, reside there as part of their life cycle, or enter the lungs through the bloodstream. After migrating to the lungs to combat the parasites, eosinophils discharge their contents into the lungs, which results in eosinophilic pneumonia. The tapeworms Echinococcus and *Taenia solium*, as well as Paragonimus lung flukes, are significant parasites that infect the lungs. Key parasites that live in the lungs as part of their regular life cycle are the hookworms *Ancylostoma duodenale* and *Necator americanus*, the worms (helminths). *Ascaris lumbricoides* and *Strongyloides stercoralis*. Eosinophilic pneumonia is commonly referred to as Löffler's syndrome when helminths are the cause. When the final group of parasite eggs enter the lungs through the bloodstream, it results in eosinophilic pneumonia. *Ascaris lumbricoides*, *Strongyloides stercoralis*, *Trichinella spiralis*, hookworms, and schistosomes are a few examples of this.

2.3.3.3. Acute and Chronic Eosinophilic Pneumonia

As of 2005, the causes of eosinophilic pneumonia, both acute and chronic, were unknown. There is some suspicion that the body's reaction to an unknown environmental agent is what causes the acute form, at the very least.

2.3.4. Diagnosis

Three situations can lead to the diagnosis of eosinophilic pneumonia: increased eosinophils on a complete blood count and abnormalities in the lungs on a chest X-ray or computed tomography; increased eosinophils in lung tissue found during a biopsy; or increased eosinophils in fluid from a bronchoscopy (bronchoalveolar lavage fluid). Examining a person's medical history usually reveals any associations with cancer or medication. After assessing a person's exposure to common parasites and running laboratory tests to rule out possible causes, specific parasitic infections are diagnosed. The following criteria are used to diagnose acute or chronic eosinophilic pneumonia if no underlying cause is identified. A chest shows changes in multiple areas and fluid surrounding the lungs, respiratory failure following an acute febrile illness lasting typically less than one week, and eosinophils comprising more than 25% of white blood cells in fluid obtained by bronchoalveolar lavage are the most common indicators of acute eosinophilic pneumonia. Elevated levels of immunoglobulin G, erythrocyte sedimentation rate, and white blood cell count are among the other common laboratory abnormalities. Testing for pulmonary function typically indicates a limited process with a lower capacity for carbon monoxide diffusion. The likelihood of chronic eosinophilic pneumonia increases if the illness has persisted for more than a month. Increased blood eosinophil counts, elevated platelet counts, iron deficiency anemia, and elevated erythrocyte sedimentation rate are laboratory tests commonly used to diagnose chronic eosinophilic pneumonia. Anywhere abnormalities can be seen on a chest X-ray, but the most specific finding is increased shadow away from the heart in the lung periphery.

2.3.4.1. Differential Diagnosis

This includes:

- Asthma.
- Environmental allergic reaction.
- Granulomatosis with polyangiitis.
- Allergic bronchopulmonary aspergillosis.
- Churg–Strauss syndrome.
- Loeffler's syndrome.
- Acute eosinophilic pneumonia.
- Chronic eosinophilic pneumonia (Carrington's disease).
- Polyarteritis nodosa.
- Parasitic infections.
- Tropical pulmonary eosinophilia.
- Tuberculosis.
- Fungal infection.
- Sarcoidosis.
- Drug reaction with eosinophilia and systemic symptoms.
- Mastocytosis.
- Lymphoproliferative hypereosinophilic syndrome.
- Myeloproliferative hypereosinophilic syndrome.

2.4. Asthma

Chronic inflammatory respiratory disease, asthma is typified by recurrent bouts of coughing, chest tightness, wheezing, and dyspnea, especially in the early morning or night. People of all ages are affected, but it usually starts in childhood and can last into adulthood. The disease known as asthma is diverse, resulting in reversible airflow obstruction due to a variety of underlying mechanisms such as bronchial hyperresponsiveness, airway inflammation, and airflow limitation.

The intricate interaction of immune dysregulation, environmental factors, and genetic predisposition is the pathophysiology of asthma. In those who are vulnerable, exposure to allergens like pollen, dust mites, animal dander, or respiratory viruses can set off an immunological reaction that causes inflammation of the airways and the release of pro-inflammatory mediators like histamine, leukotrienes, and cytokines. This inflammatory cascade contributes to the typical symptoms of asthma by causing bronchoconstriction, mucus production, and airway edema.

Clinical assessment, which includes a thorough medical history, physical examination, and pulmonary function tests, is the basis for diagnosing asthma. Recurrent respiratory symptoms like coughing, wheezing, and dyspnea, as well as evidence of reversible airflow obstruction on spirometry or peak expiratory flow rate (PEFR) measurements, are common diagnostic criteria. To assess the degree and underlying causes of asthma, further tests like imaging studies, bronchial provocation testing, and allergy testing may be carried out.

The goals of managing asthma are to reduce the likelihood of future problems, avoid exacerbations, and attain and maintain symptom control. The Global Initiative for Asthma (GINA) guidelines and other international asthma management guidelines typically call for a stepwise approach based on the severity and control of the disease. Pharmacological interventions, avoiding allergens, patient education, and routine asthma control monitoring are some possible treatment approaches. Pharmacological treatment for asthma consists of both reliever drugs to lessen symptoms and bronchoconstriction and controller drugs to lessen airway inflammation. For the majority of patients with persistent asthma, inhaled corticosteroids (ICS) are the first line of treatment and the cornerstone of asthma management. For patients whose asthma remains uncontrolled even after receiving ICS therapy, additional controller drugs such as leukotriene receptor antagonists, biologic agents that target particular inflammatory pathways, and long-acting beta-agonists (LABA) may be added.

Metered-dose inhalers (MDIs), dry powder inhalers (DPIs), and nebulizers are all examples of inhalation devices that are frequently used to administer asthma medications directly to the lungs, maximizing their effectiveness and reducing any systemic side effects. For patients with asthma to receive the best possible treatment outcomes, using inhalers correctly and following recommended dosage instructions are crucial. Apart from taking medication, avoiding allergens and controlling the environment can help lessen the symptoms of asthma and lower the chance of flare-ups. The implementation of strategies to enhance indoor air quality and lower allergen exposure at home and at work, as well as the identification and avoidance of particular allergens or triggers, such as tobacco smoke, indoor air pollutants, or occupational exposures, may fall under this category.

To effectively manage asthma, patients must be empowered to identify early warning indicators of worsening symptoms, correctly use inhaler devices, follow recommended medication regimens, and seek immediate medical attention when needed. Asthma action plans, which are created in partnership with medical professionals, offer patients and caregivers individualized advice on managing their asthma and support them in navigating a range of treatment scenarios, such as emergencies and symptom exacerbations. The common chronic respiratory illness known as asthma is characterized by reversible airflow obstruction, bronchial hyperresponsiveness, and inflammation of the airways. To improve quality of life and achieve optimal outcomes, people with asthma require a comprehensive approach that includes pharmacological therapy, allergen avoidance, patient education, and regular monitoring of asthma control Ekim (2016).

2.4.1. Allergen Control in Asthma

Asthma remains a major public health concern because it is one of the most common chronic illnesses, particularly in children. While genetics plays a significant role in asthma, environmental triggers and lifestyle choices have also been linked to a dramatic rise in asthma cases in recent years. Planning intervention strategies requires a thorough understanding of how various factors interact to cause asthma. One of the main causes of asthma morbidity is allergen exposure. For those with a genetic predisposition, environmental exposure causes allergen sensitization, and continued exposure increases the risk of developing asthma and other allergic diseases. Research indicates that avoiding and controlling environmental triggers can prevent asthma attacks, lessen symptom frequency, and reduce the need for medication. Therefore, the management of asthma should concentrate on environmental control. The key to effectively managing asthma is recognizing and avoiding environmental triggers both indoors and outdoors. Determining the rationale behind asthma development and creating primary preventive measures are essential to reducing the incidence of asthma attacks globally.

In industrialized nations, allergic diseases associated with asthma and asthma itself are the most common chronic illnesses. The prevalence of allergic diseases has been dynamically rising in recent years. The design of the home environment and the level of indoor allergens are thought to be the factors for those diseases, though the precise cause of the increase is unknown. Asthma and other allergy-related illnesses are a major public health concern and a financial strain on healthcare systems. Allergies and asthma pose a serious threat to life. Furthermore, these illnesses have detrimental effects on both adults and children. While there has been much discussion in recent years regarding the rise in asthma cases among children and adults, environmental factors are thought to be the primary cause of this increase. The main causes of asthma development include lifestyle changes, variations in ethnicity and genetic heterogeneity, and modifications in the type of housing. Taking the necessary precautions to avoid being exposed to the allergens is the first step in symptom control, as avoiding allergens is crucial for the management of allergic diseases. Disease inflammation may be avoided by successfully identifying and avoiding environmental triggers. When it comes to allergic diseases like asthma, avoiding allergens is more effective than receiving treatment. Thus, implementing environmental control measures is advised by international asthma guidelines as part of a methodical approach to treating asthma.

The importance of the environment in asthma development is becoming increasingly apparent in the pathogenesis of the disease. Asthma is influenced by a combination of genetic factors and exposure to environmental triggers. Sensitivity to allergens is a critical component, as exposure to these substances can result in the onset of asthma symptoms and inflammation. Managing asthma requires a multifaceted approach due to its complex origins. Research has shown that utilizing a combination of interventions is more effective than relying on a single method. Therefore, successful asthma management should encompass a range of strategies, including both pharmaceutical and non-pharmaceutical approaches.

When it comes to allergen control, the risk of exposure for those who are sensitive to allergens should be determined, and appropriate interventions should be planned to reduce or eliminate the risk. Numerous tactics have been developed and tested in recent years to lower the rates of morbidity and mortality associated with asthma. Numerous studies have indicated that, within the parameters of those strategies, allergen control education alone is insufficient to modify environmental control behaviors. In conclusion, one-off interventions are typically ineffective. However, avoiding allergens effectively necessitates a thorough strategy.

2.4.2. Indoor Allergens

Chronic airway inflammation brought on by the interaction of genetics and environment is the hallmark of asthma. Although it is acknowledged that certain seasons act as allergen triggers, exposure to indoor allergens and their year-round presence increases the risk of developing asthma. While there are many environmental factors that can cause asthma, indoor allergens are the main culprits. Exposure to indoor allergens occurs in indoor areas, which include not only homes but also workplaces, restaurants, schools, and automobiles. Indoor environments pose a health risk. Numerous population surveys and epidemiological cohort studies have also highlighted the strong link between indoor allergen exposure and the pathogenesis of allergic diseases like asthma. The biological activities of allergens heighten the IgE response and directly result in allergic inflammation. The development of IgE and Th2 responses is influenced by atopic predisposition and environmental allergen exposure.

Living in modern conditions and spending long hours indoors can increase exposure to allergens, leading to sensitization and symptoms of asthma. Common indoor allergens that have been identified as triggers for allergies include dust mites, cockroaches, mice, pet dander, and mold. While these allergens can be found in homes in all urban areas, their presence may vary in different geographic regions due to the climate. It requires more effort to control indoor allergens compared to seasonal allergens as they can persist throughout the year. Studies have shown that children are more likely to be sensitized to indoor allergens, and those who are sensitive to indoor allergens are also likely to be sensitive to outdoor allergens.

The most common cause of trigger exposure and allergen sensitization is poor housing conditions. Asthmatics may experience symptoms when exposed to indoor allergens. It has long been thought that dogs and cats cause the symptoms. High dust mite allergen levels in the home, however, represent the primary risk factor for those who are already sensitized. Asthma triggers include excessive moisture, improper or subpar heating and cooling systems, crowding, cockroaches, and structural issues. Reducing exposure to indoor allergens improves asthma symptoms and reduces medication use (Ekim, 2016).

2.4.3. Dust Mites

Although dust mites have been a part of human life for centuries, dust mite allergies have become much more common recently. The modern housing stock and prolonged indoor living periods have created ideal conditions for dust mites, which could account for this increase. The first known indoor allergens are dust mites. Dermatophagoides pteronyssinus (Dp) and Dermatophagoides farina are two of the most prevalent dust mites in homes. Dust from mattresses, pillows, carpets, upholstered furniture, bed linens, clothing, and plush toys may contain high concentrations of mites. Dust mite allergens, which are carried by larger substances and hang out in the air for a brief period of time, may be the cause of the IgE sensitization that 90% of children with asthma exhibit to household dust. These mites are immobile and live inside clothing. Allergen distribution varies from room to room in the house, with the bedroom—especially the bed—having the highest concentration. Humidity and heat are breeding grounds for dust mites. Exposure to dust mites can cause sensitization and act as an asthma attack trigger. The onset, severity, and morbidity of asthma are closely associated with dust mite allergy.

Several investigations have been conducted to examine the impact of eliminating dust mites on asthma symptoms. Covering the bed and pillows with dust-resistant clothing is the most efficient way to get rid of dust mites from the bed. According to a clinical study, using dust-resistant cloth to cover pillows and beds may help eliminate seven dust mite allergens. Interventions aimed at eliminating dust mites from beds, however, are insufficiently successful in lowering exposure. Rather, more successful interventions center on the patient's overall exposure during a given day. Carpets ought to be taken out and replaced, if at all possible, with porcelain flooring. According to their research, children should use semipermeable polyurethane bed and pillow coverings because they have substantial, long-term therapeutic benefits. Furthermore, toys pose a significant risk for asthma symptoms and may be a source of mites. Once a week, toys should be stored in a deep freezer or cleaned in hot water.

To temporarily get rid of dust mites in soft furnishings, acaricides are advised. On the other hand, research has indicated that it could work well in conjunction with an allergen-impermeable mattress to get rid of dust mites. Another efficient way to get rid of dust mites is by vacuuming. To reduce the amount of dust mites in the air, vacuum cleaners should be fitted with high-efficiency particulate air (HEPA) filters or a special bag. Furthermore helpful in getting rid of mites are steam cleaning and wet vacuuming. Other items, such as bedding, should be thrown away in hot water with detergent. Because colder water does not kill mites, the water temperature should be higher than 550C. The mites may be eliminated by dry cleaning.

2.4.4. Cockroaches

After dust mites, cockroach allergens are the second agent that causes indoor allergic sensitization. Old buildings, multifamily homes, urban environments, and low socioeconomic status are all risk factors for high levels of cockroach allergens and cockroach occupation. Sensitization to cockroach allergens is fairly common in some geographical areas, particularly in children. The climate in those areas plays a significant role, and spending a lot of time indoors during the winter increases the risk of being exposed to cockroach allergens. There could be cockroach allergens in every body, even split or shit. *Blattella germanica* and *Periplaneta americana* are the two species that produce the most common cockroach allergens.

In enclosed spaces, eliminating cockroach allergens is a prolonged procedure. Allergenic material remains in the enclosed space long after cockroaches have been eliminated, although this method has been said to be the best. Therefore, the material containing active allergen proteins should be thoroughly vacuumed after the cockroaches have been eradicated. A phase II study conducted by the National Cooperative Inner-City Asthma Study (NCICAS) has highlighted how difficult it is to completely eradicate cockroach allergens in enclosed spaces. While interventions such as education, cleaning, and extermination guarantee a temporary reduction, the number of allergens increases over time. Cleaning every room is necessary to eradicate the allergen reservoirs that cockroaches carry. According to studies, professional pest control teams can effectively eradicate cockroach allergens with the use of pesticides. To eradicate cockroach allergens, more potent measures or chemical agents must be investigated; however, these substances must not be harmful to human health.

2.4.5. Environmental Tobacco Smoke

A significant proportion of individuals with asthma—between 25 and 35%—regularly smoke, which is a public health concern. About 30% of children struggle to manage their asthma when exposed to secondhand tobacco smoke. Everyone is affected by ambient tobacco smoke, regardless of age. On the down side, children are more vulnerable to its effects and are unable to take appropriate preventative measures. The primary cause of indoor air pollution is passive smoking. In addition to their homes, cars, other public places, and restaurants expose children to smoke. But the most frequent location for exposure is home.

There are differences in the effects of prenatal and postnatal tobacco smoke exposure. The long-term consequences of maternal smoking exposure on a child's respiratory health occur during pregnancy. Chemicals found in smoke are harmful to fetal development and are transferred to the placenta. The baby's prenatal exposure to smoke is linked to deficiencies in the index of tidal respiratory flow and functional residual capacity. Moreover, a higher serum IgE level and a higher frequency of skin-prick test responses in children are linked to maternal smoking. Furthermore, many studies have indicated that smoking mothers raise the possibility of snarling breathing in children younger than six. The factors that lead to the development of allergies are lung irritation and the amount of smoking exposure during pregnancy. Children with asthma who have smoking parents are more likely to have frequent exacerbations and more severe symptoms. Children who were exposed to indoor tobacco smoke had a significantly worse quality of life due to asthma and a higher incidence of respiratory infections. Apart from its association with smaller airways during pregnancy and its action as a pro-inflammatory lung irritant after birth, some have suggested that ambient tobacco smoke could also have an impact on the development of allergies.

Because tobacco smoke damages the respiratory and circulatory systems and is the main cause of many illnesses and fatalities, it is a major global public health concern. While there are several interventions designed to educate and increase people's consciousness, they are not as widespread as would be ideal. Unfortunately, despite the development of numerous strategies, there is still no solution for this public health issue. Giving up tobacco use inside the home and letting parents and family members know about the required tobacco education programs offered at schools are the only ways to protect kids from secondhand smoke. This is one of the suggested methods for increasing public awareness of tobacco smoke in the environment (Ekim, 2016).

2.4.6. Outdoor Allergens

Throughout their lives, people are either directly or indirectly exposed to outdoor allergens. It is more difficult to control outdoor allergens than indoor allergens. Air pollution, fungus spores, and pollens are the most frequent sources of outdoor allergens. One significant risk factor for allergic rhinitis is pollen. Additionally, they aggravate asthma because their particulates enter the lower respiratory tract. There is evidence to suggest that airborne allergens and pollens can exacerbate asthma attacks. Sensitized individuals should stay indoors during specific times of the day with closed windows to minimize allergen inhalation and alleviate pollen-related respiratory symptoms. Additionally, mask wear in outdoor settings may help lower exposure.

Because urbanization increases air pollution, it is a significant contributing factor to asthma. One major risk factor for health and quality of life in urban areas is air pollution. Since their immune and respiratory systems are still developing and their lungs have not fully developed, children are more susceptible to infections from air pollution and weather-related factors. Although it is widely accepted that air pollution may aggravate asthma symptoms, there is disagreement over how much of an impact it has on the onset of the condition. Inflammation of the asthmatic airways, heightened bronchial sensitivity, ER admissions, and rising drug usage rates are all linked to air pollution. The kind of pollutants, their concentration in the environment, and the length of exposure to the pollutants all affect how well the lungs function. Pollutant-induced mucosal lining of the airways and impaired mucociliary clearance allow allergens to enter the immune system and spread. While the types and concentrations of air pollutants vary by region, ozone (O3), nitrogen dioxide (NO2), particulate matter (PM), sulfur dioxide (SO2), and carbon monoxide (CO) are the most prevalent.

Air pollution, vehicle emissions, and modern lifestyles are major risk factors for respiratory allergies in urban areas. Although it can be challenging to control allergens that have been classified as outdoor, limiting exposure to those allergens may be the best course of action. Since outdoor environments are the sources of outdoor allergens, individual efforts to control them may prove inadequate. Firstly, high-level ozone and PM2.5 levels should be warned of, traffic should be reduced in urban areas, and local authorities should regulate vehicle emission rates to lessen the inflammation caused by air pollution and asthma. Patients should stay indoors and incorporate asthma management activities into their plans on days when the air quality is poor. Governments, businesses, and private sector authorities must work locally, nationally, and internationally to find solutions to the global problem of air pollution.

2.4.7. Sensitization

Sensitization is the process by which particular IgE antibodies to allergens are produced, and it is the first step in the immune response. Numerous factors influence the incidence and prevalence of asthma. One of the most crucial elements is allergic sensitization, particularly for kids and teenagers. Allergy sensitization multiplies the risk of developing asthma by 4–20. The impact of lifestyle factors remains a topic of discussion. However, a family history of allergic diseases is unquestionably a significant contributing factor to the development of allergic sensitization. Numerous studies have confirmed the significance of early exposure to environmental factors and living conditions.

Proteins known as allergens can pass through the respiratory and nasal mucosa. Asthma risk factors include being sensitive to allergens in the air, though the significance of this factor is still up for debate. Furthermore, there is still more research to be done on the dose-response relationship. According to epidemiological evidence, inhaler allergen exposure at a high level is a significant risk factor for atopic bronchial asthma, particularly during the early years of life. Numerous studies have documented a direct correlation between allergen sensitization and the onset, severity, and exacerbation of asthma symptoms. In particular, allergy sensitization and exposure are linked to childhood asthma (Table 2.5).

Table 2.5. *Factors Affecting Allergic Sensitization*

Allergy History of Family	Genetic Influence on Allergic Sensitization
Gender	Under debate
Childhood environment	Rural and farming environment
	Close interaction with furry animals in early childhood
	Air pollution
	Crowded family
	Exposure to tobacco smoke

Source: Ekim, A. (2016). Allergen Control in Asthma. InTech. doi: 10.5772/62767.

Early childhood exposure to high levels of allergens increases the risk of developing asthma in children. Compared to outdoor allergens, early childhood exposure to indoor allergens is a significant factor in the development of sensitization. Studies on the population in inner cities and towns have shown that over 80% of school-aged children with asthma are sensitized to one or more indoor allergens. One of the main factors influencing the disease's persistence into later life is allergic sensitization.

The most widely used technique for diagnosing allergies is the skin prick test, which is the fundamental test procedure to demonstrate IgE-based allergic disease sensitization. During the test, tiny amounts of various allergen extracts are pricked on the upper arm, and the subject's response to these extracts is evaluated. It confirms the type of allergy for sensitization and allows for the simultaneous testing of multiple allergens. The test guarantees objective confirmation of allergen sensitization. In addition to the patient's history, the National Asthma Education and Prevention Program (NAEPP) advises using the test to evaluate exposure to allergens. It is useful for targeted immunotherapy because it accurately interprets a child's sensitization from birth. If a child's symptoms change or new environmental allergens become available, the test can be administered again. Skilled medical practitioners conduct the test using internationally recognized allergens. In the test, ≥3 mm swollen tissue is accepted as a positive allergen reaction (Figure 2.5) Ekim (2016).

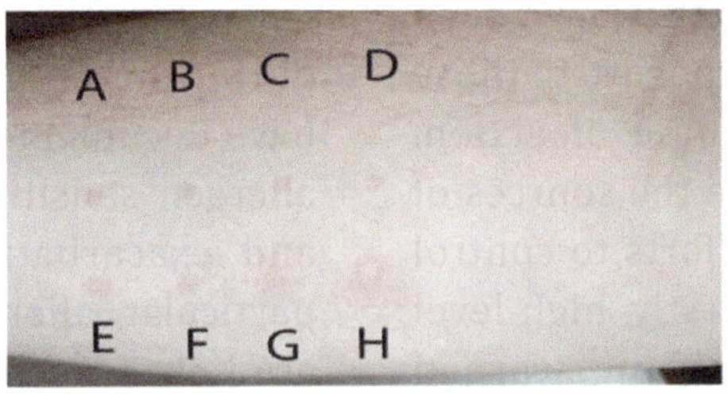

Figure 2.5. *Skin prick test.*

Another sensitization test is the measuring of specific IgE antibodies for a certain antigen such as Enzyme-Linked Immunosorbent Assay (ELISA) or Radioallergosorbent test (RAST). ELISA identifies IgE with a colored reaction product whereas RAST uses radioactively labelled allergen.

Source: Ekim, A. (2016). Allergen Control in Asthma. InTech. doi: 10.5772/62767.

A Closer Look

Asthma

Asthma is a chronic inflammation of the lungs that causes breathing problems. As many as 15 million Americans suffer from asthma and many more probably have it and don't know it. Asthma is not contagious. While there is no cure yet, asthma can be controlled, usually through medications prescribed by a doctor and by avoiding the things that trigger an asthma attack.

Typical symptoms of asthma include wheezing, coughing, chest tightness, shortness of breath, and excess mucus. These conditions result from the underlying inflammation of the airways of the lungs. The airway muscles contract at the same time that the lung tissue swells, constricting the flow of air in and out of the lungs. Further, mucus is excreted, and it plugs up the tiny airways.

Symptoms of asthma may appear as a result of respiratory infections or exposure to a wide range of irritants, as well as exposure to certain medications, emotional stress, weather changes, exercise, and physical conditions. Among the irritants that can trigger asthma are pollen, mold, dust, cockroach, animal dander, urine, saliva, workplace chemicals, smoke, perfume, hair spray, vapors, paint, cleaners, food additives, cosmetics, air pollutants, gases, fumes, and aerosols.

Emotions such as fear, anger, frustration, crying, and laughing can cause asthma in some people. People with asthma often have to be careful about exercise, sometimes by taking medication before exertion. Menstrual period, pregnancy, and thyroid conditions also are known to trigger asthma problems.

Certain food additives and medicines are asthma triggers, too. These include sulfites in tuna, lemon juice, grape juice, dried apples and raisins, and wine. Medication irritants include aspirin, ibuprofen, indomethacin, and naproxen.

When an irritant is inhaled or swallowed, the body reacts by releasing extra antibodies, known as immune globulin E, to fend off the noxious substance by generating a substance called histamine. This substance swells tissue, constricts muscles, and produces mucus. While these three effects are part of the body's defense system for keeping out foreign irritants, an overreaction can cause asthma symptoms.

Each asthma sufferer must devise a plan to manage the condition according to a physician's advice. The idea is to prevent inflammation of the lungs and keep the airways from constricting. An individual, even a child, can learn when the lungs are starting to react to irritants. Avoiding the irritants is a primary means of preventing the airways of the lungs from reacting. Quick use of medication also can stave off an asthma attack.

Many asthma sufferers monitor the air flow through their lungs with a device that measures the peak air flow. Using such a self-test, they can know their relative susceptibility to an asthma attack and gauge the need for a medicated breathing therapy. Physicians prescribe a wide variety of drugs to help reduce lung inflammation and dilate the airways.

Parents of children with asthma must seek the continued care of a health care professional, usually a physician. The doctor will administer one or more tests to make a firm diagnosis that the condition really is asthma and not another bronchial problem. The parents and child will work to learn which irritants to avoid, often by keeping a journal of the foods and medicines ingested and the environment encountered. Usually, the doctor will prescribe medication, such as steroids and antibiotics, to tackle the lung inflammation, as well as a regimen of inhaling a drug to open the airways of the lungs.

Parents will help the child "get in tune" with his or her body to recognize when the symptoms of an asthma attack are imminent. Parents also will develop a positive plan of action--based on a physician's recommendations--for an acute asthma attack.

Summary

- Management of allergic conditions in pediatric pulmonology involves a multifaceted approach aimed at controlling symptoms, reducing inflammation, and preventing exacerbations.
- Bronchopulmonary aspergillosis (BPA) is a spectrum of diseases caused by the fungus *Aspergillus* affecting the lungs and airways.
- The diagnosis of IPA requires a high index of suspicion and is based on a combination of clinical, radiological, and microbiological findings.
- Allergic bronchopulmonary aspergillosis (ABPA) is an immune-allergic disease of the lung due to a hypersensitivity reaction to antigens of *Aspergillus* fumigatus after colonization into the airways.
- Posttreatment recurrences of ABPA are commonly seen, whether using oral corticosteroids, antifungal therapy or a combination of both, and prolonged treatment can result in adverse effects.
- Hypersensitivity pneumonitis (HP) or extrinsic allergic alveolitis (EAA) is a syndrome caused by the repetitive inhalation of antigens from the environment in susceptible or sensitized people.
- Management of HP involves identifying and removing the offending antigen from the patient's environment to prevent further exposure and halt disease progression.
- Eosinophilic pneumonia (EP) is a rare but potentially serious respiratory condition characterized by the accumulation of eosinophils within the lung parenchyma and airways, leading to inflammation, tissue damage, and impaired gas exchange.
- Parasites cause eosinophilic pneumonia in three different ways. Parasites can either invade the lungs, live in the lungs as part of their life cycle, or be spread to the lungs by the bloodstream.
- Asthma is a chronic inflammatory respiratory condition characterized by recurrent episodes of wheezing, breathlessness, chest tightness, and coughing, particularly at night or early in the morning.
- Cockroach allergens are the second agent of indoor allergic sensitization after dust mites. Urban environment, low socio economic status, old buildings, and multifamily homes are all risk factors for cockroach occupation and high level cockroach allergens.

References

1. Asano, K., Hebisawa, A., Ishiguro, T., Takayanagi, N., Nakamura, Y., Suzuki, J., et al. (2021). New clinical diagnostic criteria for allergic bronchopulmonary aspergillosis/mycosis and its validation. *The Journal of Allergy and Clinical Immunology, 147*(4), 1261–1268.e5.
2. Beasley, R., Semprini, A., & Mitchell, E. A. (2015). Risk factors for asthma: Is prevention possible? *The Lancet, 386*(9998), 1075–1085.
3. Boaventura, R., Sibila, O., Agusti, A., & Chalmers, J. D. (2018). Treatable traits in bronchiectasis. *The European Respiratory Journal, 52*(3), 1801269.

4. Caminati, M., Feleszko, W., Michel, M., Annesi-Maesano, I., Vitte, J., Task Force Diagnosis EAACI, et al. (2022). *Aspergillus* fumigatus and personalized medicine: Toward a clinically reliable algorithm. *Allergy, 77*(11), 3476–3477.

5. Chaudhary, N., Datta, K., Askin, F. B., Staab, J. F., & Marr, K. A. (2012). Cystic fibrosis transmembrane conductance regulator regulates epithelial cell response to *Aspergillus* and resultant pulmonary inflammation. *American Journal of Respiratory and Critical Care Medicine, 185*, 301–310.

6. Chauhan, B., Santiago, L., Hutcheson, P. S., Schwartz, H. J., Spitznagel, E., Castro, M., et al. (2000). Evidence for the involvement of two different MHC class II regions in susceptibility or protection in allergic bronchopulmonary aspergillosis. *The Journal of Allergy and Clinical Immunology, 106*(4), 723–729.

7. Chishimba, L., Niven, R. M., Cooley, J., & Denning, D. W. (2012). Voriconazole and posaconazole improve asthma severity in allergic bronchopulmonary aspergillosis and severe asthma with fungal sensitization. *The Journal of Asthma, 49*(4), 423–433.

8. Cockcroft, D. W. (2014). Allergen-induced asthma. *Canadian Respiratory Journal, 21*(5), 279–282.

9. Cohen-Cymberknoh, M., Blau, H., Shoseyov, D., Mei-Zahav, M., Efrati, O., Armoni, S., et al. (2009). Intravenous monthly pulse methylprednisolone treatment for ABPA in patients with cystic fibrosis. *Journal of Cystic Fibrosis, 8*(4), 253–257.

10. Denning, D. W., Pleuvry, A., & Cole, D. C. (2013). Global burden of allergic bronchopulmonary aspergillosis with asthma and its complication chronic pulmonary aspergillosis in adults. *Medical Mycology, 51*, 361–370.

11. Dick, S., Doust, E., Cowie, H., Ayres, J. G., & Turner, S. (2014). Associations between environmental exposures and asthma control and exacerbations in young children: A systematic review. *BMJ Open, 4*, e003827.

12. Ekim, A. (2016). Allergen control in asthma. *InTech.*

13. Gago, S., Denning, D. W., & Bowyer, P. (2019). Pathophysiological aspects of *Aspergillus* colonization in disease. *Medical Mycology, 57*(Supplement_2), S219–S227.

14. Greenberger, P. A. (2002). Allergic bronchopulmonary aspergillosis. *The Journal of Allergy and Clinical Immunology, 110*(5), 685–692.

15. Halken, S., Høst, A., Niklassen, U., Hansen, L. G., Nielsen, F., Pedersen, S., Osterballe, O., Veggerby, C., & Poulsen, L. K. (2003). Effect of mattress and pillow encasings on children with asthma and house dust mite allergy. *The Journal of Allergy and Clinical Immunology, 111*(1), 169–176.

16. Hohl, T. M., & Feldmesser, M. (2007). *Aspergillus* fumigatus: Principles of pathogenesis and host defense. *Eukaryotic Cell, 6*(11), 1953–1963.

17. Howieson, S. G., Lawson, A., McSharry, C., Morris, G., McKenzie, E., & Jackson, J. (2003). Domestic ventilation rates, indoor humidity and dust mite allergens–Are our homes causing the asthma pandemic? *Building Services Engineering, Research and Technology, 24*(3), 137–147.

18. Jin, M., Douglass, J. A., Elborn, J. S., Agarwal, R., Calhoun, W. J., Lazarewicz, S., et al. (2023). Omalizumab in allergic bronchopulmonary aspergillosis: A systematic review and meta-analysis. *The Journal of Allergy and Clinical Immunology: In Practice, 11*(3), 896–905.

19. Knutsen, A. P., & Slavin, R. G. (2011). Allergic bronchopulmonary aspergillosis in asthma and cystic fibrosis. *Clinical & Developmental Immunology, 2011*, 843763.

20. Knutsen, A. P., Bush, R. K., Demain, J. G., Denning, D. W., Dixit, A., Fairs, A., et al. (2012). Fungi and allergic lower respiratory tract diseases. *The Journal of Allergy and Clinical Immunology, 129*(2), 280–291.

21. Lukaszewicz, R., Mahay, G., Boyer, O., & Martinet, J. (2022). Medical algorithm: *Aspergillus* fumigatus components in the diagnosis of allergic bronchopulmonary aspergillosis. *Allergy, 77*(1), 327–330.

22. Matsui, E. C. (2013). Environmental control for asthma: Recent evidence. *Current Opinion in Allergy and Clinical Immunology, 13*(4), 417–425.

23. Maturu, V. N., & Agarwal, R. (2015). Prevalence of *Aspergillus* sensitization and allergic bronchopulmonary aspergillosis in cystic fibrosis: Systematic review and meta-analysis. *Clinical and Experimental Allergy, 45*(12), 1765–1778.

24. Menzies-Gow, A., Corren, J., Bourdin, A., Chupp, G., Israel, E., Wechsler, M. E., et al. (2021). Tezepelumab in adults and adolescents with severe, uncontrolled asthma. *The New England Journal of Medicine, 384*, 1800–1809.

25. Mikura, S., Saraya, T., Yoshida, Y., Oda, M., Ishida, M., Honda, K., et al. (2021). Successful treatment of Mepolizumab- and prednisolone-resistant allergic bronchopulmonary aspergillosis with Dupilumab. *Internal Medicine, 60*(17), 2839–2842.

26. Milián, E., & Díaz, A. M. (2004). Allergy to house dust mites and asthma. *P R Health Sci J, 23*(1), 47–57.

27. Muthu, V., Sehgal, I. S., Dhooria, S., Aggarwal, A. N., & Agarwal, R. (2018). Utility of recombinant *Aspergillus* fumigatus antigens in the diagnosis of allergic bronchopulmonary aspergillosis: A systematic review and diagnostic test accuracy meta-analysis. *Clinical and Experimental Allergy, 48*, 1107–1136.

28. Muthu, V., Sehgal, I. S., Prasad, K. T., Dhooria, S., Aggarwal, A. N., Garg, M., et al. (2020). Allergic bronchopulmonary aspergillosis (ABPA) sans asthma: A distinct subset of ABPA with a lesser risk of exacerbation. *Medical Mycology, 58*, 260–263.

29. National Asthma Education and Prevention Program (NAEPP). (2007). Expert panel report 3: Guidelines for the diagnosis and management of asthma.

30. Nishimura, T., Okano, T., Naito, M., Tsuji, C., Iwanaka, S., & Sakakura, Y. (2021). Complete withdrawal of glucocorticoids after dupilumab therapy in allergic bronchopulmonary aspergillosis: A case report. *World Journal of Clinical Cases, 9*(23), 6922–6928.

31. Ogata, H., Sha, K., Kotetsu, Y., Enokizu-Ogawa, A., Katahira, K., Ishimatsu, A., et al. (2023). Tezepelumab treatment for allergic bronchopulmonary aspergillosis. *Respirology Case Reports, 11*(5), e01147.

32. Oliveira Rodrigues Valle, S., Sarquis Serpa, A., & Sarquis Serpa, F. (2023). Allergic bronchopulmonary aspergillosis/mycosis: An underdiagnosed disease. *IntechOpen*.

33. Ramonell, R. P., Lee, F. E., Swenson, C., & Kuruvilla, M. (2020). Dupilumab treatment for allergic bronchopulmonary aspergillosis: A case series. *The Journal of Allergy and Clinical Immunology: In Practice, 8*(2), 742–743.

34. Raulf, M., Marcus, J., Ingrid, S., Hoffmeyer, F., Nowak, D., Ochmann, U., et al. (2019). Update of reference values for IgG antibodies against typical antigens of hypersensitivity pneumonia. *Allergo Journal International, 28*, 192–206.

35. Richardson, G., Eick, S., & Jones, R. (2005). How is the indoor environment related to asthma? Literature review. *Journal of Advanced Nursing, 52*(3), 328–339.

36. Roboubi, A., Audousset, C., Fréalle, É., Brun, A. L., Laurent, F., Vitte, J., et al. (2023). Allergic bronchopulmonary aspergillosis: A multidisciplinary review. *Journal of Medical Mycology, 33*(3), 101392.

37. Schönberger, H. J., Maas, T., Dompeling, E., Knottnerus, J. A., van Weel, C., & van Schayck, C. P. (2004). Compliance of asthmatic families with a primary prevention programme of asthma and effectiveness of measures to reduce inhalant allergens: A randomized trial. *Clinical and Experimental Allergy, 34*(7), 1024–1031.

38. Sheehan, W. J., & Phipatanakul, W. (2005). Difficult to control asthma: Epidemiology and its link with environmental factors. *Current Opinion in Allergy and Clinical Immunology, 15*(5), 397–401.

39. Singh Sehgal, I., & Agarwal, R. (2014). Pulse methylprednisolone in allergic bronchopulmonary aspergillosis exacerbations. *European Respiratory Review, 23*(131), 149–152.

40. Tomomatsu, K., Yasuba, H., Ishiguro, T., Imokawa, S., Hara, J., Soeda, S., et al. (2023). Real-world efficacy of anti-IL-5 treatment in patients with allergic bronchopulmonary aspergillosis. *Scientific Reports, 13*(1), 5468.

41. Van de Veerdonk, F. L., Gresnigt, M. S., Romani, L., Netea, M. G., & Latgé, J. P. (2017). *Aspergillus* fumigatus morphology and dynamic host interactions. *Nature Reviews Microbiology, 15*(11), 661–674.

42. Warm, K., Lindberg, A., Lundbäck, B., & Rönmark, E. (2013). Increase in sensitization to common airborne allergens among adults: Two population-based studies 15 years apart. *Allergy Asthma Clinical Immunology, 9*(1), 20.

Chapter

ANATOMICAL DISORDERS

3

Contents

Introduction

Anatomical disorders encompass a broad spectrum of conditions that involve structural abnormalities or malformations in the body's anatomical components. These disorders can affect various systems and organs, leading to a diverse range of clinical manifestations and health implications. From congenital anomalies to acquired deformities, anatomical disorders pose significant challenges to affected individuals and healthcare providers alike.

Congenital anatomical disorders are present at birth and often arise due to genetic factors, environmental exposures, or a combination of both. These conditions may involve abnormal development or formation of organs, tissues, or body structures during embryonic or fetal growth. Examples of congenital anatomical disorders include congenital heart defects, neural tube defects, cleft lip and palate, limb abnormalities, and chromosomal abnormalities such as Down syndrome. These disorders may result in functional limitations, developmental delays, and lifelong disabilities, necessitating early detection, multidisciplinary management, and supportive care to optimize outcomes.

In contrast, acquired anatomical disorders develop later in life and may result from trauma, injury, infection, inflammation, degeneration, or neoplastic growth affecting the body's anatomical structures. Traumatic injuries such as fractures, dislocations, and soft tissue injuries can disrupt the normal integrity and function of bones, joints, ligaments, and muscles, leading to pain, deformity, and functional impairment. Inflammatory conditions such as arthritis, tendonitis, and bursitis involve inflammation of joint structures, tendons, or bursae, causing pain, swelling, and restricted mobility.

Furthermore, infectious agents such as bacteria, viruses, fungi, and parasites can invade and damage anatomical structures, leading to infectious anatomical disorders such as osteomyelitis, cellulitis, abscesses, and septic arthritis. Degenerative disorders such as osteoarthritis, degenerative disc disease, and age-related changes in bone density and joint cartilage commonly occur with aging and may result in chronic pain, stiffness, and functional decline.

Moreover, neoplastic growths such as benign tumors, malignant tumors, and metastatic lesions can arise in various anatomical structures, posing diagnostic and therapeutic challenges. Tumors may compress adjacent structures, invade surrounding tissues, or metastasize to distant sites, causing local symptoms and systemic complications. Early detection, accurate diagnosis, and timely intervention are essential for managing neoplastic anatomical disorders and optimizing patient outcomes.

Overall, anatomical disorders encompass a wide range of conditions affecting the body's structural integrity and function, with congenital anomalies, acquired deformities, traumatic injuries, inflammatory conditions, infectious diseases, degenerative changes, and neoplastic growths contributing to the complexity of these disorders. Multidisciplinary approaches involving medical, surgical, rehabilitative, and supportive interventions are crucial for addressing the diverse needs of individuals with anatomical disorders and improving their quality of life.

Orientation and Directional Terms

Term	Definition	Illustration
Down Syndrome	Down syndrome is a condition in which a person has an extra chromosome or an extra piece of a chromosome. This extra copy changes how a baby's body and brain develop. It can cause both mental and physical challenges during their lifetime.	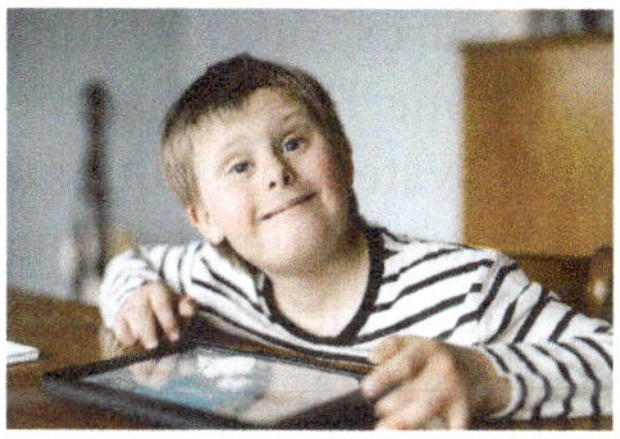
Osteoarthritis	Osteoarthritis is a degenerative joint disease, in which the tissues in the joint break down over time. It is the most common type of arthritis and is more common in older people.	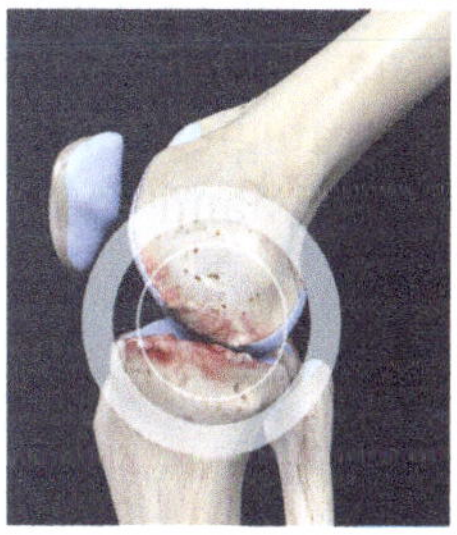
Rheumatoid Arthritis (RA)	Rheumatoid arthritis, or RA, is an autoimmune and inflammatory disease, which means that your immune system attacks healthy cells in your body by mistake, causing inflammation (painful swelling) in the affected parts of the body.	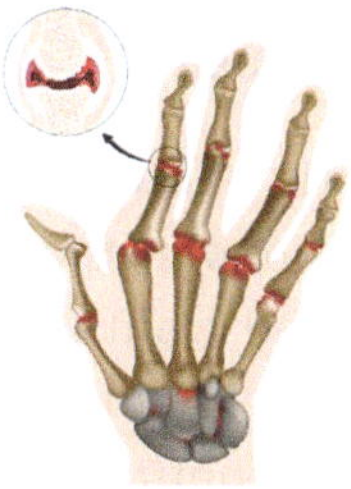 Rheumatoid Arthritis
Carpal Tunnel Syndrome (CTS	It is a common acquired compressive neuropathy of the median nerve that presents with symptoms of numbness and tingling in the median nerve distribution of the hand.	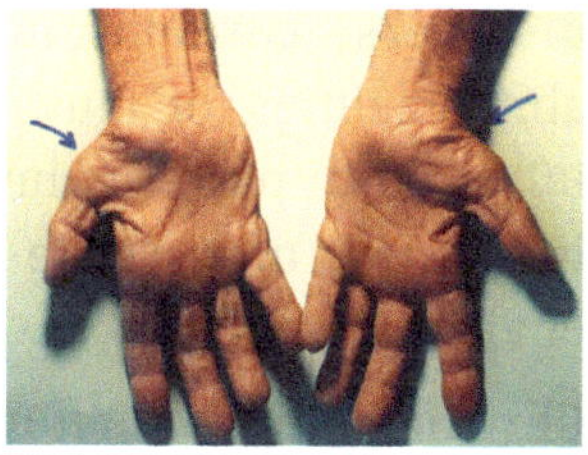
Peripheral Nervous System (PNS)	Your peripheral nervous system (PNS) is that part of your nervous system that lies outside your brain and spinal cord. It plays a key role in both sending information from different areas of your body back to your brain, as well as carrying out commands from your brain to various parts of your body.	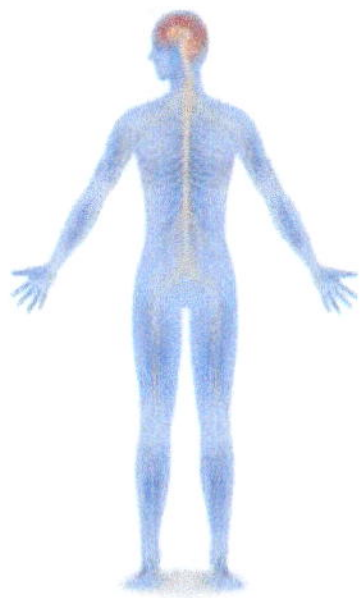

3.1. Congenital Disorders

Congenital disorders are conditions present at birth, often resulting from genetic abnormalities, prenatal exposures, or developmental factors during gestation. These disorders can affect various organ systems, leading to structural or functional abnormalities that may impact an individual's health, development, and quality of life. In this comprehensive exploration, we will delve into the diverse spectrum of congenital disorders, their etiology, classification, clinical manifestations, diagnostic approaches, management strategies, and implications for affected individuals and their families.

3.1.1. Etiology of Congenital Disorders

Congenital disorders can arise from a multitude of factors, including:

- **Genetic Factors:** Mutations or alterations in the DNA sequence inherited from one or both parents can lead to congenital disorders. These genetic abnormalities may involve single genes (monogenic disorders), chromosomal abnormalities, or multifactorial inheritance patterns involving the interaction of multiple genes and environmental factors.
- **Chromosomal Abnormalities:** Errors in chromosomal number or structure can result in congenital disorders such as Down syndrome (trisomy 21), Turner syndrome (monosomy X), Klinefelter syndrome (XXY), and chromosomal deletions, duplications, or translocations.
- **Environmental Exposures:** Prenatal exposure to teratogenic agents such as drugs, alcohol, tobacco, radiation, infections, toxins, and maternal illnesses can disrupt normal fetal development and increase the risk of congenital anomalies.
- **Maternal Health:** Maternal age, nutritional status, preexisting medical conditions (e.g., diabetes, hypertension), maternal infections (e.g., rubella, cytomegalovirus, Zika virus), and prenatal care can influence fetal development and the risk of congenital disorders.
- **Developmental Factors:** Abnormalities in embryonic development, organogenesis, or fetal growth may occur due to intrinsic or extrinsic factors, leading to congenital malformations or functional deficits in affected organs or systems.

3.1.2. Classification of Congenital Disorders

Congenital disorders encompass a broad spectrum of conditions classified based on various criteria, including:

- **Anatomical Classification:** Congenital disorders can affect virtually any organ system, including the central nervous system, cardiovascular system, musculoskeletal system, gastrointestinal system, genitourinary system, respiratory system, sensory organs, and integumentary system.
- **Etiological Classification:** Congenital disorders can be categorized based on their underlying etiology, such as genetic disorders (e.g., Down syndrome, cystic fibrosis), chromosomal

abnormalities (e.g, trisomy 18), teratogenic exposures (e.g., fetal alcohol syndrome), or multifactorial inheritance patterns (e.g., cleft lip and palate).

- **Clinical Manifestations:** Congenital disorders may manifest with a wide range of clinical features, including structural anomalies (e.g., limb abnormalities, cardiac defects), developmental delays, intellectual disabilities, growth disturbances, sensory impairments, metabolic disorders, and functional limitations.
- **Severity and Prognosis:** Congenital disorders vary in severity, ranging from mild conditions with minimal impact on health and function to life-threatening anomalies requiring intensive medical intervention and lifelong support. Prognosis depends on factors such as the nature of the disorder, associated complications, availability of treatments, and supportive care.

3.1.3. Clinical Manifestations of Congenital Disorders

The clinical manifestations of congenital disorders are diverse and can affect multiple organ systems. Common features include:

- **Structural Anomalies:** Congenital malformations involving the musculoskeletal system (e.g., clubfoot, polydactyly), cardiovascular system (e.g, congenital heart defects), central nervous system (e.g., neural tube defects), gastrointestinal system (e.g., cleft lip and palate), genitourinary system (e.g., hypospadias), and other organ systems.
- **Developmental Delays:** Delayed milestones in motor, cognitive, language, or social-emotional development may occur in individuals with congenital disorders affecting the central nervous system, such as intellectual disabilities, autism spectrum disorders, and cerebral palsy.
- **Intellectual Disabilities:** Impairments in cognitive function, learning abilities, adaptive skills, and social interactions may be present in individuals with genetic syndromes (e.g., Down syndrome, fragile X syndrome), chromosomal abnormalities, or brain malformations.
- **Growth Abnormalities:** Congenital disorders may lead to growth restriction (e.g., intrauterine growth restriction), growth acceleration (e.g., macrosomia), short stature (e.g., Turner syndrome), or dysmorphic features associated with specific genetic syndromes.
- **Sensory Impairments:** Hearing loss, vision impairment, and other sensory deficits may occur due to congenital abnormalities affecting the auditory system (e.g., congenital deafness), visual system (e.g., congenital cataracts), or other sensory pathways.
- **Metabolic Disorders:** Inborn errors of metabolism, such as phenylketonuria (PKU), galactosemia, and congenital adrenal hyperplasia, can result in metabolic disturbances, biochemical abnormalities, and systemic complications if left untreated.

- **Cardiopulmonary Complications:** Congenital heart defects (e.g., ventricular septal defect, tetralogy of Fallot) and respiratory abnormalities (e.g., tracheoesophageal fistula, congenital diaphragmatic hernia) may lead to cardiopulmonary compromise, respiratory distress, cyanosis, and feeding difficulties in newborns.
- **Genitourinary Abnormalities:** Congenital disorders affecting the genitourinary system may result in renal anomalies (e.g., renal agenesis, polycystic kidney disease), urinary tract malformations (e.g., vesicoureteral reflux), or genital abnormalities (e.g., ambiguous genitalia).

3.1.4. Diagnostic Approaches for Congenital Disorders

Diagnosing congenital disorders involves a comprehensive evaluation of the individual's medical history, family history, prenatal exposures, physical examination findings, and appropriate diagnostic tests, including:

- **Prenatal Screening:** Prenatal screening tests such as maternal serum screening, cell-free DNA testing, ultrasound imaging, and prenatal diagnostic procedures (e.g., chorionic villus sampling, amniocentesis) may be used to detect fetal anomalies, chromosomal abnormalities, or genetic disorders during pregnancy.
- **Newborn Screening:** Newborn screening programs aim to detect certain congenital disorders early in life through blood tests, hearing tests, and other screening modalities. Common conditions screened include phenylketonuria, congenital hypothyroidism, cystic fibrosis, and hearing loss.
- **Imaging Studies:** Radiographic imaging modalities such as X-rays, ultrasound, magnetic resonance imaging (MRI), and computed tomography (CT) scans may be used to visualize structural anomalies, assess organ morphology, and guide further diagnostic evaluation.
- **Genetic Testing:** Molecular genetic testing, cytogenetic analysis, chromosomal microarray analysis (CMA), and next-generation sequencing techniques may be employed to identify specific genetic mutations, chromosomal abnormalities, or gene variants associated with congenital disorders.
- **Metabolic Testing:** Biochemical assays, metabolic screening tests, and specialized laboratory analyses may be performed to detect metabolic abnormalities, enzymatic deficiencies, or metabolic markers indicative of inborn errors of metabolism.
- **Electrophysiological Studies:** Electrophysiological tests such as electroencephalography (EEG), electromyography (EMG), nerve conduction studies, and auditory brainstem response (ABR) testing may be used to assess neurological function, sensory pathways, and neuromuscular integrity.
- **Cardiac Evaluation:** Echocardiography, electrocardiography (ECG), and other cardiac imaging studies may

be indicated to evaluate congenital heart defects, arrhythmias, or cardiopulmonary abnormalities in affected individuals.

3.1.5. Management Strategies for Congenital Disorders

The management of congenital disorders is multifaceted and often requires a multidisciplinary approach involving medical specialists, allied healthcare professionals, educators, and support services. Treatment strategies may include:

- **Medical Interventions:** Pharmacological therapies, nutritional supplementation, hormone replacement therapy, enzyme replacement therapy, and other medical interventions may be used to manage symptoms, prevent complications, or address underlying metabolic abnormalities in individuals with congenital disorders.
- **Surgical Procedures:** Surgical interventions such as corrective surgeries, organ transplants, reconstructive procedures, and palliative surgeries may be necessary to address structural anomalies, repair congenital defects, or improve functional outcomes in affected individuals.
- **Rehabilitative Services:** Physical therapy, occupational therapy, speech therapy, and other rehabilitative services play a vital role in optimizing mobility, independence, communication skills, and activities of daily living in individuals with congenital disorders.
- **Educational Support:** Special education programs, individualized education plans (IEPs), early intervention services, and developmental support services are essential for addressing the learning needs, cognitive impairments, and developmental delays associated with congenital disorders.
- **Genetic Counseling:** Genetic counseling services provide information, guidance, and support to individuals and families affected by congenital disorders, including risk assessment, family planning options, carrier testing, and psychosocial counseling.
- **Psychosocial Support:** Counseling, psychotherapy, support groups, and community resources can help individuals and families cope with the emotional, social, and practical challenges associated with living with a congenital disorder, including stigma, grief, adjustment issues, and caregiving responsibilities.
- **Long-Term Follow-Up:** Regular medical monitoring, disease surveillance, and long-term follow-up care are essential for managing chronic conditions, monitoring disease progression, assessing treatment outcomes, and addressing evolving needs throughout the lifespan of individuals with congenital disorders.

3.1.6. Prevention and Public Health Strategies

Preventing congenital disorders and reducing their burden on affected individuals, families, and healthcare systems require a multifaceted approach involving:

- **Preconception Care:** Optimizing maternal health, addressing modifiable risk factors (e.g., smoking, alcohol use, obesity), and promoting healthy lifestyle behaviors before conception can help reduce the risk of congenital disorders and improve pregnancy outcomes.
- **Prenatal Care:** Access to comprehensive prenatal care, early detection of fetal anomalies through prenatal screening and diagnostic testing, and appropriate management of maternal conditions can minimize the risk of congenital disorders and facilitate timely interventions.
- **Newborn Screening Programs:** Expanded newborn screening programs, early detection of treatable conditions, timely initiation of interventions, and follow-up care are essential for preventing morbidity and mortality associated with congenital metabolic disorders, endocrine disorders, and other heritable conditions.
- **Genetic Counseling and Testing:** Providing accessible genetic counseling services, carrier screening, preimplantation genetic diagnosis (PGD), and prenatal genetic testing options can help individuals make informed reproductive choices, reduce the transmission of genetic disorders, and prevent recurrence in future pregnancies.
- **Health Education and Awareness:** Public health campaigns, educational initiatives, and community outreach efforts aimed at raising awareness about congenital disorders, promoting prenatal health, and advocating for supportive services can empower individuals, families, and healthcare providers to address the needs of affected individuals and reduce disparities in care.
- **Research and Innovation:** Continued investment in biomedical research, genetic studies, developmental biology, and translational research is critical for advancing our understanding of congenital disorders, identifying novel therapeutic targets, developing innovative treatments, and improving outcomes for affected individuals.

3.2. Musculoskeletal Disorders

Musculoskeletal disorders (MSDs) encompass a wide range of conditions affecting the bones, muscles, tendons, ligaments, and joints. These disorders can result from various factors including injury, overuse, genetic predisposition, aging, and underlying medical conditions. MSDs are prevalent worldwide and can significantly impact an individual's quality of life, work productivity, and overall health. In this comprehensive exploration, we will delve into the various types of musculoskeletal disorders, their causes, symptoms, diagnosis, treatment options, and preventive measures.

3.2.1. Types of Musculoskeletal Disorders

- **Osteoarthritis (OA):** Osteoarthritis is the most common form of arthritis, characterized by the gradual degeneration of joint cartilage and the underlying bone.

It primarily affects weight-bearing joints such as the knees, hips, and spine. Common symptoms include joint pain, stiffness, swelling, and reduced range of motion. Risk factors for OA include aging, obesity, joint injury, and genetics.

- **Rheumatoid Arthritis (RA):** Rheumatoid arthritis is an autoimmune disorder where the body's immune system mistakenly attacks the synovium (joint lining), leading to chronic inflammation, joint damage, and systemic symptoms. It commonly affects the small joints of the hands and feet but can involve multiple joints throughout the body. Symptoms include joint pain, swelling, stiffness, fatigue, and systemic inflammation.
- **Osteoporosis:** Osteoporosis is a condition characterized by low bone density and deterioration of bone tissue, leading to an increased risk of fractures. It is more prevalent in postmenopausal women due to hormonal changes that affect bone density. Risk factors include aging, gender, family history, low calcium intake, sedentary lifestyle, and certain medications.
- **Muscle Strains and Sprains:** Muscle strains and sprains occur when muscles or ligaments are stretched or torn due to sudden movements, overuse, or trauma. Common sites of injury include the back, neck, shoulders, and lower extremities. Symptoms include pain, swelling, bruising, and limited range of motion.
- **Tendinitis:** Tendinitis is inflammation or irritation of a tendon, usually caused by repetitive motions, overuse, or improper technique during physical activity. Common types include Achilles tendinitis, tennis elbow (lateral epicondylitis), golfer's elbow (medial epicondylitis), and rotator cuff tendinitis. Symptoms include pain, tenderness, swelling, and stiffness around the affected tendon.
- **Carpal Tunnel Syndrome (CTS):** Carpal tunnel syndrome occurs when the median nerve, which runs from the forearm into the palm, becomes compressed or squeezed at the wrist. It is often associated with repetitive hand and wrist movements, prolonged typing, and activities that require gripping or vibrating tools. Symptoms include numbness, tingling, weakness, and pain in the hand and fingers, especially at night.
- **Fibromyalgia:** Fibromyalgia is a chronic disorder characterized by widespread musculoskeletal pain, fatigue, sleep disturbances, and tender points in the body. The exact cause of fibromyalgia is unknown, but it is believed to involve abnormalities in pain processing in the central nervous system. Other symptoms may include cognitive difficulties, headaches, irritable bowel syndrome (IBS), and mood disorders.
- **Scoliosis:** Scoliosis is a sideways curvature of the spine, often diagnosed during adolescence or childhood. While most cases of scoliosis are mild, severe curvature

can cause back pain, breathing difficulties, spinal deformity, and impaired organ function. The cause of scoliosis is often idiopathic, but it can also be congenital or neuromuscular in nature.

- **Herniated Disc (Herniated Nucleus Pulposus, HNP):** A herniated disc occurs when the soft, gel-like center (nucleus pulposus) of an intervertebral disc protrudes through the tough outer layer (annulus fibrosus), compressing nearby spinal nerves. This can cause pain, numbness, tingling, or weakness in the back, neck, arms, or legs, depending on the location of the herniation.
- **Ankylosing Spondylitis (AS):** Ankylosing spondylitis is a chronic inflammatory condition that primarily affects the spine, causing pain, stiffness, and progressive fusion of the vertebrae. It belongs to a group of disorders known as spondyloarthropathies and can also affect other joints, tendons, ligaments, and organs such as the eyes and heart. AS typically develops in early adulthood and has a strong genetic component.

3.2.2. Causes of Musculoskeletal Disorders

Musculoskeletal disorders can arise from a variety of factors, including:

- **Trauma:** Acute injuries such as fractures, dislocations, muscle strains, and ligament sprains can lead to musculoskeletal disorders.
- **Overuse:** Repetitive movements, improper ergonomics, and prolonged or excessive physical activity can strain muscles, tendons, and ligaments, contributing to injuries and chronic conditions.
- **Age-related Changes:** Aging is associated with natural wear and tear of the musculoskeletal system, including degenerative changes in joints, loss of bone density, and decreased muscle mass and strength.
- **Genetics:** Genetic factors can predispose individuals to certain musculoskeletal conditions such as osteoarthritis, rheumatoid arthritis, and ankylosing spondylitis.
- **Autoimmune Disorders:** Autoimmune diseases like rheumatoid arthritis and systemic lupus erythematosus involve immune-mediated inflammation that targets the joints and connective tissues.
- **Hormonal Changes:** Hormonal fluctuations, particularly in women during menopause, can affect bone density and increase the risk of osteoporosis.
- **Obesity:** Excess body weight can place added stress on joints, leading to accelerated wear and tear, osteoarthritis, and other musculoskeletal problems.
- **Occupational Hazards:** Certain occupations involving repetitive tasks, heavy lifting, awkward postures, or exposure to vibrations or ergonomic stressors can increase the risk of developing musculoskeletal disorders.

- **Poor Posture:** Incorrect body mechanics, prolonged sitting, and poor ergonomics at workstations can contribute to muscle imbalances, spinal misalignment, and chronic pain.
- **Underlying Medical Conditions:** Systemic diseases such as diabetes, hyperparathyroidism, Paget's disease, and certain infections can affect the musculoskeletal system and increase the risk of complications.

3.2.3. Symptoms of Musculoskeletal Disorders

The symptoms of musculoskeletal disorders vary depending on the specific condition but may include:

- **Pain:** Persistent or intermittent pain localized to a specific joint, muscle, or area of the body.
- **Stiffness:** Reduced flexibility and range of motion in affected joints or muscles, especially after periods of inactivity.
- **Swelling:** Inflammation and swelling around affected joints or soft tissues, often accompanied by warmth and redness.
- **Weakness:** Reduced muscle strength and endurance, leading to difficulty performing daily activities or maintaining proper posture.
- **Tenderness:** Sensitivity or pain upon palpation of tender points, muscles, or joints.
- **Numbness and Tingling:** Altered sensation such as numbness, tingling, or pins-and-needles sensation in the affected area, indicating nerve involvement.
- **Fatigue:** Generalized fatigue, weakness, or malaise, especially in chronic conditions like fibromyalgia or autoimmune disorders.
- **Limited Mobility:** Difficulty moving or performing certain movements due to pain, stiffness, or mechanical restrictions.
- **Deformity:** Visible deformities, misalignments, or asymmetries in the skeletal or soft tissue structures.
- **Systemic Symptoms:** In autoimmune or inflammatory conditions, systemic symptoms such as fever, fatigue, weight loss, and skin rashes may occur.

3.2.4. Diagnosis of Musculoskeletal Disorders

Diagnosing musculoskeletal disorders typically involves a comprehensive evaluation by a healthcare professional, including:

- **Medical History:** A detailed history of symptoms, previous injuries, family history of musculoskeletal disorders, and relevant medical conditions.
- **Physical Examination:** A thorough physical examination to assess range of motion, joint stability, muscle strength, reflexes, and presence of tender points or swelling.
- **Imaging Studies:** Radiographic imaging such as X-rays, magnetic resonance imaging

(MRI), computed tomography (CT), or ultrasound may be ordered to visualize structural abnormalities, fractures, joint damage, and soft tissue injuries.

- **Laboratory Tests:** Blood tests to assess markers of inflammation, autoimmune antibodies, rheumatologic factors, and metabolic parameters may be useful in diagnosing specific conditions such as rheumatoid arthritis, osteoporosis, or systemic lupus erythematosus.
- **Electrophysiological Studies:** Nerve conduction studies and electromyography (EMG) may be performed to evaluate nerve function, and muscle activity, and identify nerve compression or dysfunction in conditions like carpal tunnel syndrome or radiculopathy.
- **Diagnostic Procedures:** Invasive procedures such as arthroscopy, joint aspiration, or biopsy may be necessary in certain cases to obtain tissue samples, assess joint inflammation, or rule out other underlying conditions.

3.2.5. Treatment Options for Musculoskeletal Disorders

The treatment approach for musculoskeletal disorders depends on the underlying cause, severity of symptoms, functional limitations, and individual patient factors. Treatment modalities may include:

1. Medications:
   - Analgesics and anti-inflammatory drugs to relieve pain and inflammation (e.g., NSAIDs, acetaminophen).
   - Disease-modifying antirheumatic drugs (DMARDs) and biologic agents for autoimmune disorders like rheumatoid arthritis.
   - Muscle relaxants for muscle spasms and tension.
   - Osteoporosis medications (e.g., bisphosphonates, calcium, vitamin D) to improve bone density and reduce fracture risk.
2. **Physical Therapy:** Individualized exercise programs, manual therapy techniques, stretching, strengthening exercises, and modalities such as heat, cold, ultrasound, and electrical stimulation to improve mobility, reduce pain, and restore function.
3. **Occupational Therapy:** Adaptive equipment, ergonomic modifications, and strategies to optimize activities of daily living, work tasks, and joint protection techniques.
4. **Orthotic Devices:** Splints, braces, orthopedic supports, and shoe inserts to stabilize joints, correct alignment, and alleviate pressure on affected structures.
5. **Injections:** Corticosteroid injections, hyaluronic acid injections, platelet-rich plasma (PRP) therapy, or prolotherapy may be used to reduce inflammation, lubricate joints, and alleviate pain.
6. **Surgical Intervention:** In cases of severe joint damage, instability, or failure of conservative treatments, surgical options such as arthroscopy, joint replacement (arthroplasty), spinal fusion, or tendon repair may be considered to restore function and alleviate pain.
7. **Lifestyle Modifications:** Weight management, smoking cessation,

dietary modifications, ergonomic adjustments, and activity modifications to reduce stress on joints and promote overall musculoskeletal health.

8. **Complementary and Alternative Therapies:** Acupuncture, chiropractic care, massage therapy, herbal supplements, and mind-body interventions such as yoga, tai chi, and meditation may provide adjunctive benefits in managing pain, and stress, and improving overall well-being.

3.2.6. Prevention of Musculoskeletal Disorders

Preventive measures play a crucial role in reducing the risk of musculoskeletal disorders and promoting musculoskeletal health. Strategies include:

- **Regular Exercise:** Engage in regular physical activity to strengthen muscles, improve flexibility, and maintain joint mobility. Incorporate a combination of aerobic exercise, strength training, and flexibility exercises tailored to individual fitness levels and preferences.
- **Proper Body Mechanics:** Practice good posture, body mechanics, and ergonomic principles during daily activities, work tasks, and recreational pursuits to minimize strain on muscles, joints, and ligaments.
- **Healthy Lifestyle Habits:** Maintain a balanced diet rich in calcium, vitamin D, and other nutrients essential for bone health. Avoid smoking, limit alcohol intake, and manage stress to reduce inflammation and support overall musculoskeletal well-being.
- **Workplace Ergonomics:** Ensure ergonomic workstations, proper lifting techniques, frequent breaks, and use of supportive equipment to reduce the risk of work-related musculoskeletal injuries.
- **Safety Precautions:** Wear appropriate protective gear, adhere to safety guidelines, and use proper equipment during sports, recreational activities, and occupational tasks to prevent accidents and traumatic injuries.
- **Regular Health Screenings:** Undergo regular medical check-ups, bone density screenings, and musculoskeletal assessments to detect early signs of conditions such as osteoporosis, arthritis, or spinal disorders and initiate timely interventions.
- **Weight Management:** Maintain a healthy weight through balanced nutrition and regular exercise to reduce the load on weight-bearing joints and decrease the risk of osteoarthritis, back pain, and other obesity-related musculoskeletal issues.
- **Stress Management:** Practice stress-reduction techniques such as mindfulness, relaxation exercises, deep breathing, and hobbies to alleviate muscle tension, promote relaxation, and improve overall resilience to physical and emotional stressors.

3.3. Neurological Disorders

Neurological disorders encompass a broad spectrum of conditions affecting the central nervous system (CNS), peripheral nervous system (PNS), and neuromuscular junction. These disorders can result from various causes, including genetic factors, autoimmune processes, infections, traumatic injuries, degenerative changes, vascular events, and metabolic abnormalities. In this comprehensive exploration, we will delve into the diverse array of neurological disorders, their classification, etiology, clinical manifestations, diagnostic approaches, treatment modalities, and implications for affected individuals and their families.

3.3.1. Classification of Neurological Disorders

Neurological disorders can be classified based on various criteria, including:

- **Anatomical Location:** Neurological disorders may affect specific regions of the CNS (e.g., brain, spinal cord) or PNS (e.g., peripheral nerves, neuromuscular junction), leading to localized or diffuse symptoms and impairments.
- **Pathophysiological Mechanisms:** Neurological disorders can result from diverse pathophysiological processes, including neurodegeneration (e.g., Alzheimer's disease, Parkinson's disease), inflammation (e.g., multiple sclerosis, encephalitis), ischemia (e.g, stroke), demyelination (e.g, Guillain-Barré syndrome), genetic mutations (e.g., Huntington's disease, muscular dystrophy), and traumatic injuries (e.g., traumatic brain injury, spinal cord injury).
- **Clinical Manifestations:** Neurological disorders manifest with a wide range of symptoms and signs, including motor deficits (e.g., weakness, tremors), sensory disturbances (e.g., numbness, tingling), cognitive impairment (e.g., memory loss, confusion), autonomic dysfunction (e.g., urinary incontinence, orthostatic hypotension), and psychiatric symptoms (e.g., depression, anxiety).
- **Temporal Course:** Neurological disorders may be acute (e.g., stroke, traumatic brain injury), chronic progressive (e.g., Alzheimer's disease, amyotrophic lateral sclerosis), relapsing-remitting (e.g., multiple sclerosis), or episodic (e.g., migraine, epilepsy) in nature, with variable patterns of symptom onset, progression, and remission.

3.3.2. Etiology of Neurological Disorders

Neurological disorders can arise from a multitude of factors, including:

- **Genetic Factors:** Inherited genetic mutations, chromosomal abnormalities, and gene variants can predispose individuals to various neurological disorders, including neurodegenerative diseases, neuromuscular disorders, and neurodevelopmental conditions.
- **Environmental Exposures:** Prenatal exposures to teratogenic agents (e.g., alcohol, drugs, toxins), maternal infections (e.g., Zika virus, cytomegalovirus), and perinatal complications (e.g., prematurity, birth trauma) can disrupt normal brain development and increase the risk of neurological disorders.
- **Autoimmune Processes:**

Autoimmune disorders such as multiple sclerosis, neuromyelitis optica, and myasthenia gravis involve immune-mediated inflammation and damage to the CNS, PNS, or neuromuscular junction, leading to neurological dysfunction and clinical symptoms.

- **Infectious Agents:** Viral, bacterial, fungal, and parasitic infections can cause neurological complications such as encephalitis, meningitis, myelitis, neuropathy, and neurocognitive impairment through direct neural invasion, inflammatory responses, and immune-mediated mechanisms.
- **Vascular Events:** Ischemic strokes, hemorrhagic strokes, transient ischemic attacks (TIAs), and cerebral venous thrombosis can disrupt cerebral blood flow, oxygenation, and perfusion, leading to neuronal injury, infarction, and neurological deficits.
- **Traumatic Injuries:** Head injuries, spinal cord injuries, peripheral nerve injuries, and traumatic brain injuries resulting from motor vehicle accidents, falls, sports injuries, and assaults can cause structural damage, axonal injury, and functional impairments in the nervous system.
- **Degenerative Processes:** Neurodegenerative diseases such as Alzheimer's disease, Parkinson's disease, Huntington's disease, and amyotrophic lateral sclerosis involve progressive loss of neurons, protein aggregation, and synaptic dysfunction, leading to cognitive decline, movement disorders, and functional decline.
- **Metabolic Abnormalities:** Metabolic disorders such as metabolic encephalopathies, mitochondrial diseases, lysosomal storage disorders, and vitamin deficiencies can impair energy metabolism, neurotransmitter synthesis, and neuronal function, resulting in neurological symptoms and systemic complications.

3.3.3. Clinical Manifestations of Neurological Disorders

The clinical manifestations of neurological disorders vary widely depending on the underlying pathology, affected neural structures, and individual patient factors. Common symptoms include:

- **Motor Symptoms:** Weakness, paralysis, spasticity, tremors, rigidity, dystonia, ataxia, gait disturbances, and abnormal movements (e.g., chorea, myoclonus) may occur due to dysfunction of the motor pathways, corticospinal tracts, basal ganglia, cerebellum, or neuromuscular junction.
- **Sensory Symptoms:** Numbness, tingling, sensory loss, paresthesia, hypersensitivity, and pain (e.g., neuropathic pain, radicular pain) may result from sensory nerve damage, spinal cord lesions, peripheral neuropathy, or central sensory processing abnormalities.
- **Cognitive Symptoms:** Memory impairment, attention deficits, executive dysfunction, language disturbances, visuospatial difficulties, and perceptual

disturbances may occur in neurological disorders affecting cognition, such as Alzheimer's disease, vascular dementia, frontotemporal dementia, and traumatic brain injury.

- **Autonomic Dysfunction:** Orthostatic hypotension, urinary retention, urinary incontinence, constipation, sweating abnormalities, and sexual dysfunction may arise from dysregulation of autonomic nervous system function in conditions such as autonomic neuropathy, multiple system atrophy, and spinal cord injury.
- **Psychiatric Symptoms:** Depression, anxiety, psychosis, personality changes, agitation, and behavioral disturbances may occur as primary features of certain neurological disorders (e.g., major depressive disorder, generalized anxiety disorder) or as secondary manifestations of brain pathology (e.g., frontal lobe lesions, temporal lobe epilepsy).
- **Seizures and Epilepsy:** Seizures manifest as paroxysmal alterations in behavior, consciousness, motor activity, sensation, or autonomic function due to abnormal electrical activity in the brain. Epilepsy is characterized by recurrent unprovoked seizures and may be idiopathic or secondary to underlying brain lesions, genetic factors, or metabolic disturbances.
- **Neurogenic Pain:** Neuropathic pain, trigeminal neuralgia, postherpetic neuralgia, and other forms of neurogenic pain result from nerve damage, dysfunctional pain processing pathways, or abnormal sensory input, leading to chronic pain syndromes and functional impairment.
- **Sleep Disorders:** Insomnia, hypersomnia, sleep apnea, restless legs syndrome, and parasomnias may occur in neurological disorders affecting sleep-wake regulation, circadian rhythms, or sleep architecture, such as narcolepsy, Parkinson's disease, and REM sleep behavior disorder.

3.3.4. Diagnostic Approaches for Neurological Disorders

Diagnosing neurological disorders requires a comprehensive evaluation of the patient's medical history, neurological examination findings, and appropriate diagnostic tests, including:

- **Neurological Examination:** A thorough neurological examination assesses mental status, cranial nerve function, motor strength and coordination, sensory perception, reflexes, gait, and other neurological signs to localize pathology and identify specific deficits.
- **Neuroimaging Studies:** Structural imaging modalities such as magnetic resonance imaging (MRI), computed tomography (CT), and positron emission tomography (PET) scans provide detailed visualization of brain and spinal cord anatomy, identify structural abnormalities (e.g., tumors, hemorrhages, infarctions), and guide surgical planning.
- **Electrophysiological Tests:**

Electrophysiological studies such as electroencephalography (EEG), nerve conduction studies (NCS), electromyography (EMG), and evoked potentials assess electrical activity, nerve conduction velocities, muscle function, and sensory responses to evaluate neuromuscular integrity, peripheral nerve function, and central nervous system excitability.

- **Laboratory Investigations:** Blood tests, cerebrospinal fluid (CSF) analysis, genetic testing, metabolic panels, autoimmune serologies, and infectious disease screening may be performed to detect biochemical abnormalities, identify specific biomarkers, and evaluate underlying etiologies such as infections, autoimmune disorders, metabolic disturbances, or genetic mutations.
- **Neuropsychological Testing:** Neuropsychological assessments evaluate cognitive function, memory, attention, executive function, language skills, and emotional well-being to detect subtle cognitive deficits, neurobehavioral changes, and functional impairments associated with neurological disorders.
- **Neurodiagnostic Procedures:** Invasive procedures such as lumbar puncture (spinal tap), nerve biopsy, muscle biopsy, electrocorticography (ECoG), and intracranial pressure monitoring may be indicated to obtain tissue samples, assess CSF parameters, localize epileptic foci, or monitor intracranial dynamics in selected cases.

3.3.5. Treatment Modalities for Neurological Disorders

The management of neurological disorders aims to alleviate symptoms, optimize functional outcomes, prevent disease progression, and improve quality of life through various treatment modalities, including:

- **Medications:** Pharmacological therapies such as analgesics, anticonvulsants, antidepressants, anxiolytics, antipsychotics, dopaminergic agents, cholinesterase inhibitors, and immunomodulators target specific symptoms, underlying pathology, or disease mechanisms in neurological disorders.
- **Surgical Interventions:** Surgical procedures such as tumor resection, neurostimulation (e.g., deep brain stimulation, spinal cord stimulation), epilepsy surgery, neurovascular interventions (e.g., thrombectomy, embolization), and shunting procedures may be indicated to relieve compression, remove lesions, restore neural function, or manage complications in selected cases.
- **Rehabilitative Therapies:** Physical therapy, occupational therapy, speech therapy, and rehabilitation programs focus on improving mobility, strength, coordination, balance, cognitive function, communication skills, and activities of daily living in individuals with neurological impairments.
- **Psychotherapy and Counseling:** Psychological interventions, cognitive-behavioral therapy (CBT), supportive counseling, and psychoeducation address emotional distress, coping strategies,

adjustment issues, caregiver stress, and psychosocial challenges associated with neurological disorders and their impact on individuals and families.

- **Symptomatic Management:** Symptomatic treatments such as pain management, spasticity management, bladder, and bowel management, sleep hygiene measures, and assistive devices (e.g., mobility aids, orthotics, communication devices) alleviate distressing symptoms, enhance functional independence, and improve quality of life.
- **Disease-Modifying Therapies:** Disease-modifying treatments such as disease-modifying antirheumatic drugs (DMARDs), disease-modifying antiepileptic drugs (AEDs), disease-modifying therapies for multiple sclerosis (DMTs), and neuroprotective agents aim to slow disease progression, reduce relapses, and preserve neurological function in chronic neurological conditions.
- **Palliative Care and Supportive Services:** Palliative care teams provide comprehensive symptom management, psychosocial support, advance care planning, and end-of-life care for individuals with advanced neurological disorders, focusing on improving comfort, dignity, and quality of life for patients and their families.

3.3.6. Prevention and Public Health Strategies

Preventing neurological disorders and reducing their burden on individuals, families, and communities require a multifaceted approach involving:

- **Primary Prevention:** Primary prevention strategies focus on reducing modifiable risk factors for neurological disorders, such as promoting healthy lifestyle behaviors (e.g., regular exercise, balanced diet, smoking cessation), preventing traumatic injuries (e.g., helmet use, fall prevention), and addressing environmental exposures (e.g., lead abatement, pesticide regulation).
- **Early Detection and Intervention:** Early detection programs, screening initiatives, and public awareness campaigns raise awareness about warning signs and symptoms of neurological disorders, promote timely diagnosis and treatment, and facilitate access to healthcare services for at-risk populations.
- **Vaccination Programs:** Immunization programs targeting vaccine-preventable diseases (e.g., measles, mumps, rubella, polio, influenza) reduce the incidence of neurological complications such as encephalitis, meningitis, and demyelinating disorders associated with viral infections.
- **Maternal and Child Health Initiatives:** Improving maternal health, prenatal care, maternal nutrition, and perinatal services can prevent congenital neurological disorders, birth injuries, and developmental disabilities through early detection, preventive interventions, and supportive care

during pregnancy and childbirth.

- **Environmental Health Policies:** Implementing environmental regulations, occupational safety standards, and pollution control measures can minimize exposure to neurotoxic substances (e.g., heavy metals, pesticides, air pollutants) and mitigate the risk of neurological disorders associated with environmental hazards.
- **Neurological Research and Innovation:** Investing in neuroscience research, neuroimaging technologies, biomarker discovery, genetic studies, and drug development initiatives is essential for advancing our understanding of neurological disorders, identifying novel therapeutic targets, and developing innovative treatments to prevent, treat, and cure neurological conditions.

3.4. Cardiovascular Disorders

Cardiovascular disorders encompass a wide range of conditions affecting the heart and blood vessels, including coronary artery disease, hypertension, heart failure, arrhythmias, valvular heart disease, congenital heart defects, peripheral vascular disease, and vascular inflammation. These disorders represent a leading cause of morbidity and mortality worldwide, posing significant public health challenges and socioeconomic burdens. In this comprehensive exploration, we will delve into the diverse spectrum of cardiovascular disorders, their classification, etiology, risk factors, clinical manifestations, diagnostic approaches, treatment modalities, and implications for affected individuals and healthcare systems.

3.4.1. Classification of Cardiovascular Disorders

Cardiovascular disorders can be classified based on various criteria, including:

- **Anatomical Location:** Cardiovascular disorders may affect the heart (e.g., coronary artery disease, myocardial infarction, cardiomyopathy), blood vessels (e.g., atherosclerosis, peripheral artery disease), or both (e.g., ischemic heart disease, stroke).
- **Pathophysiological Mechanisms:** Cardiovascular disorders can result from diverse pathophysiological processes, including atherogenesis, endothelial dysfunction, inflammation, thrombosis, vascular remodeling, myocardial ischemia, fibrosis, and arrhythmogenesis.
- **Clinical Presentation:** Cardiovascular disorders manifest with a wide range of symptoms and signs, including chest pain, dyspnea, palpitations, fatigue, syncope, edema, cyanosis, claudication, and neurological deficits, depending on the underlying pathology and affected organ systems.
- **Etiological Factors:** Cardiovascular disorders may be classified based on their underlying etiology, including genetic factors (e.g., familial hypercholesterolemia, hypertrophic cardiomyopathy), lifestyle factors (e.g., smoking, sedentary lifestyle, unhealthy diet), environmental exposures (e.g., air pollution, toxins), and comorbid conditions (e.g., diabetes, obesity, chronic kidney disease).

3.4.2. Etiology and Risk Factors of Cardiovascular Disorders

Cardiovascular disorders arise from a complex interplay of genetic, environmental, behavioral, and physiological factors, including:

- **Genetic Factors:** Inherited genetic mutations, polymorphisms, and familial predispositions contribute to the development of cardiovascular disorders such as familial hypercholesterolemia, hypertrophic cardiomyopathy, familial dilated cardiomyopathy, and hereditary arrhythmias.
- **Modifiable Risk Factors:** Lifestyle factors such as smoking, physical inactivity, unhealthy diet (e.g, high intake of saturated fats, sodium, and refined carbohydrates), excessive alcohol consumption, and psychosocial stress contribute to the development of cardiovascular disorders by promoting atherosclerosis, hypertension, obesity, insulin resistance, and metabolic syndrome.
- **Medical Conditions:** Comorbid conditions such as diabetes mellitus, hypertension, dyslipidemia, chronic kidney disease, obstructive sleep apnea, and autoimmune disorders increase the risk of cardiovascular disorders through mechanisms such as endothelial dysfunction, inflammation, oxidative stress, and dysregulated metabolism.
- **Environmental Exposures:** Environmental factors such as air pollution, secondhand smoke, industrial chemicals, heavy metals (e.g., lead, mercury), and psychosocial stressors contribute to cardiovascular disorders by promoting endothelial injury, oxidative damage, systemic inflammation, and sympathetic activation.
- **Age and Sex:** Advancing age, male sex, and hormonal factors (e.g., estrogen, testosterone) influence the prevalence, severity, and clinical outcomes of cardiovascular disorders, with age-related changes in vascular function, myocardial structure, and hemodynamic regulation contributing to increased cardiovascular risk in older adults.
- **Family History:** A family history of cardiovascular disorders, premature coronary artery disease, stroke, or sudden cardiac death increases the risk of developing similar conditions due to shared genetic susceptibilities, environmental exposures, and lifestyle patterns within families.

3.4.3. Clinical Manifestations of Cardiovascular Disorders

Cardiovascular disorders present with a wide range of symptoms and signs depending on the underlying pathology, affected organ systems, and individual patient factors. Common manifestations include:

- **Chest Pain:** Angina pectoris, a symptom of myocardial ischemia, presents as retrosternal chest discomfort or pressure that may radiate to the neck, jaw, shoulder, or arm and is typically precipitated by exertion or emotional stress.
- **Dyspnea:** Shortness of breath, exertional dyspnea, orthopnea,

paroxysmal nocturnal dyspnea, and breathlessness on lying flat (platypnea) may occur in cardiovascular disorders such as heart failure, pulmonary edema, pulmonary hypertension, or acute coronary syndromes.

- **Palpitations:** Awareness of abnormal or irregular heartbeats, skipped beats, palpable pulsations, or rapid heart rates may occur in arrhythmias such as atrial fibrillation, ventricular tachycardia, supraventricular tachycardia, or premature ventricular contractions.
- **Edema:** Peripheral edema, dependent edema, ankle swelling, jugular venous distention, ascites, and hepatomegaly may indicate fluid retention, congestive heart failure, venous insufficiency, or right-sided heart failure.
- **Fatigue:** Generalized fatigue, weakness, lethargy, malaise, and exercise intolerance may result from reduced cardiac output, myocardial dysfunction, anemia, deconditioning, or systemic effects of chronic illness in cardiovascular disorders.
- **Syncope:** Loss of consciousness, presyncope, dizziness, lightheadedness, or near-fainting episodes may occur due to transient reductions in cerebral perfusion secondary to arrhythmias, vasovagal syncope, orthostatic hypotension, or cardiac causes.
- **Neurological Symptoms:** Neurological deficits such as weakness, numbness, tingling, visual disturbances, aphasia, dysarthria, and cognitive impairment may occur in cardiovascular disorders associated with embolic events, transient ischemic attacks (TIAs), or cerebrovascular accidents (CVAs).
- **Peripheral Symptoms:** Claudication, rest pain, skin changes (e.g., pallor, rubor, cyanosis), nonhealing ulcers, diminished peripheral pulses, and cool extremities may indicate peripheral arterial disease, arterial occlusion, or microvascular insufficiency in the lower extremities.

3.4.4. Diagnostic Approaches for Cardiovascular Disorders

Diagnosing cardiovascular disorders involves a comprehensive evaluation of the patient's medical history, cardiovascular risk factors, physical examination findings, and appropriate diagnostic tests, including:

- **Electrocardiography (ECG):** A standard 12-lead ECG assesses cardiac rhythm, conduction intervals, ST-T wave changes, QRS morphology, and evidence of myocardial ischemia, infarction, or arrhythmias.
- **Echocardiography:** Transthoracic echocardiography (TTE) and transesophageal echocardiography (TEE) provide real-time imaging of cardiac chambers, valves, wall motion, ejection fraction, cardiac output, and structural abnormalities to evaluate cardiac structure and function.
- **Cardiac Biomarkers:** Serum biomarkers such as troponin, creatine kinase-MB (CK-MB), brain natriuretic peptide (BNP), and pro-BNP levels are measured to assess myocardial injury, ischemia, necrosis, and heart

failure in patients with acute coronary syndromes or heart failure.

- **Cardiac Imaging:** Noninvasive cardiac imaging modalities such as coronary computed tomography angiography (CTA), cardiac magnetic resonance imaging (MRI), nuclear perfusion imaging (e.g, myocardial SPECT), and coronary angiography evaluate coronary artery anatomy, stenosis severity, myocardial perfusion, and cardiac function.
- **Stress Testing:** Exercise treadmill testing, pharmacological stress testing (e.g., dobutamine stress echocardiography, myocardial perfusion imaging), and stress cardiac MRI assess myocardial ischemia, exercise capacity, and hemodynamic response to stress in patients with suspected coronary artery disease.
- **Ambulatory Monitoring:** Holter monitoring, event recording, implantable loop recorders, and mobile cardiac telemetry monitor cardiac rhythm over extended periods to detect arrhythmias, monitor response to treatment, and correlate symptoms with rhythm disturbances.
- **Invasive Procedures:** Invasive diagnostic procedures such as cardiac catheterization, coronary angiography, intravascular ultrasound (IVUS), fractional flow reserve (FFR), and optical coherence tomography (OCT) assess coronary anatomy, stenosis severity, and hemodynamic significance of lesions in patients with suspected or known coronary artery disease.

3.4.5. Treatment Modalities for Cardiovascular Disorders

The management of cardiovascular disorders aims to reduce cardiovascular risk, relieve symptoms, improve quality of life, and prevent adverse cardiovascular events through various treatment modalities, including:

- **Lifestyle Modifications:** Lifestyle interventions such as smoking cessation, regular physical activity, healthy diet (e.g., DASH diet, Mediterranean diet), weight management, stress reduction, and alcohol moderation are recommended to reduce cardiovascular risk factors and promote cardiovascular health.
- **Pharmacological Therapies:** Pharmacotherapy with medications such as antiplatelet agents, statins, beta-blockers, ACE inhibitors, angiotensin receptor blockers (ARBs), diuretics, calcium channel blockers, nitrates, anticoagulants, and antiarrhythmic drugs targets specific cardiovascular risk factors, underlying pathophysiology, or symptomatic relief in cardiovascular disorders.
- **Revascularization Procedures:** Revascularization strategies such as percutaneous coronary intervention (PCI), coronary artery bypass grafting (CABG), peripheral artery angioplasty, and carotid endarterectomy restore blood flow, relieve ischemia, and improve outcomes in patients with obstructive coronary artery disease, peripheral arterial disease, or carotid artery stenosis.
- **Implantable Devices:** Implantable cardiac devices such as pacemakers, implantable cardioverter-defibrillators

(ICDs), cardiac resynchronization therapy (CRT) devices, and left ventricular assist devices (LVADs) regulate cardiac rhythm, prevent sudden cardiac death, and improve cardiac function in selected patients with arrhythmias, heart failure, or conduction disorders.

- **Cardiac Rehabilitation:** Multidisciplinary cardiac rehabilitation programs provide supervised exercise training, education, risk factor modification, psychosocial support, and lifestyle counseling to optimize cardiovascular health, functional capacity, and adherence to secondary prevention strategies in patients with cardiovascular disorders.
- **Surgical Interventions:** Surgical procedures such as coronary artery bypass surgery, valve repair or replacement, cardiac transplantation, atrial fibrillation ablation, and aneurysm repair address structural heart defects, valvular abnormalities, arrhythmias, or end-stage heart failure in selected patients with advanced cardiovascular disease.

3.5. Respiratory Disease

Respiratory disease are any of the diseases and disorders of the airways and the lungs that affect human respiration (Figure 3.1). Any part of the respiratory system may become infected or diseased and the effects may have a wide variety of complications.

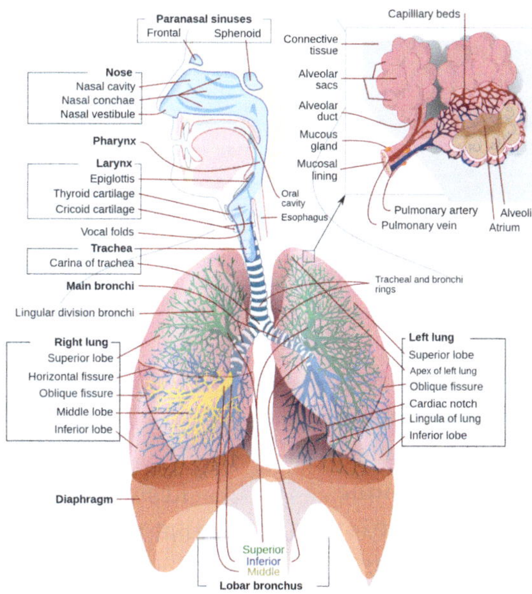

Figure 3.1. *Respiratory disorders affect the lung.*

Source: By LadyofHats, Jmarchn – Own work using:Sobotta, Johannes (1982). Atlas der Anatomie des Menschen / 2 Brust, Bauch, Becken, untere Extremitäten, Haut. (18th ed.), Munich: Urban & Schwarzenberg ISBN: 3-541-02828-9. OCLC: 260005032.Gray, Henry (1980) Gray's Anatomy (36th ed.), Edinburgh: Churchill Livingstone ISBN: 0-443-01505-8. OCLC: 7775214.Yokochi, Chihiro (1991) Atlas fotográfico de anatomía del cuerpo humano (3rd ed.), Mexico: Interamericana/McGraw-Hill ISBN: 968-25-1677-3. OCLC: 33318149. Also used several online diagrams like:[1][2], Public Domain, https://commons.wikimedia.org/w/index.php?curid=3945169.

The response to infection in the body, is an inflammatory reaction. As a result, hyperemia, and swelling of the mucous lining occur causing difficulty in respiration and a degree of hypoventilation. Fibrosis occurs if the condition becomes chronic, resulting in a loss of elasticity, with a possible permanent decrease in ventilation. The oxygen uptake is impaired and carbon dioxide accumulates. The tissues no longer perform as well and general health is impaired, with the patient easily fatiguing.

Alongside the inflammatory reaction, there is increased mucus secretion, resulting in obstruction of the airways with the collapse of the lung tissue distal to the block. It is of paramount importance to regain expansion of the area as soon as possible because the collapsed tissue becomes fibrotic, with a permanent reduction of the ventilation capacity of the lungs.

3.5.1. Types of Respiratory Disorders

There are two types of respiratory diseases and disorders: Infectious and Chronic.

- Pulmonary infections are most commonly bacterial or viral. In the viral type, a pathogen replicates inside a cell and causes a disease, such as the flu. People with weakened lungs and immune systems are more vulnerable to infectious respiratory conditions.
- Chronic lung diseases, fall into one of two main classes: Obstructive or Restrictive.

3.5.1.1. Chronic Respiratory Disorders

Chronic respiratory diseases (CRDs) are a group of chronic diseases affecting the airways and the other structures of the lungs. Hundreds of millions of people around the world suffer from preventable chronic respiratory diseases.

Alongside tobacco smoke, other risk factors include air pollution, occupational chemicals and dusts, and frequent lower respiratory infections during childhood. CRDs are not curable; however, various forms of treatment that help open the air passages and improve shortness of breath can help control symptoms and improve daily life for people living with these conditions. Obstructive Conditions: involve blocked or narrowed airways, making it difficult for the lungs to exhale and exchange old air for fresh air. Examples include-

- Chronic obstructive pulmonary disease: an estimated 65 million people have moderate to severe chronic obstructive pulmonary disease (COPD), from which about 3 million die each year.
- Alpha-1 antitrypsin deficiency.
- Asthma: about 334 million people suffer from asthma, which is the most common chronic disease of childhood, affecting 14% of children globally. The prevalence of asthma in children is rising.
- Bronchiectasis.
- Cystic fibrosis.

Restrictive Conditions: reduce the volume of air that the lungs can hold. Lungs can lose their elasticity or the ability to expand. Examples include:

- Pulmonary fibrosis,
- Sarcoidosis,
- Lung cancer: the most common lethal neoplasm in the world is lung cancer, which kills 1.6 million people each year; and the numbers are growing.

3.5.1.2. Infectious Conditions

Infectious lung conditions are usually temporary, although some respiratory infections can become chronic or frequently recur. For decades, acute lower respiratory tract infections have been among the top three causes of death and disability among both children and adults. Pulmonary infections are common and are caused by a wide range of organisms. Causes include:

1. Pulmonary viral infection
2. Pulmonary bacterial infection: bacterial pneumonia
3. Pulmonary mycobacterial infection: pulmonary tuberculosis; pulmonary nontuberculous mycobacterial infection
4. Pulmonary fungal infection: pulmonary aspergillosis

3.5.2. Treatment Modalities for Respiratory Disorders

The management of respiratory disorders aims to alleviate symptoms, improve lung function, prevent disease progression, and optimize quality of life through various treatment modalities, including:

- **Medications:** Pharmacological therapies such as bronchodilators (e.g., beta-agonists, anticholinergics), corticosteroids, leukotriene modifiers, mast cell stabilizers, mucolytics, antibiotics, antivirals, antifungals, and anticoagulants target specific respiratory disorders, underlying pathophysiology, or symptomatic relief.
- **Oxygen Therapy:** Supplemental oxygen therapy provides oxygen supplementation to correct hypoxemia, improve tissue oxygenation, alleviate dyspnea, and prevent complications in patients with respiratory failure, hypoxemic respiratory disorders, or acute exacerbations of chronic respiratory conditions.
- **Mechanical Ventilation:** Invasive mechanical ventilation (e.g., endotracheal intubation, mechanical ventilators) and noninvasive ventilation (e.g., bilevel positive airway pressure [BiPAP], continuous positive airway pressure [CPAP]) support respiratory function, assist ventilation, and maintain oxygenation in patients with acute respiratory failure, respiratory distress, or neuromuscular respiratory disorders.
- **Pulmonary Rehabilitation:** Pulmonary rehabilitation programs combine exercise training, breathing exercises, education, and psychosocial support to improve functional capacity, respiratory muscle strength, dyspnea perception, and health-related quality of life in patients with chronic respiratory disorders such as COPD, interstitial lung diseases, and pulmonary hypertension.
- **Airway Clearance Techniques:** Airway clearance techniques such as chest physiotherapy, postural drainage, percussion, vibration, coughing techniques, and mechanical devices (e.g., oscillatory positive expiratory pressure [PEP] devices, high-frequency chest wall oscillation [HFCWO] devices) facilitate the mobilization and clearance of respiratory secretions in patients

with impaired mucociliary clearance, bronchiectasis, or cystic fibrosis.

- **Surgical Interventions:** Surgical procedures such as lung resection (e.g., lobectomy, pneumonectomy), lung transplantation, bronchial thermoplasty, lung volume reduction surgery, bullectomy, and pleurodesis may be indicated for selected patients with advanced respiratory disorders, severe emphysema, end-stage lung disease, or recurrent pneumothorax unresponsive to conservative management.
- **Interventional Procedures:** Interventional pulmonology procedures such as bronchoscopic interventions (e.g., endobronchial biopsy, airway stent placement, laser therapy, cryotherapy, photodynamic therapy) and thoracic procedures (e.g., thoracentesis, pleural biopsy, pleurodesis, pleural catheter placement) provide diagnostic and therapeutic options for patients with airway lesions, pleural effusions, or mediastinal masses.

3.5.3. Prevention and Public Health Strategies

Preventing respiratory disorders and reducing their burden on individuals, families, and communities require a multifaceted approach involving:

- **Immunization Programs:** Vaccination against respiratory pathogens such as influenza, pneumococcus, pertussis, measles, mumps, rubella, and *Haemophilus influenzae* type b (Hib) reduces the incidence, severity, and complications of vaccine-preventable respiratory infections, protecting vulnerable populations and promoting herd immunity.
- **Smoking Cessation Initiatives:** Tobacco control measures, smoking cessation programs, public awareness campaigns, and regulatory policies (e.g., tobacco taxes, smoke-free laws, graphic health warnings) reduce smoking prevalence, prevent tobacco-related diseases, and promote respiratory health by addressing the leading modifiable risk factor for respiratory disorders.
- **Environmental Regulations:** Implementing air quality standards, pollution control measures, emission reduction policies, clean energy initiatives, and sustainable transportation strategies mitigate environmental exposures to air pollutants, allergens, industrial emissions, and indoor contaminants, reducing the risk of respiratory disorders and respiratory exacerbations.
- **Occupational Health and Safety:** Occupational health programs, workplace regulations, personal protective equipment (PPE), engineering controls, and exposure monitoring initiatives minimize occupational hazards, respiratory exposures, and work-related lung diseases in high-risk industries (e.g., mining, construction, agriculture, manufacturing).
- **Respiratory Hygiene Practices:** Promoting respiratory hygiene practices such as hand hygiene, cough etiquette, mask-wearing,

and social distancing reduces the transmission of respiratory pathogens, prevents respiratory infections, and protects vulnerable individuals, particularly during outbreaks of infectious diseases (e.g., COVID-19).

- **Indoor Air Quality:** Improving indoor air quality through ventilation, air filtration, humidity control, mold remediation, and reduction of indoor allergens (e.g., dust mites, pet dander, mold) creates healthy indoor environments, reduces respiratory symptoms, and prevents indoor air pollution-related respiratory disorders.

3.6. Gastrointestinal Diseases

Gastrointestinal diseases affect your gastrointestinal (GI) tract, from mouth to anus. There are two types: functional and structural. Some examples include colitis, food poisoning, lactose intolerance and diarrhea.

3.6.1. What Are Functional Gastrointestinal Diseases?

Functional diseases are those in which the GI tract looks normal when examined but doesn't function properly. They are the most common problems affecting the GI tract (including your colon and rectum). Constipation, irritable bowel syndrome (IBS), nausea, gas, bloating, and diarrhea are common examples.

Many factors can upset your GI tract and its motility (ability to keep moving), including:

- Eating a diet low in fiber.
- Not getting enough exercise.
- Traveling or other changes in routine.
- Eating large amounts of dairy products.
- Stress.
- Resisting the urge to have a bowel movement, possibly because of hemorrhoids.
- Overusing anti-diarrheal medications that, over time, weaken the bowel muscle movements called motility.
- Taking antacid medicines containing calcium or aluminum.
- Taking certain medicines (especially antidepressants, iron pills and strong pain medicines such as narcotics).
- Pregnancy.

Some people also have heightened sensitivity in the organs of their GI tract (visceral hypersensitivity). This can make them feel pain or discomfort even when the organs are functioning normally.

3.6.2. What Are Structural Gastrointestinal Diseases?

Structural gastrointestinal diseases are those where your bowel looks abnormal upon examination and also doesn't work properly. Sometimes, the structural abnormality needs to be removed surgically. Common examples of structural GI diseases include strictures, stenosis, hemorrhoids, diverticular disease, colon polyps, colon cancer and inflammatory bowel disease.

3.6.3. Common Gastrointestinal Diseases That Healthcare Providers Treat

Healthcare providers who specialize in gastrointestinal diseases are called gastroenterologists. Surgeons who specialize in gastrointestinal diseases are called colorectal surgeons (proctologists). Some of the most common conditions they treat include:

3.6.3.1. Constipation

Constipation, which is a functional problem, makes it hard for you to have a bowel movement (or pass stools), the stools are infrequent (less than three times a week), or incomplete. Constipation is often related to inadequate "roughage" or fiber in your diet, or a disruption of your routine or diet.

Constipation causes you to strain during a bowel movement. It may cause small, hard stools and sometimes anal problems such as fissures or hemorrhoids. Constipation is rarely a sign that you have a more serious medical condition.

You can treat your constipation at home by:

- Increasing the amount of fiber and water in your diet.
- Exercising regularly and increasing the intensity of your exercises as tolerated.
- Moving your bowels when you have the urge (resisting the urge causes constipation).

If these treatment methods don't work, laxatives can be useful. Always follow the instructions on your laxative medicine, as well as the advice of your healthcare provider.

3.6.3.2. Irritable Bowel Syndrome (IBS)

Irritable bowel syndrome (also called spastic colon, irritable colon, IBS, or nervous stomach) is a functional condition where your intestinal muscles contract more or less often than "normal." Certain foods, medicines, and emotional stress are some factors that can trigger IBS.

Symptoms of IBS include:

- Abdominal pain and cramps.
- Excess gas.
- Bloating.
- Change in bowel habits such as harder, looser, or more urgent stools than normal.
- Constipation and/or diarrhea.

You can treat IBS at home by:

- Avoiding excessive caffeine.
- Increasing fiber in your diet.
- Monitoring which foods trigger your IBS (and avoiding these foods).
- Minimizing stress or learning different ways to cope with stress.
- Taking medicines as prescribed by your healthcare provider.
- Avoiding dehydration, and hydrating well throughout the day.
- Getting high-quality rest/sleep.

3.6.3.4. Hemorrhoids

Hemorrhoids are dilated veins in your anal canal. This is a structural disease. They're caused by chronic excess pressure from straining during a bowel movement, persistent diarrhea, or pregnancy. There are two types of hemorrhoids: internal and external.

Internal hemorrhoids are blood vessels on the inside of your anal opening. When they fall down into the anus as a result of straining, they become irritated and start to bleed. Ultimately, internal hemorrhoids can fall down enough to prolapse (sink or stick) out of the anus.

Treatment includes:

- Improving bowel habits (such as avoiding constipation, not straining during bowel movements and moving your bowels when you have the urge).
- Your healthcare provider using ligating bands to eliminate the vessels.
- Your healthcare provider removing them surgically. Surgery is needed only for a small number of people with very large, painful, and

persistent hemorrhoids. External hemorrhoids are veins that lie just under the skin on the outside of the anus. Sometimes, after straining, the external hemorrhoidal veins burst and a blood clots form under the skin. This very painful condition is called a "pile."

Treatment includes removing the clot and vein under local anesthesia and/or removing the hemorrhoid itself.

3.6.3.5. Anal Fissures

Anal fissures are also a structural disease. They are splits or cracks in the lining of your anus. The most common cause of an anal fissure is the passage of very hard or watery stools. The crack in the anal lining exposes the underlying muscles that control the passage of stool through the anus and out of the body. An anal fissure is one of the most painful problems you can have because the exposed muscles become irritated from exposure to stool or air. This leads to intense burning pain, bleeding, or spasms after bowel movements.

Initial treatment for anal fissures includes pain medicine, dietary fiber to reduce the occurrence of large, bulky stools and sitz baths (sitting in a few inches of warm water). If these treatments don't relieve your pain, surgery might be needed to repair the fissure.

3.6.3.6. Perianal Abscesses

Perianal abscesses, also a structural disease, can occur when the tiny anal glands that open on the inside of your anus become blocked, and the bacteria always present in these glands cause an infection. When pus develops, an abscess forms. Treatment includes draining the abscess, usually under local anesthesia in the healthcare provider's office.

3.6.3.7. Anal Fistula

An anal fistula – again, a structural disease – often follows drainage of an abscess. It's an abnormal, tube-like passageway from the anal canal to a hole in the skin near the opening of your anus. Body wastes traveling through your anal canal are diverted through this tiny channel and out through the skin, causing itching and irritation. Fistulas also cause drainage, pain, and bleeding. They rarely heal by themselves and usually need surgery to drain the abscess and "close off" the fistula.

3.6.3.8. Diverticular Disease

Diverticulosis is the presence of small outpouchings (diverticula) in the muscular wall of your large intestine that form in weakened areas of the bowel. They usually occur in the sigmoid colon, the high-pressure area of the lower large intestine. Diverticular disease is very common and occurs in 10% of people over age 40 and in 50% of people over age 60 in Western cultures. It is often caused by too little roughage (fiber) in the diet. Diverticulosis can sometimes develop/progress into diverticulitis

Complications of diverticular disease happen in about 10% of people with outpouchings. They include infection or inflammation in the pouches (diverticulitis), which can lead to bleeding and obstruction. Treatment of diverticulitis includes treating constipation and sometimes antibiotics if really severe. Surgery is needed as a last resort in those who have significant complications to remove the involved diseased segment of the colon.

3.6.3.9. Colon Polyps and Cancer

Each year, 130,000 Americans are diagnosed with colorectal cancer, the second most common form of cancer in the United States. Fortunately, with advances in early detection and treatment, colorectal cancer is one of the most curable forms of the disease. By using a variety of screening tests, it is possible to prevent, detect, and treat the disease long before symptoms appear.

3.6.3.9.1. The Importance of Colorectal Cancer Screening

Almost all colorectal cancers begin as colon polyps, benign (non-cancerous) growths in the tissues lining your colon and rectum. Cancer develops when these polyps grow and abnormal cells develop and start to invade surrounding tissue. Removal of polyps can prevent the development of colorectal cancer. Almost all precancerous polyps can be removed painlessly during a colonoscopy screening. If not caught in the early stages, colorectal cancer can spread throughout the body. More advanced cancer requires more complicated surgical techniques.

Most early forms of colorectal cancer do not cause symptoms, which makes screening especially important. When symptoms do occur, the cancer might already be quite advanced. Symptoms include blood on or mixed in with the stool, a change in normal bowel habits, narrowing of the stool, abdominal pain, weight loss, or constant tiredness.

Most cases of colorectal cancer are detected in one of four ways:

- By screening people at average risk for colorectal cancer beginning at age 45.
- By screening people at higher risk for colorectal cancer (e.g., those with a family history or a personal history of colon polyps or cancer).
- By investigating the bowel in patients with symptoms.
- A chance finding at a routine check-up.

Early detection is the best chance for a cure.

3.6.3.10. Colitis

There are several types of colitis, which are conditions that cause inflammation of the bowel. These include:

- Infectious colitis.
- Ulcerative colitis (cause unknown).
- Crohn's disease (cause unknown).
- Ischemic colitis (caused by not enough blood going to the colon).
- Radiation colitis (after radiotherapy).

Colitis can cause diarrhea, rectal bleeding, abdominal cramps and urgency (frequent and immediate need to empty the bowels). Treatment depends on the diagnosis, which is made by colonoscopy and biopsy.

3.7. Endocrine Disorders

The endocrine system is a network of glands that produce and release hormones. These hormones help control many important body functions, including the body's ability to change calories into energy that powers cells and organs. The endocrine system affects how your heart beats, how your bones and tissues grow, and even your ability to make a baby.

Disorders of the endocrine system happen if your hormone levels are too high or too low, or if your body doesn't respond to hormones in the expected way. You may develop diabetes, thyroid disease, growth disorders, sexual dysfunction, and a host of other hormone-related disorders.

3.7.1. Glands of the Endocrine System

Each gland of the endocrine system releases specific hormones into your bloodstream. These hormones travel through your blood to other cells and help control or coordinate many body processes.

Endocrine glands include:

- **Adrenal glands:** Two glands that sit on top of the kidneys that release the hormone cortisol.
- **Hypothalamus:** A part of the lower middle brain that tells the pituitary gland when to release hormones.
- **Islet cells in the pancreas:** Cells in the pancreas that control the release of the hormones insulin and glucagon.
- **Ovaries:** The female reproductive organs that release eggs and produce sex hormones.
- **Parathyroid:** Four tiny glands in the neck that play a role in bone development.
- **Pineal gland**: A gland located near the center of the brain that may be linked to sleep patterns.
- **Pituitary gland:** It's present at the base of the brain behind the sinuses. It is often called the "master gland" because it influences many other glands, especially the thyroid. Problems with the pituitary gland can affect bone growth, a woman's menstrual cycles, and the release of breast milk.
- **Testes:** The male reproductive glands that produce sperm and sex hormones.
- **Thymus:** A gland in the upper chest that helps develop the body's immune system early in life.
- **Thyroid:** A butterfly-shaped gland in the front of the neck that controls metabolism.

Even the slightest hiccup with the function of one or more of these glands can throw off the delicate balance of hormones in your body and lead to an endocrine disorder, or endocrine disease.

3.7.2. Endocrine Disorder Causes

Endocrine disorders are typically grouped into two categories:

- Endocrine diseases that result when a gland produces too much or too little of an endocrine hormone, called a hormone imbalance.
- Endocrine diseases that result due to the development of lesions (such as nodules or tumors) in the endocrine system, which may or may not affect hormone levels.

The endocrine feedback system helps control the balance of hormones in the bloodstream. If your body has too much or too little of a certain hormone, the feedback system signals the proper gland or glands to correct the problem. A hormone imbalance may occur if this feedback system has trouble keeping the right level of hormones in the bloodstream, or if your body doesn't clear them out of the bloodstream properly.

Increased or decreased levels of endocrine hormone may be caused by:

- A problem with the endocrine feedback system.
- Disease.
- Failure of a gland to stimulate another gland to release hormones (e.g., a problem with the hypothalamus can disrupt hormone production in the pituitary gland).
- A genetic disorder, such as multiple endocrine neoplasia (MEN) or congenital hypothyroidism.
- Infection.

- Injury to an endocrine gland.
- Tumor of an endocrine gland.

Most endocrine tumors and nodules (lumps) are noncancerous. They usually don't spread to other parts of the body. However, a tumor or nodule on the gland may interfere with the gland's hormone production.

3.7.3. Symptoms of Endocrine Disorders

The symptoms of an endocrine disorder vary widely and depend on the specific gland involved. However, most people with endocrine disease complain of fatigue and weakness. Certain symptoms may make you think you have a different disease or disorder. Some symptoms that are worth talking to your doctor about include:

- Changes in your heart rate.
- Changes to your skin or eyes.
- Bone fractures.
- High blood sugar levels.
- High calcium levels.
- Low or high blood pressure.
- Unexplained changes in your weight.
- Loss of sex drive.
- Infertility.
- Menstrual cycle disorders.

3.7.4. Types of Endocrine Disorders

There are many different types of endocrine disorders. Diabetes is the most common endocrine disorder diagnosed in the U.S.

Other endocrine disorders include:

- **Adrenal insufficiency.** The adrenal gland releases too little of the hormone cortisol and sometimes, aldosterone. Symptoms include fatigue, stomach upset, dehydration, and skin changes. Addison's disease is a type of adrenal insufficiency.
- **Cushing's disease.** The overproduction of a pituitary gland hormone leads to an overactive adrenal gland. A similar condition called Cushing's syndrome may occur in people, particularly children, who take high doses of corticosteroid medications.
- **Gigantism (acromegaly) and other growth hormone problems.** If the pituitary gland produces too much growth hormone, a child's bones and body parts may grow abnormally fast. If growth hormone levels are too low, a child can stop growing in height.
- **Hyperthyroidism.** The thyroid gland produces too much thyroid hormone, leading to weight loss, fast heart rate, sweating, and nervousness. The most common cause for an overactive thyroid is an autoimmune disorder called Grave's disease.
- **Hypothyroidism.** The thyroid gland does not produce enough thyroid hormone, leading to fatigue, constipation, dry skin, and depression. The underactive gland can cause slowed development in children. Some types of hypothyroidism are present at birth.
- **Hypopituitarism.** In this condition, the pituitary gland releases little or no hormones. It may be caused by several different diseases. Women with this condition may stop getting their periods.
- **Multiple endocrine neoplasia type 1 and 2 (MEN1 and MEN2).** These

rare, genetic conditions are passed down through families. They cause tumors of the parathyroid, adrenal, and thyroid glands, leading to overproduction of hormones.

- **Polycystic ovary syndrome (PCOS).** The overproduction of androgens interferes with the development of eggs and their release from the female ovaries. PCOS is a leading cause of infertility.
- **Precocious puberty.** This refers to abnormally early puberty that occurs when glands tell the body to release sex hormones too soon in life.

A Closer Look

Dermatological disorders

Dermatological disorders encompass a broad spectrum of conditions affecting the skin, hair, and nails, often presenting with a wide array of symptoms and manifestations. Taking a closer look at these disorders reveals the intricate interplay of genetic, environmental, and immunological factors that contribute to their development and progression.

One category of dermatological disorders includes inflammatory conditions such as eczema, psoriasis, and acne. These disorders are characterized by abnormal immune responses, leading to inflammation, redness, itching, and discomfort. Eczema, also known as atopic dermatitis, is a chronic inflammatory skin condition characterized by dry, itchy patches that can appear anywhere on the body. Psoriasis, on the other hand, is characterized by thick, red patches of skin covered with silvery scales, resulting from an accelerated skin cell turnover. Acne, a common dermatological disorder, arises from the blockage of hair follicles by oil and dead skin cells, leading to the formation of pimples, blackheads, and cysts.

Another category of dermatological disorders includes infectious conditions such as fungal, bacterial, and viral infections. Fungal infections, such as athlete's foot and ringworm, are caused by fungi that thrive in warm, moist environments, leading to symptoms like itching, redness, and flaking of the skin. Bacterial infections, such as cellulitis and impetigo, occur when bacteria enter the skin through cuts, wounds, or breaks in the skin barrier, resulting in redness, swelling, and sometimes pus-filled lesions. Viral infections, such as herpes simplex and warts, are caused by viruses that infect the skin and mucous membranes, leading to the formation of painful blisters, ulcers, or raised growths.

Furthermore, dermatological disorders may also include neoplastic conditions such as skin cancer. Skin cancer, including melanoma, basal cell carcinoma, and squamous cell carcinoma, arises from the uncontrolled growth of abnormal cells in the skin. Risk factors for skin cancer include excessive sun exposure, genetic predisposition, and immunosuppression. Early detection and treatment of skin cancer are crucial for favorable outcomes, highlighting the importance of regular skin examinations and sun protection practices.

Summary

- Congenital disorders can be defined as structural or functional anomalies that occur during intrauterine life. Also called birth defects, congenital anomalies or congenital malformations, these conditions develop prenatally and may be identified before or at birth, or later in life. An estimated 6% of babies worldwide are born with a congenital disorder, resulting in hundreds of thousands of associated deaths. However, the true number of cases may be much higher because statistics do not often consider terminated pregnancies and stillbirths
- Musculoskeletal disorders are conditions that affect muscles, bones, joints, and connective tissue. They can be present at birth or develop as a result of injury or disease.
- Neurological disorders are medically defined as disorders that affect the brain as well as the nerves found throughout the human body and the spinal cord. Structural, biochemical or electrical abnormalities in the brain, spinal cord or other nerves can result in a range of symptoms. Examples of symptoms include paralysis, muscle weakness, poor coordination, loss of sensation, seizures, confusion, pain, and altered levels of consciousness.
- Cardiovascular disease is a group of diseases affecting your heart and blood vessels. These diseases can affect one or many parts of your heart and/or blood vessels. A person may be symptomatic (physically experiencing the disease) or asymptomatic (not feeling anything at all).
- Respiratory diseases may be caused by infection, by smoking tobacco, or by breathing in secondhand tobacco smoke, radon, asbestos, or other forms of air pollution. Respiratory diseases include asthma, chronic obstructive pulmonary disease (COPD), pulmonary fibrosis, pneumonia, and lung cancer.
- GERD, diarrhea, and colorectal cancer are examples of gastrointestinal diseases. When examined, some diseases show nothing wrong with the GI tract, but there are still symptoms. Other diseases have symptoms, and there are also visible irregularities in the GI tract. Most gastrointestinal diseases can be prevented and/or treated.

References

1. Felson, D. T., & LaValley, M. P. (2014). The ACR20 and defining a threshold for response in rheumatic diseases: Too much of a good thing. *Arthritis Research & Therapy*, *16*(1), 101.
2. Filipovic, I., Walker, D., Forster, F., & Curry, A. S. (2011). Quantifying the economic burden of productivity loss in rheumatoid arthritis. *Rheumatology (Oxford, England)*, *50*(6), 1083–1090.
3. Greenberg, J. D., Harrold, L. R., Bentley, M. J., Kremer, J., Reed, G., & Strand, V. (2009). Evaluation of composite measures of treatment response without acute-phase reactants in patients with rheumatoid arthritis. *Rheumatology (Oxford, England)*, *48*(6), 686–690.
4. Gu, B. K., Choi, D. J., Park, S. J., Kim, Y. J., & Kim, C. H. (2018). 3D bioprinting technologies for tissue engineering applications. In H. Chun, C. Park, I. Kwon, & G. Khang (Eds.), *Cutting-Edge Enabling Technologies for Regenerative Medicine* (Vol. 1078, pp. 15–28). Singapore: Springer.
5. Haddad, A., & Chandran, V. (2013). Arthritis mutilans. *Current Rheumatology Reports*, *15*(4), 321.

6. Hagen, K. B., Byfuglien, M. G., Falzon, L., Olsen, S. U., & Smedslund, G. (2009). Dietary interventions for rheumatoid arthritis. *Cochrane Database of Systematic Reviews, 2009*(1), CD006400.

7. Harirforoosh, S., Asghar, W., & Jamali, F. (2013). Adverse effects of nonsteroidal anti-inflammatory drugs: An update of gastrointestinal, cardiovascular and renal complications. *Journal of Pharmacy & Pharmaceutical Sciences, 16*(5), 821–847.

8. Harris, E. C., & Coggon, D. (2015). Hip osteoarthritis and work. *Best Practice and Research: Clinical Rheumatology, 29*(3), 462–482.

9. Hartvigsen, J., Hancock, M. J., Kongsted, A., Louw, Q., Ferreira, M. L., Genevay, S., Hoy, D., Karppinen, J., Pransky, G., Sieper, J., Smeets, R. J., & Underwood, M. (2018). What low back pain is and why we need to pay attention. *Lancet, 391*(10137), 2356–2367.

10. Marieb, E. N., & Hoehn, K. (2016). *Human Anatomy & Physiology* (10th ed., Global ed.). Harlow: Pearson Education.

11. Marieb, E. N., & Smith, L. A. (2018). *Human Anatomy & Physiology: Laboratory Manual* (13th ed.). Upper Saddle River: Pearson.

12. Marieb, E. N., Keller, S. M., & ProQuest (Firm). (2018). *Essentials of Human Anatomy & Physiology* (12th ed., Global ed.). New York, NY: Pearson.

13. Martini, F., Ober, W. C., Nath, J. L., Bartholomew, E. F., & Petti, K. (2017). *Visual Anatomy & Physiology* (3rd ed.). Upper Saddle River: Pearson.

14. Pack, P. E., & Bassett, S. E. (2011). *Anatomy & Physiology Quick Review* (2nd ed., Vol. CliffsNotes). Hoboken, NJ: Wiley.

15. Patton, K. T., & Thibodeau, G. A. (2018). *The Human Body in Health & Disease* (7th ed.). St. Louis, MO: Elsevier.

16. Tortora, G. J., & Derrickson, B. (2014). *Principles of Anatomy and Physiology* (14th ed.). New York: Wiley.

Chapter

UPPER AND LOWER AIRWAY INFECTIONS

4

Contents

Introduction

A range of respiratory tract diseases, including viruses, bacteria, and fungi, can be attributed to upper and lower airway infections. Numerous anatomical areas of the respiratory system are impacted by these infections, which can cause a broad range of clinical presentations and symptoms.

The pharynx, larynx, sinuses, and nasal passages are the main organs affected by upper airway infections. Common examples include sinusitis, pharyngitis (sore throat), laryngitis, and the common cold (caused by rhinovirus). Common symptoms include runny nose, sore throat, coughing, and hoarseness in the nasal passages. Upper airway infections can cause severe discomfort and may result in complications in certain individuals, such as those with compromised immune systems or underlying respiratory conditions, even though they typically resolve on their own in a matter of days to weeks.

Lower airway infections, on the other hand, impact the lungs, trachea, and bronchi. Bronchitis, bronchiolitis, and pneumonia are a few examples. More severe symptoms, such as fever, shortness of breath, chest pain, and coughing up sputum, are frequently present with lower airway infections. Both bacterial and viral pathogens can cause these infections; untreated bacterial pneumonia has the potential to be fatal. Antibiotics, antiviral drugs, supportive care, and, in extreme situations, hospitalization are possible forms of treatment for lower airway infections. Comprehending the differentiation between upper and lower respiratory tract infections is imperative for precise diagnosis and suitable handling of respiratory ailments.

Orientation and Directional Terms

Term	Definition	Illustration
Retropharyngeal abscesses	A retropharyngeal abscess is a collection of pus in the back of the throat caused by bacteria growing in the lymph nodes. It's an uncommon but potentially life-threatening condition that's most common in children under the age of five, but can also occur in adults.	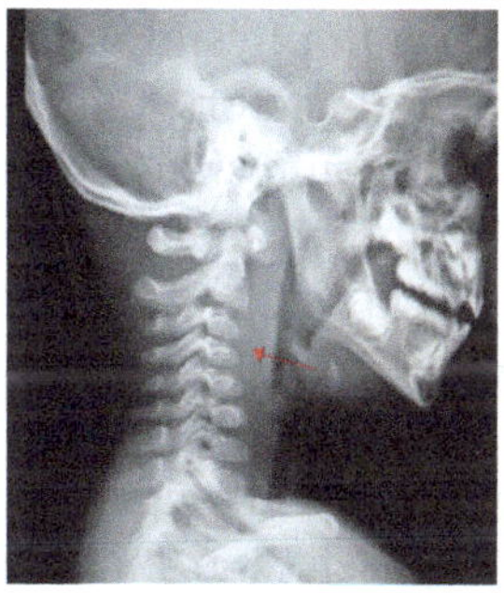
Gastroesophageal reflux disease (GERD)	Gastroesophageal reflux disease (GERD) occurs when stomach acid repeatedly flows back into the tube connecting your mouth and stomach (esophagus).	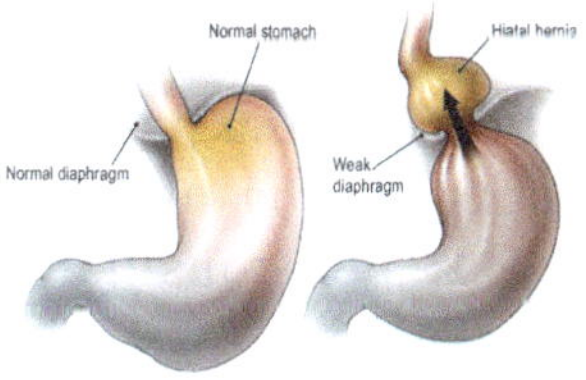
Laryngomalacia	Laryngomalacia is a congenital condition that causes the soft tissues above a child's vocal cords to partially block their airway.	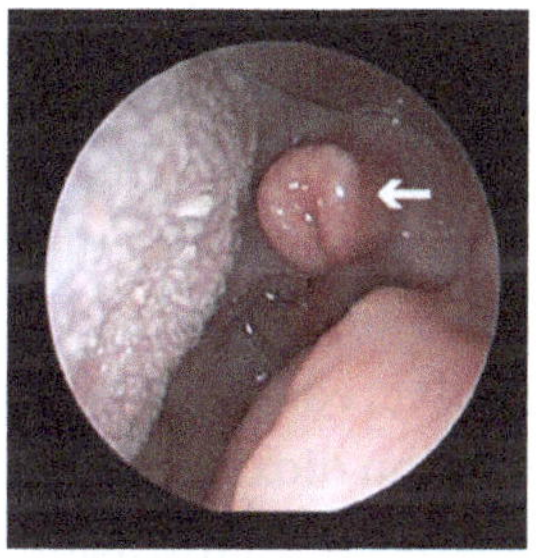
Epiglottis	The epiglottis is a small, leaf-shaped flap of cartilage in the throat that acts as a lid to prevent food and drink from entering the windpipe.	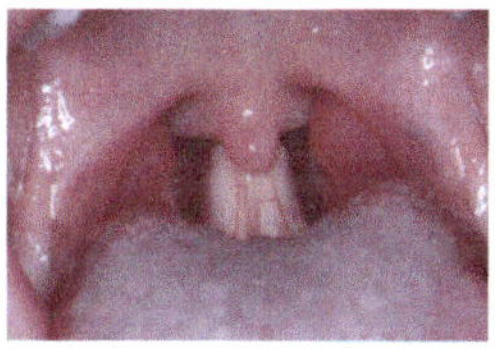
Bacterial tracheitis	Bacterial tracheitis is a rare infection that causes inflammation in the trachea, larynx, and bronchi. It can occur as a result of a secondary bacterial infection of the trachea, or as a complication of a respiratory infection after a virus.	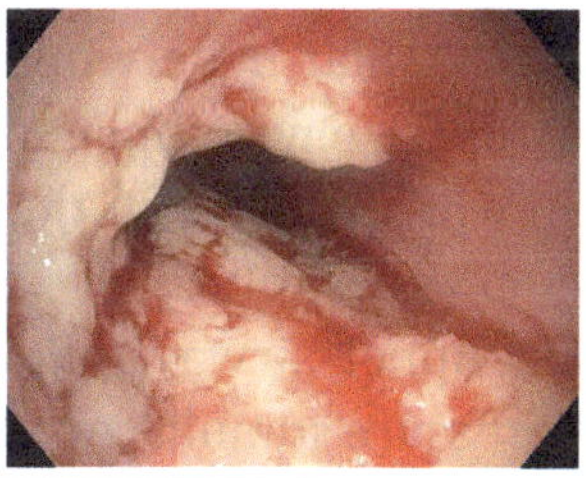

4.1. The Pediatric Airway

Many illnesses and congenital abnormalities can result in structural abnormalities, in addition to the normal physiological processes and developmental factors that affect the airway. A lot of these could show signs of upper airway blockage. Obstacles of the nasal passages, oropharynx, larynx, and glottis are all included in the wide differential diagnosis for extra-thoracic airway obstruction. Blockage may result from chin and tongue anatomic anomalies like macroglossia and micrognathia. As in the cases of nasal piriform aperture stenosis and choanal atresia, obstruction of the nasopharynx is brought on by nasal polyps and a persistent bucconasal membrane. Adenoid-tonsillar enlargement, peri-tonsillar abscesses, and retropharyngeal abscesses can all obstruct the airway within the oropharynx.

The condition known as obstructive sleep apnea (OSA) is characterized by partial or complete collapse of the upper airway during inspiration, which results in a significant (more than 50%) decrease in airflow. The increase in end tidal carbon dioxide ($ETCO_2$) and decrease in hemoglobin oxygen saturation (SaO_2) during the obstructive event(s) cause autonomic, physical, and electroencephalographic (EEG) arousals. Numerous short- and long-term behavioral and metabolic deficiencies and disorders have been linked to OSA.

Adenotonsillar hypertrophy, gastric reflux disease (GERD), environmental tobacco smoke exposure, which results in the compromise of the upper airway's soft tissues, low muscle tone, attenuated upper airway reflexes to PCO_2 and negative pressure stimuli, craniofacial dysplasia, and mandibular hypoplasia are among the numerous causes of open airway disease (OSA), many of which act in combination. Approximately 2% of children have OSA, which is more common in obese children, children with craniofacial abnormalities, and children with central hypotonia. Polysomnography, another name for a sleep study, is used to diagnose OSA by simultaneously measuring several physiological parameters, such as EEG, EKG, EMG, breathing effort, air flow, eye movements, pulse oximetry, $ETCO_2$ levels, and respiratory effort during sleep. Although a lateral neck film can be used to look for signs of tonsillar or adenoidal hypertrophy, it is not thought to be a sensitive method for diagnosing OSA because it does not take into consideration the dynamic changes in airway patency that occur during sleep.

The removal of the tonsils and adenoids is the initial course of treatment for OSA in children. In as many as 85–90% of children with OSA, this is curative (Ray et al., 1993; Stroud and Friedman, 2001; Samuels M, Wieteska, 2011; Wald, 2014) (Figures 4.1 and 4.2).

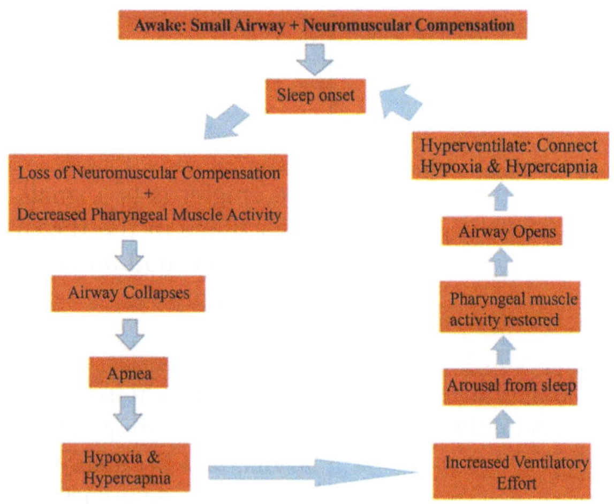

Figure 4.1. *Pathophysiology of OSA.*

Source: Jyothi, I, Renuka Prasad, K, Rajalakshmi, R, Satish Kumar, R, Ramphanindra, T, Vijayakumar, T, & Kaliappan, I. (2019). Obstructive Sleep Apnea: A Pathophysiology and Pharmacotherapy Approach. IntechOpen. doi: 10.5772/intechopen.77981.

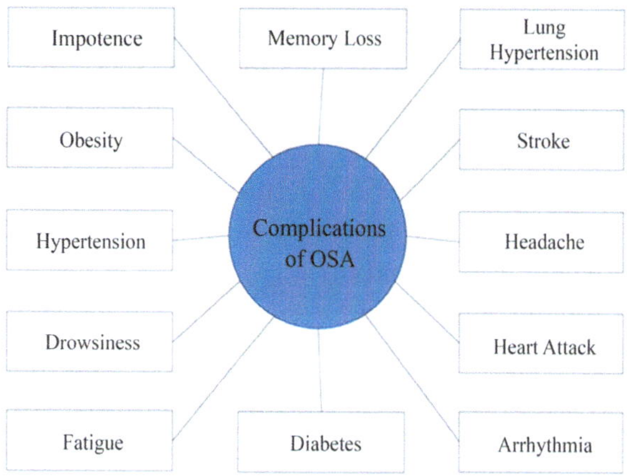

Figure 4.2. *OSA complications.*

Source: Jyothi, I, Renuka Prasad, K, Rajalakshmi, R, Satish Kumar, R, Ramphanindra, T, Vijayakumar, T, & Kaliappan, I. (2019). Obstructive Sleep Apnea: A Pathophysiology and Pharmacotherapy Approach. IntechOpen. doi: 10.5772/intechopen.77981.

However, this surgery is insufficient in some pediatric populations, including older children, obese children, children with chromosomal disorders, craniofacial abnormalities, central hypotonia, and some otherwise healthy children, necessitating further treatment. Continuous positive airway pressure (CPAP) is typically recommended in these situations for sleeping.

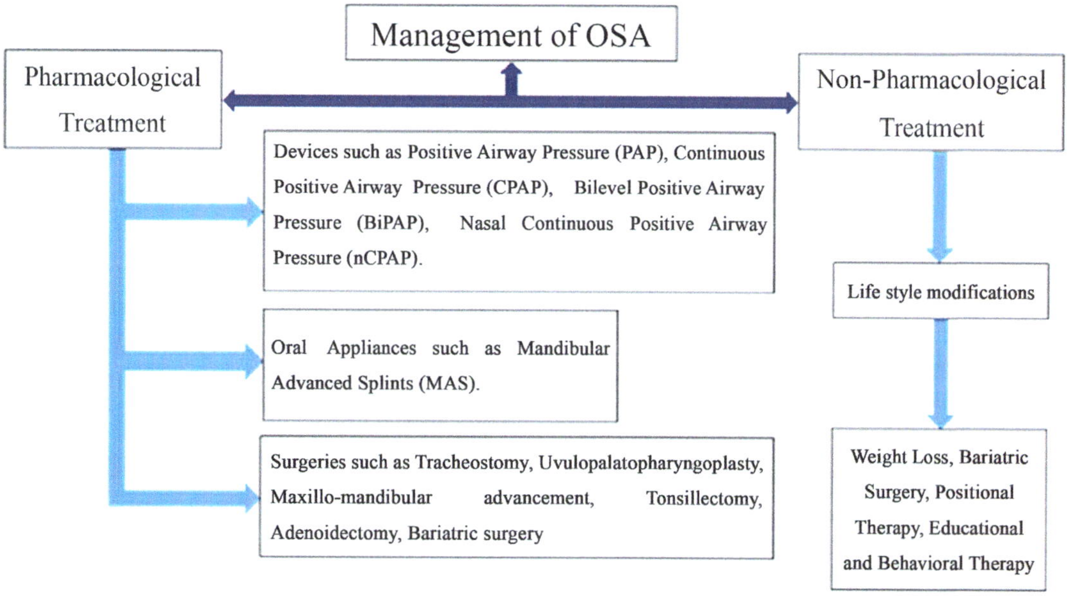

Figure 4.3. *OSA treatment.*

Source: Jyothi, I, Renuka Prasad, K, Rajalakshmi, R, Satish Kumar, R, Ramphanindra, T, Vijayakumar, T, & Kaliappan, I. (2019). Obstructive Sleep Apnea: A Pathophysiology and Pharmacotherapy Approach. IntechOpen. doi: 10.5772/intechopen.77981.

Laryngomalacia and laryngostenosis are two common causes of extra-thoracic obstruction at the larynx. Laryngomalacia, which is more prevalent in children under two, occurs when the supporting structures of the larynx are underdeveloped. This causes the epiglottis, arytenoids, and aryepiglottic folds to collapse into the airway during inhalation, leading to a stridor. Diagnosis is typically done through laryngoscopy as radiologic imaging can be inconclusive. Laryngostenosis, also known as subglottic stenosis, is a narrowing of the airway that can be either congenital or acquired. Endotracheal intubation is a common cause of acquired laryngostenosis (Figure 4.3).

A lingual thyroid may obstruct the midline as a result of thyroid descent failure. When the tongue protrudes, remnants of the thyroglossal duct may form a cyst, which appears as a smooth mass in the neck's midline and usually moves upward. Less common causes of midline obstruction include cysts, webs, and laryngoceles. A web forms when the embryonic airway is unable to reacanalize, and a cyst, which is located in the aryepiglottic fold, is filled with salivary gland mucus. The laryngeal ventricle's saccule dilates, resulting in a laryngocele.

Rare causes of upper airway obstruction include vallecular cysts. Usually, they appear within the first week of life or at birth. The range of symptoms that present include chest retractions, feeding difficulties, reflux, failure to thrive, hoarse cry, inspiratory stridor, apnea, and cyanosis. Laryngomalacia is frequently linked to. Vallecular cysts are typically detected on the lingual surface of the epiglottis obstructing the upper airway and are evaluated by laryngoscopy. Cross-sectional imaging or ultrasound are two methods that can identify them. To see the cyst, the base of the tongue must be visualized carefully. Thyro-glossal cysts, dermoid cysts, hemangiomas, and lymphatic malformations (cystic hygromas) are among the differential diagnoses. A hemangioma is a collection of blood vessels submucosally in the subglottic region, whereas lymphatic malformations are collections of lymphatic sacs containing clear, colorless lymph.

Only a portion of the intrathoracic trachea may collapse with expiration when there is the incomplete development of the elastic and connective tracheal tissue (tracheomalcia); the remaining airway remains normal in caliber during inspiration and expiration. Conventional fluoroscopy-guided airway studies are generally recommended for the diagnosis of tracheomalacia in infants and children. However, by using a paired inspiratory expiratory airway protocol that images the central airway at the end of inspiration and expiration, computed tomography (CT) may be more useful in illustrating the location, extent, and degree of tracheomalacia. Moreover, 3D central airway reconstruction combined with multi-detector CT (MDCT) yields incredibly detailed images of the entire central airway. The pressure inside the lumen of the cervical trachea influences its size. An excellent example of this is when there is partial or complete obstruction of the extrathoracic airway (e.g., croup). In these conditions, a forceful inspiration may cause the cervical trachea to collapse completely. Furthermore, when the vocal cords close, there may be a marked enlargement of the cervical trachea and an increase in positive pressure in the chest (Figure 4.4).

Adenopathy, tumors, and prevertebral abscesses are a few disease processes that can affect airway coagulation. The soft tissues in these pathologies are often prominent, but they do not have the angled configuration that occurs during normal expiration. The most common tumors to develop here are rhabdosarcoma, lymphoma, primitive neuroectodermal tumors (PNET), and mesenchymal cell sarcomas, which include germ cell and yolk sac tumors.

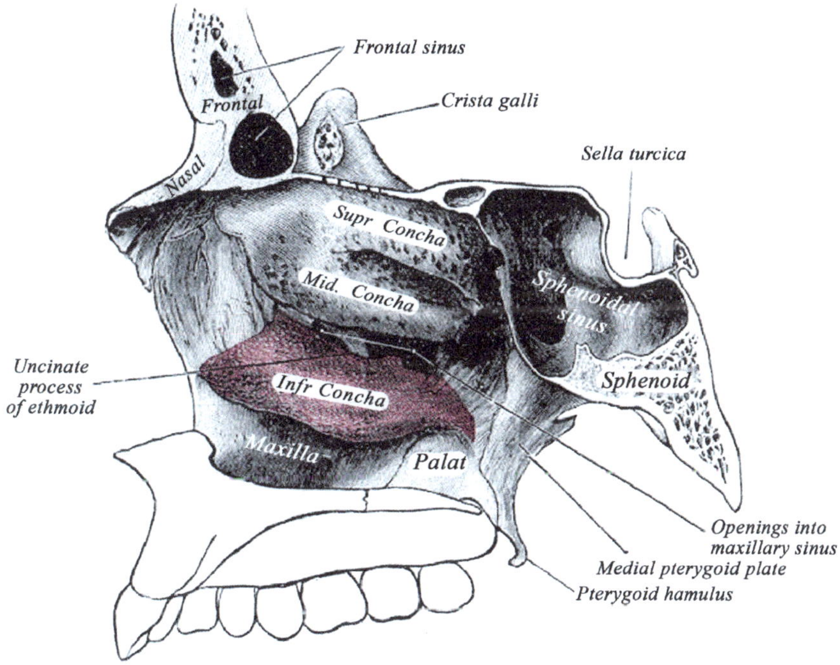

Figure 4.4. *Inferior turbinate position in the nasal cavity.*

Source: (Brian) Sun, H.-H, & Sun, S. (2021). Diagnosis and Management of Obstructive Sleep Apnea. IntechOpen. doi: 10.5772/intechopen.95072.

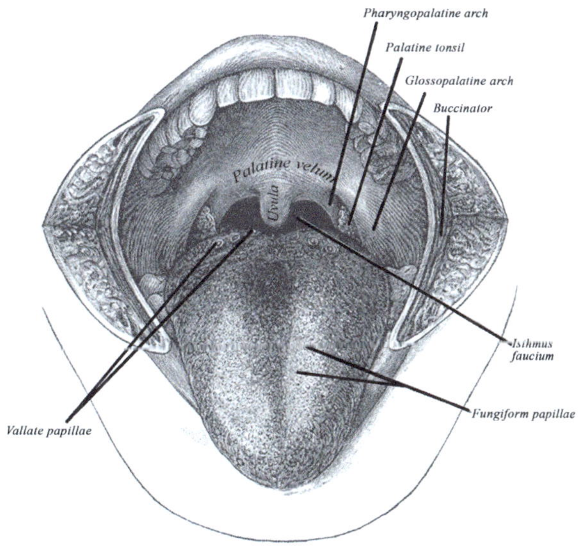

Figure 4.5. *An anatomic depiction of the uvula, tonsils, and their surrounding pillars.*

Source: (Brian) Sun, H.-H, & Sun, S. (2021). Diagnosis and Management of Obstructive Sleep Apnea. IntechOpen. doi: 10.5772/intechopen.95072.

The typical prevertebral soft tissue plains are typically obscured by these lesions. Furthermore, pathology is probably present if the retropharyngeal soft tissue fullness is more prominent superiorly than inferiorly. When retropharyngeal pathology is suspected using conventional imaging, a CT scan should be carried out to determine the disease's extent and whether a drainable abscess is present (Figure 4.5).

4.1.1. Laryngeal and Subglottic Airway

Normal subglottic "shoulder" effect is less noticeable in infants and young children due to less acute junction of the underside of the true vocal cords and infraglottic larynx than in older children and adults. Nonetheless, it is possible to differentiate between subglottic narrowing and the typical infraglottic larynx sloping. Furthermore, the vocal cords are abducted during active breathing, resulting in a typical loss of the infraglottic "shoulders," which is identified by the absence of vocal cord apposition.

The symptoms of the edema that results in subglottic narrowing, also known as "croup," include hoarse, brassy coughing and difficulty breathing. It is typically linked to parainfluenza virus infection. However, the expanded complex of laryngotracheobronchitis is also referred to as croup. During the winter, this disease mainly affects children between the ages of six months and three years. Croup is usually less serious than epiglottitis, which has a higher risk of causing a life-threatening obstruction of the airway. There may be situations where intubation is required. In the worst circumstances, pulmonary edema may arise from intrathoracic pressure that is higher than oncotic pressure during inspiration.

Epiglottitis, or inflammation of the epiglottis, is traditionally linked to hemophilus influenza type b (HIB) infection. Fortunately, since HIB vaccinations are generally accessible and highly recommended, comparatively few cases of this illness are currently being reported. On the other hand, non-type B hemophilus influenza infections do happen sometimes. Other kinds of bacteria can cause epigottitis. The edema brought on by consuming hot liquids or meals may be similar to epiglottitis. Edema brought on by hypersensitivity (e.g., an allergic reaction) can also resemble an infection anatomically. Usually occurring in the winter, epiglottitis mainly affects children between the ages of three and six. While there may be signs of inflammation in the subglottic larynx and aryepiglottic folds, epiglottic swelling is the most clinically noticeable symptom.

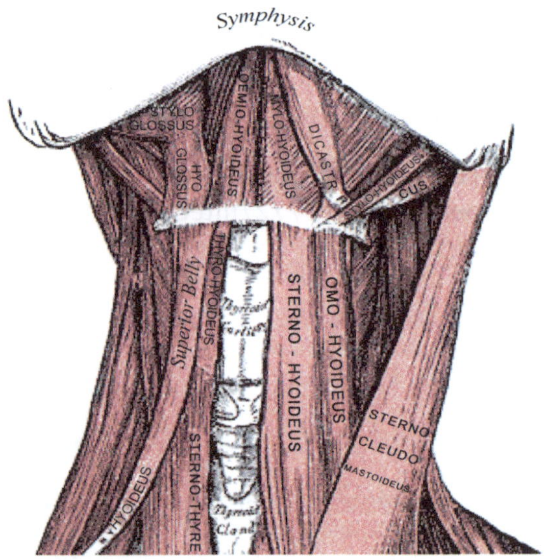

Figure 4.6. *Main anatomic landmarks for HGNS surgery including the hyoid bone and the digastric muscles.*

Source: (Brian) Sun, H.-H, & Sun, S. (2021). Diagnosis and Management of Obstructive Sleep Apnea. IntechOpen. doi: 10.5772/intechopen.95072.

A child's airway may become totally obstructed during imaging, so great caution must be used and should be avoided if at all possible. Imaging by plain film or fluoroscopy may be used to definitively diagnose a suspected case of epiglottitis. The airway may become totally obstructed if the head and neck are moved or straightened. An imaging study can become more complex when the subglottic airway or aryepiglottic folds are involved. The aryepiglottic folds and/or the subglottic airway may be impacted in some circumstances, but the epiglottis may be largely unaffected (Figures 4.6 and 4.7).

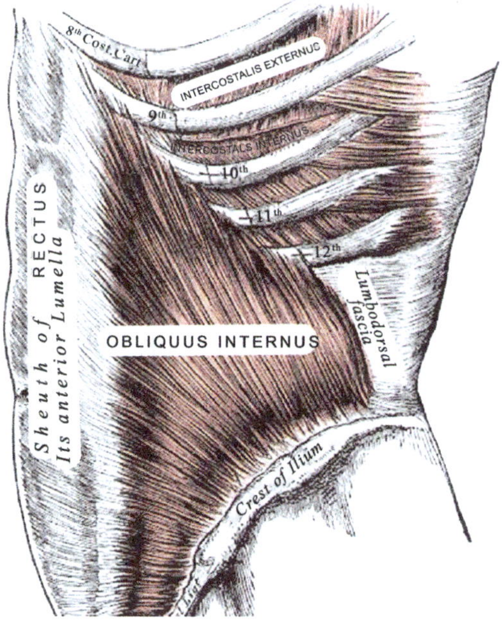

Figure 4.7. *Intercostal muscles.*

Source: (Brian) Sun, H.-H, & Sun, S. (2021). Diagnosis and Management of Obstructive Sleep Apnea. IntechOpen. doi: 10.5772/intechopen.95072.

Pseudomembraneous tracheitis and bacterial croup are two tracheal bacterial infections that can be caused by bacterial organisms, most commonly staphylococci. Clup-like symptoms and pseudomembrane formation are possible presentations of this process (Figure 4.8).

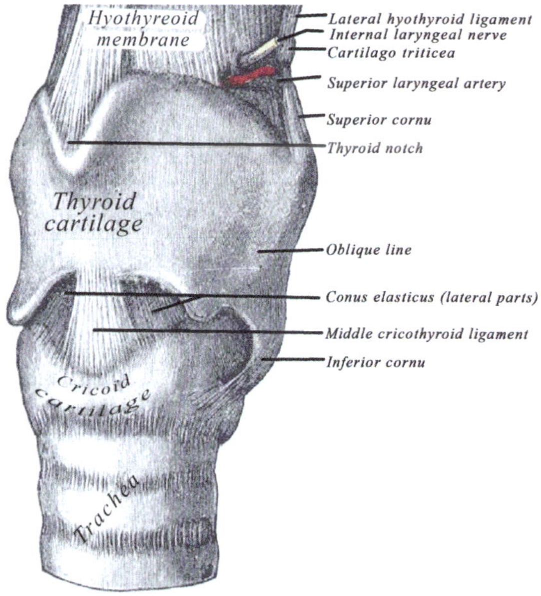

Figure 4.8. *The concerned anatomy.*

Source: (Brian) Sun, H.-H, & Sun, S. (2021). Diagnosis and Management of Obstructive Sleep Apnea. IntechOpen. doi: 10.5772/intechopen.95072.

In infants and children, focal masses can be seen in the subglottic airway. Granulation tissue may develop as a result of previous intubation or tracheotomy. These lesions can also be caused by a subglottic hemangioma, which may occur alongside cutaneous hemangiomata on the head or neck. Subglottic hemangiomas are typically found posterolaterally, about 1–1.5 cm below the vocal cords, and often resolve on their own by age 5 or 6. While plain radiographs or conventional fluoroscopy can detect subglottic hemangiomas, CT imaging, particularly MDCT with its advanced capabilities, can be beneficial in diagnosis.

Table 4.1. *OSA Analyses: Epworth Sleepiness Scale(Johns MW. 1991)*

How likely are you to doze off or fall asleep in the following scenarios?
0 = Never
1 = Slight chance of dozing off
2 = Moderate chance of dozing off
3 = High chance of dozing off
Total Score – A score of greater than 10 denotes a higher risk of OSA
0 – 5: Lower normal daytime sleepiness
6 – 10: Higher normal daytime sleepiness
11 – 12: Mild excessive daytime sleepiness
13 – 15: Moderate excessive daytime sleepiness
16 – 24: Severe excessive daytime sleepiness
Scenario Score
Sitting and reading______
Watching TV______
Sitting inactive in a public place (i.e., theater)______
As a passenger in a car for an hour______
Lying down to rest in the afternoon______
Sitting and talking to someone______
Sitting quietly after lunch without alcohol______
While stopped in traffic for a few minutes______

Source: (Brian) Sun, H.-H, & Sun, S. (2021). Diagnosis and Management of Obstructive Sleep Apnea. IntechOpen. doi: 10.5772/intechopen.95072.

Table 4.2. *OSA Risk Assessment: Berlin Questionnaire – Frequency-Based Criteria(Netzer NC et al. 1999)*

Item 1: if "Yes," a point is added.
Item 2: if "c" or "d," a point is added
Item 3: if "a" or "b," a point is added
Item 4: if "a," a point is added
Item 5: if "a" or "b," two points are added.
Category 1 is "positive" if the total points above are 2 or higher.
Item 6: if "a" or "b," a point is added
Item 7: if "a" or "b," a point is added
Item 8: if "a," a point is added
Category 2 is "positive" if the total points above are 2 or higher.

Category 3 is "positive" if the answer to item 10 is "Yes" or if the patient BMI is greater than 30kg/m²	
Patients are considered high risk of 2 or more categories are deemed positive.	
Item 1: Do you snore?	Item 6: How often do you feel tired or fatigued after sleep?
Yes A.	Nearly every day A.
No B.	3–4 times per week B.
Do not know C.	1–2 times per week C.
	1–2 times per month D.
	Never or nearly never E.
Item 2: Your snoring is	Item 7: During your waking time, do you feel tired or fatigued?
Slightly louder than breathing. A.	Nearly every day A.
As loud as talking B.	3–4 times per week B.
Louder than talking C.	1–2 times per week C.
Can be heard in adjacent rooms D.	1–2 times per month D.
I do not snore E.	Never or nearly never E.
Item 3: How often do you snore?	Item 8: Have you ever nodded off or fallen asleep while driving a vehicle?
Nearly every day A.	Yes A.
3–4 times per week B.	No B.
1–2 times per week C.	
1–2 times per month D.	
Never or nearly never E.	
Item 4: Has your snoring ever bothered other people?	Item 9: How often do you nod off while driving?
Yes A.	Nearly every day A.
No B.	3–4 times per week B.
Do not know C.	1–2 times per week C.
	1–2 times per month D.
	Never or nearly never E.
Item 5: Has anyone noticed that you stop breathing during sleep?	Item 10: Do you have high blood pressure?
Nearly every day A.	Yes A.
3–4 times per week B.	No B.
1–2 times per week C.	Do not know C.
1–2 times per month D.	
Never or nearly never E.	

Source: (Brian) Sun, H.-H, & Sun, S. (2021). Diagnosis and Management of Obstructive Sleep Apnea. IntechOpen. doi: 10.5772/intechopen.95072.

Table 4.3. *OSA Risk Assessment: Berlin Questionnaire - Demographic and Physical Health Indicators(Vasu TS et al. 2010)*

A point is added for each question that is answered with a "yes."
Snoring: Do you snore loudly?
Tired: Do you often feel tired, fatigued, or sleepy during the daytime?
Observed choking: Has anyone observed you choking during sleep?
Pressure: Do you have or are being treated for high blood pressure?
Body mass index: Is your BMI more than 35kg/m^2?
Age: Are you older than 50 years of age?
Neck size: Is your shirt collar size >17 in for males or >16 in for females?
Gender: Are you biologically male?
In general, patients with a score of 2 or below are considered low risk, 3 to 4 intermediate risk, and 5 or greater high risk.

Source: (Brian) Sun, H.-H, & Sun, S. (2021). Diagnosis and Management of Obstructive Sleep Apnea. IntechOpen. doi: 10.5772/intechopen.95072.

Since virtual tracheobronchoscopy has been shown to correlate well with conventional tracheobronchoscopy, it is especially helpful for assessing the degree of airway obstruction. An isolated subglottic mass after the age of five is more likely to be a papilloma than a hemangioma. Inoculation with the human papilloma virus, contracted during vaginal delivery, is the cause of the papillomata. Up to 20% of patients may experience nodule, and cavitary lung lesions as a result of the viral infection spreading into the lung parenchyma and down the airway. Rarely do children present with other tracheal and subglottic airway tumors (Ray et al., 1993; Stroud and Friedman, 2001; Samuels M, Wieteska, 2011; Wald, 2014).

4.2. Upper Airway Infections

A variety of respiratory conditions affecting the organs above the vocal cords, such as the larynx, trachea, and bronchi, are referred to as upper airway infections. Croup, epiglottitis, and bacterial tracheitis are three prominent upper airway infections that have different clinical manifestations and possible side effects.

Laryngotracheobronchitis, another name for croup, is mainly brought on by viral infections, most frequently the parainfluenza virus. Children between the ages of six months and three years old are usually affected, and symptoms include respiratory distress, hoarseness, barking cough, and inspiratory stridor. Most cases of croup resolve on their own and are treated with supportive measures like corticosteroids and humidified air; however, severe cases may need to be hospitalized and treated with nebulized epinephrine.

Haemophilus influenzae type b (Hib) bacteria are frequently the cause of epiglottitis, a potentially fatal infection marked by a sharply rising temperature, sore throat, dysphagia, drooling, and respiratory distress. Epiglottitis is more common in older children and adults than croup. To avoid airway blockage and respiratory failure, prompt identification, treatment with intravenous antibiotics, and airway management—including potential intubation—are crucial.

A common side effect of viral upper respiratory tract infections, like croup, is bacterial tracheitis, an uncommon but dangerous infection of the trachea. It manifests as respiratory distress, purulent secretions, fever, and severe cough. To avoid airway compromise and systemic complications, bacterial tracheitis necessitates aggressive management with intravenous antibiotics, airway support, and potentially surgical intervention in severe cases.

In general, to avoid respiratory compromise and guarantee positive results, prompt diagnosis and effective treatment of upper airway infections, such as croup, epiglottitis, and bacterial tracheitis, are essential. In severe cases, close observation and quick action might be required to minimize risks and improve patient care.

4.2.1. Croup

Although the term "croup" is often used to describe a variety of pathologies, including laryngotracheobronchitis and "spasmodic croup," which is characterized by nocturnal paroxysms of stridor without fever or inflammation, the true cause of the condition is viral laryngotracheitis. The swelling and edema of the epithelium of the upper airway cause croup.

4.2.1.1. Etiology

Epidemics caused by parainfluenza virus (types 1–3) are the most frequent cause of croup. Croup may also be caused by human coronavirus, adenovirus, or respiratory syncytial virus.

4.2.1.2. Presentation

Fever, stridor, "barking" cough, and hoarseness are the typical symptoms of croup in children between the ages of six months and three years (Figure 4.9).

Commonly, symptoms begin as coryza and nasal congestion, which may get worse over the course of 48 hours until respiratory distress and airway blockage take over.

The key to assessing severity is the presence of stridor, which, when present, especially while at rest, indicates a serious airway blockage. Suprasternal, subcostal, and intercostal recessions can all be observed at this level of airway blockage. In this situation, hypoxia could occur, so intervention is required.

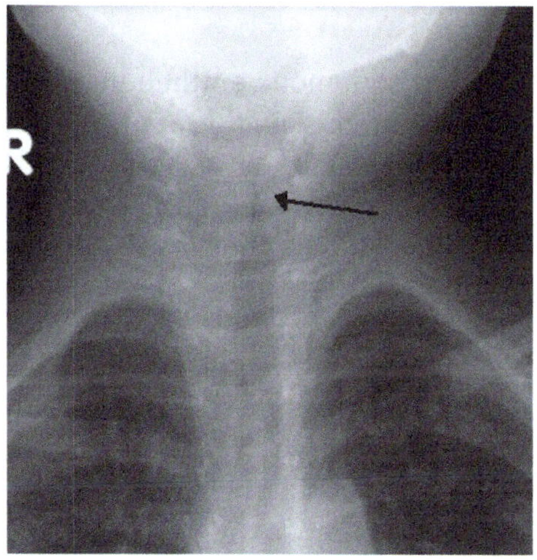

Figure 4.9. *Croup-the classic steeple.*

Source: By Frank Gaillard – Own work, CC BY-SA 3.0, https://commons.wikimedia.org/w/index.php?curid=6792682.

4.2.1.3. Management

Supportive therapies may be the cornerstone of care, with tracheal intubation used when necessary. The Westley Croup Scores, a scoring system frequently used in research that categorizes the severity of croup based on the presence of recession, stridor, cyanosis, level of consciousness, and air entry, show improvement as soon as 6 hours after administration when dexamethasone (oral or intramuscular injection, 0.15 mg kg^{-1}) and nebulized budesonide (2 mg) are administered. Steroid use also lowers readmission and hospital stay rates. It is significant to remember that the ideal dosage and method of administration are still to be established.

When compared to no treatment, nebulized adrenaline produces a significant clinical improvement 30 minutes after administration; however, this improvement is only temporary. Two hours after administration, there is no benefit.

4.2.2. Epiglottitis

The stratified squamous epithelium covers the thin cartilage of the epiglottis on its anterior (superior) surface. This epithelium extends onto the upper third of the posterior (inferior) surface, where it is replaced by the larynx's respiratory epithelium. In contrast to the posterior surface, the anterior surface of the epiglottis has only loosely adherent epithelium. When epiglottitis occurs, edema accumulates beneath the anterior surface epithelium, narrowing the airway and resulting in stridor.

4.2.2.1. Etiology

Since *Haemophilus influenzae* type b (Hib) is the most common cause of infectious epiglottitis, the number of cases has decreased in nations like the UK that have implemented childhood vaccination programs. Eight cases still arise, either from Hib itself due to the phenomenon of vaccination failure or from other pathogens such as Streptococcus species or other Haemophilus subgroups.

4.2.2.2. Presentation

To maximize their airway patency, children with infectious epiglottitis often present with a brief history of respiratory distress, drooling, stridor, and possibly a "sniffing" posture. Cough is rarely present. The child is usually very ill with a high fever and odynophagia; this is a clinical emergency.

4.2.2.3. Management

The fundamentals of early respiratory distress management in conjunction with timely antimicrobial medication administration will constitute the management guidelines. Delays in antimicrobial therapy and microbiological culture may be necessary until after attempts at venous cannulation have produced definitive control of the airway due to the additional respiratory distress that these procedures may cause. Intravenous co-amoxiclav 30 mg kg^{-1} would be a suitable starting agent when antibiotics are started.

An edematous epiglottis can narrow the airway, making traditional tracheal intubation challenging. If a tracheostomy is necessary, an ENT surgeon should ideally be present for definitive airway management. It has been demonstrated that children with epiglottitis who receive routine intubation have much lower mortality rates than those who receive medical care without an artificial airway. Usually, two to three days must pass after intubation before extubation is allowed. Apyrexia, the capacity to swallow, and a discernible cuff leak around the tracheal tube are required conditions for extubation.

4.2.3. Uvulitis

4.2.3.1. Etiology

Acute uvula infections can happen at any age and are primarily brought on by Group A Streptococcus, though Hib and other infectious organisms have also been linked to these infections. Numerous non-infectious causes of uvula inflammation have also been reported; these include allergic reactions, trauma, thermal injury, and vasculitis, all of which may result in comparable clinical manifestations.

4.2.3.2. Presentation

Inflammation of the uvula, known as uvulitis, can lead to symptoms such as fever, pain, difficulty swallowing, and drooling. However, respiratory distress is rare unless epiglottitis is also present. An infected uvula may appear swollen, red, and may have a discharge.

4.2.3.3. Management

The cause determines the course of treatment. The fundamental ideas mentioned throughout this article are applicable to all airway infections that pose a risk to airway patency. Antimicrobial therapy is the cornerstone of treatment for infective uvulitis and should be guided by sensitivities and culture.

4.2.4. Tonsillitis, Peritonsillar, and Retropharyngeal Abscess

While tonsillitis alone can cause acute airway compromise, this is uncommon unless there is also extra-tonsillar infection spread. A notable degree of airway narrowing due to tonsillitis is seen (Figure 4.10).

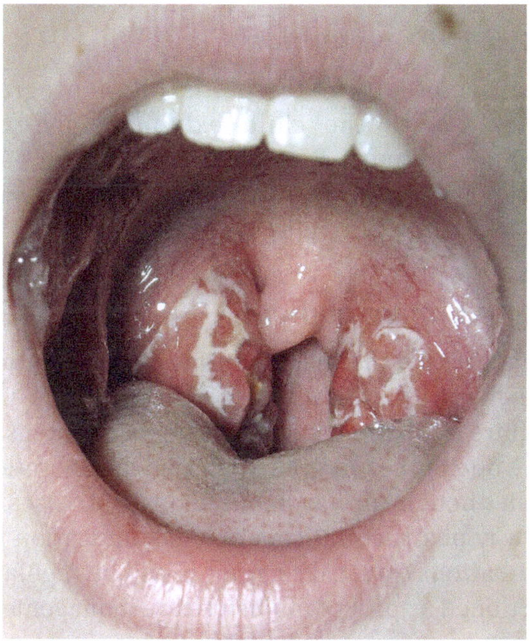

Figure 4.10. *Tonsillitis.*

Source: By James Heilman, MD – Own work, CC BY-SA 3.0, https://commons.wikimedia.org/w/index.php?curid=11596322.

4.2.4.1. Etiology

Multiple organisms are often the cause of tonsil and surrounding structure infections. Group A Streptococcus, *Staphylococcus aureus*, and respiratory anaerobes like Fusobacteria and Prevotella species are primarily to blame.

A fibrous capsule covering the palatine tonsils divides them from the superior and middle constrictor muscles. The tonsils are located between the palatoglossal and palatopharyngeal arches. There is a potential space that is bounded by the arches and the superior constrictor because of loose connective tissue in this area.

The layers of deep cervical fascia define the boundaries of the retropharyngeal space, which stretches from the base of the skull to the posterior mediastinum. This area contains the lymph nodes that drain the middle ear, adenoids, sinuses, and nasopharynx.

Peritonsillar infection typically develops after tonsillitis, progressing from localized cellulitis to the formation of an organized abscess. Retropharyngeal abscess is a much rarer disease process that is linked to upper respiratory tract infections, which may be as much as 50% of cases the abscess's precursor. However, additional causative mechanisms are mentioned, such as trauma (especially from laryngoscopy or dental procedures).

4.2.4.2. Presentation

It should come as no surprise that these infections present in remarkably similar ways given the close proximity of the structures involved and the similarity of their disease processes. While a CT scan with contrast should be able to show the infection site, it might not be necessary or even wise to perform one on a child who is experiencing respiratory distress.

4.2.4.3. Peritonsillar Abscess

A peritonsillar abscess frequently manifests as severe unilateral sore throat, fever, and voice change; however, trismus, which is brought on by a spasm of the medial pterygoid muscle, may be the characteristic that sets it apart from simple tonsillitis. A swollen tonsil with a possible gross deviation of the surrounding palatal or uvula structures will probably be found upon examination.

4.2.4.4. Retropharyngeal Abscess

A retropharyngeal abscess may cause neck swelling, dysphagia, fever, and voice changes. A serious infection may cause drooling, and severe neck pain from movement may result in torticollis. Chest pain could indicate whether the infection has spread to the mediastinum, as trismus has been reported. A rare result of a serious infection is obstruction of the airway.

4.2.4.5. Management

The cornerstones of management should be supportive care, antibiotics, and surgical drainage of the abscess. Antimicrobial therapy will be necessary and governed by local policy; however, given the high probability of both Gram-positive and anaerobe presence, caution should be exercised.

Due to the significant risk of bleeding, surgical removal of the tonsils during the acute stage of peritonsillar abscess is controversial. However, if pus has formed, tonsillectomy is generally recommended to reduce the risk of aspiration or local vascular erosion following spontaneous rupture.

Because of anatomical distortion, airway obstruction is an emergency and can be difficult to treat. A retropharyngeal abscess can make it difficult to see the glottis, so any attempt to open the airway should be done with the assistance of an ENT surgeon. Lower airway soiling can be avoided with the use of a cuffed tracheal tube and inhalation induction, as suggested (Ray et al., 1993; Stroud and Friedman, 2001; Samuels M, Wieteska, 2011; Wald, 2014).

4.2.5. Bacterial Tracheitis

Bacterial tracheitis is an invasive, exudative bacterial infection of the trachea that was originally reported to have characteristics similar to both epiglottitis and croup. A normal epiglottis with significant subglottic edema was described in the first case series.

4.2.5.1. Etiology

Streptococcus species and *H. influenzae* are among the other organisms linked to the illness, although *Staphylococcus aureus* appears to be the most frequent cause.

4.2.5.1. Presentation

The symptoms of tracheitis often progress quickly, with the child exhibiting pyrexia, stridor, and cough. Because of the infection's fast progression, airway obstruction should always be taken into account.

4.2.5.2. Management

Regardless of their clinical state at presentation, the majority of children with tracheitis will require intubation and management on intensive care due to the possibility of rapid deterioration, even though airway maintenance in cases of airway obstruction is an obvious indication for intubation. Tracheal secretions will be regularly suctioned as part of intensive care management.

By eliminating pseudomembranous exudates, endoscopy plays a crucial role in both diagnosis and treatment, potentially leading to a marked improvement in symptoms. Additionally, it offers a chance to send samples for culture. For a child who is breathing on their own, a rigid bronchoscopy under general anesthesia may be possible before tracheal intubation and transfer to intensive care, depending on the child's clinical status. This can be extremely difficult for a sick or hypoxemic child, though, and if bronchoscopy and airway toilet attempts compromise the patient, they should be intubated and have suction catheters used to remove airway debris.

Again, local advice should be followed when choosing an antibiotic agent, but the frequency of Staphylococcus and other Gram-positive organisms as the cause should direct the first course of treatment with broad-spectrum antibiotics. Both ceftriaxone and intravenous co-amoxiclav 30 mg kg1 are appropriate first-line medications. The use of glucocorticoids has no evidence to support it because they have no effect on the outcome (Ray et al., 1993; Stroud and Friedman, 2001; Samuels M, Wieteska, 2011; Wald, 2014).

4.3. Lower Respiratory Tract Infections

Relatively speaking, 45% of all community-acquired infections and 25% of all nosocomial infections are lower respiratory trace infections (LRTIs), making them one of the most prevalent infections in humans. To avoid the severe morbidity and hospitalization risk associated with many LRTIs, early diagnosis is often crucial. However, it is still difficult to identify the relevant pathogens before starting antibiotic therapy, so treatment is frequently empirical. Therefore, it is generally preferred to use antibiotics with a spectrum tailored to the variety of pulmonary pathogens.

The ideal antimicrobial agent for treating lung respiratory tract infections (LRTIs) should possess the capacity to infiltrate pulmonary tissues, cells, and fluids to reach concentrations that either inhibit or kill the causative organisms. However, the clinical relevance of this ability in humans has not yet been thoroughly evaluated. Fluoroquinolones can reach bronchial and pulmonary concentrations that are equal to or higher than serum concentrations due to their excellent lung penetration. Additionally, for most intracellular pathogens causing LRTIs, intracellular concentrations are also within the therapeutic range. As an example, aminoglycosides only reach 30–40% of their serum level in the lung and less in the inter- and intracellular milieu. In contrast, the majority of β-lactam antibiotics do not exceed 50% of their serum level within bronchial secretions.

Reducing the length of therapy is currently the general trend to improve treatment cost-effectiveness and shorten hospital stays, as well as to lessen the likelihood of resistance and adverse events developing while maintaining clinical efficacy. The growing use of step-down or switch therapy, in which an intravenous formulation is initially used to initiate treatment and an oral formulation is subsequently used to continue it, is also significant. Improved patient compliance and pharmacoeconomic benefits are two benefits of this.

The pathogens responsible for LRTs, current treatment modalities, and fluoroquinolone experience to date are the main topics of this paper. The treatment of infections in adult patients was the main focus of this meeting; although the use of some fluoroquinolones, especially ciprofloxacin, in the treatment of cystic fibrosis is well documented, the topic was not covered.

4.3.1. Chronic Bronchitis (Acute Exacerbations)

4.3.1.1. Definition and Diagnosis

The classic definition of chronic bronchitis is persistent inflammation and irritation of the bronchial tree, characterized by symptoms of coughing up phlegm for three consecutive months for two years, interspersed with occasional acute exacerbations that worsen symptoms. It is usually a progressive condition most commonly found in older men (>40 years old), and it is closely associated with smoking.

As much as 25% of adults suffer from chronic bronchitis, making it a highly prevalent condition. Antibiotic therapy is typically started during times of acute exacerbation when infection and inflammation are at their worst. A change in the quantity, consistency, and color of the sputum; increased dyspnea; productive cough; tachypnea; tightness in the chest; increased fatigue; and, particularly in the elderly, confusion are indications and symptoms of acute exacerbations. Physical examination may also reveal rales, ronchi, and occasionally prolonged exhalation.

4.3.1.2. Etiology

The bacterial species that are frequently linked to acute flare-ups of chronic bronchitis are typically not very pathogenic and are found in the upper respiratory tract's normal flora. Approximately 70% of isolates from patients experiencing acute exacerbations of chronic bronchitis are non-typeable *Haemophilus influenzae*. It is believed that certain bacterial adhesions interact with epithelial cell receptors to cause colonization of the airways. As soon as *H. influenzae* enters the respiratory system, mucociliary clearance usually removes it quickly. However, in people who are impaired in this host defense mechanism, it adheres to pooled mucus longer, allowing surface contact with areas of damaged bronchial epithelium. Bacterial toxins and metabolic products may cause additional epithelium damage, which could facilitate the bacterium's spread through the respiratory tract. *Moraxella catarrhalis* may also be involved in a smaller number of cases of purulent exacerbation, but *Streptococcus pneumoniae* is another frequently encountered bacterium that causes it. Rare causes include *Pseudomonas aeruginosa*, *Staphylococcus aureus*, and *Klebsiella pneumoniae*. *Neisseria* spp. are among the other bacteria that may be exclusively predominant or mixed pathogens in acute exacerbations of chronic bronchitis. Bordetella species. Rhodococci species. and anaerobes. It is important to take into account how Mycoplasma and *Chlamydia pneumoniae* contribute to chronic bronchitis.

4.3.1.3. Treatment

Adults and children with infections caused by streptococci and pneumococci susceptible to penicillin are treated with oral penicillins, which are effective against Gram-positive cocci and bacilli. They have no effect on "atypical" pathogens or microorganisms that produce β-lactamase. Ceramycin-susceptible Gram-positive organisms can be effectively treated with oral cephalosporins, such as cefalexin, cefadroxil, cefradine, and cefaclor. However, their effectiveness against penicillin-resistant *Streptococcus pneumoniae*, Enterobacteriaceae, and β-lactamase-positive *H. influenzae*. Other well-known therapies include amoxicillin/clavulanic acid, trimethoprim, and sulfamethoxazole.

4.3.1.4. Fluoroquinolones

In a study involving 218 outpatients, ciprofloxacin (500 mg twice daily) was found to be equally effective as amoxicillin/clavulanic acid (875 mg/125 mg twice daily) or cefixime (400 mg once daily) in treating acute exacerbations of chronic bronchitis. There have been reports of eradication rates of 81%, 82%, and 78% with cefixime, ciprofloxacin, and amoxicillin/clavulanic acid, respectively. Additionally, 86% of patients treated with ciprofloxacin, 91% of cases treated with amoxicillin/clavulanic acid, and 81% of the cefixime group experienced clinical success.

It has also been demonstrated that ofloxacin works well. In Chodosh's review, ciprofloxacin, ofloxacin, temafloxacin, and enoxacin were found to be more effective than enoxacin in treating acute exacerbations of chronic bronchitis. In a double-blind study, DeAbate et al. contrasted ofloxacin and sparfloxacin. The overall response rates were 85.4% and 88.8%, respectively, for the two categories of eradication or presumed eradication of pathogens and cure or improvement of clinical signs and symptoms. The rates of presumed eradication and combined eradication were 92.5% and 89.9%, respectively.

Table 4.2 summarizes the findings of two multicenter studies using levo-floxacin to treat acute bacterial exacerbations of chronic bronchitis Levofloxacin had eradication rates of 90% and 89% for *Streptococcus pneumoniae* and *Staphylococcus aureus*, respectively, while cefaclor had rates of 86% and 67%, respectively. Furthermore, the cefaclor group had an overall rate of bacteriologic resistance of 24%, while the levofloxacin group had an overall rate of 2%. In the second study, levofloxacin was found to be as effective as cefuroxime axetil, with 95% of patients treated with levofloxacin and 93% of patients treated with cefuroxime axetil experiencing clinical success (Table 4.4).

Table 4.4. *The Most Relevant FDA-Approved Syndromic Panels for the Diagnosis of Respiratory Illnesses for Both the Upper and the Lower Respiratory Tracts*

Assay	Company	Target	Time-to-Result	Type of Amplification	References
QIAstat-Dx Respiratory SARS-CoV-2 Panel	QIAGEN GmbH	22 Pathogens (FLU A, FLU A subtype H1N1/2009, H1, and H3; FLU B; CoV 229E, HKU1, NL63, OC43; SARS-CoV-2; PIV 1, 2, 3, and 4; RSV A/B; h-MPV A/B; ADV; h-BocaV; RV/Enterovirus; *Mycoplasma pneumoniae*; *Legionella pneumophila*; *Bordetella pertussis*)	About 1 h	Multiplex real-time RT-PCR	[Cassidy, H. et al. 2022, Lebourgeois, S. et al. 2021]
BioCode Respiratory Pathogen Panel (RPP)	Applied BioCode, Inc.	17 Pathogens (ADV; CoV 229E, OC43, HKU1, NL63; h-MPV A/B; FLU A, FLU A subtype H1N1/2009, H1, and H3; FLU B; PIV 1, 2, 3, and 4; RSV A/B; RV/Enterovirus; *Bordetella pertussis*; *Chlamydia pneumoniae*; *Mycoplasma pneumoniae*)	About 5 h	RT-PCR	[Yu, C.Y. et al. 2021]
ePlex Respiratory Pathogen Panel 2	GenMarkDiagnostics, Inc.	18 Pathogens (ADV; CoV 229E, OC43, HKU1, NL63; SARS-CoV-2; h-MPV A/B; FLU A, FLU A subtype H1N1/2009, H1, and H3; FLU B, PIV 1, 2, 3, and 4; RSV A, B; RV/Enterovirus; *Chlamydia pneumoniae*; *Mycoplasma pneumoniae*)	About 2 h	RT-PCR	[Couturier, M.R. et al. 2019, Cassidy, H. et al. 2021]

Assay	Company	Target	Time-to-Result	Type of Amplification	References
eSensor Respiratory Viral Panel (RVP)	Clinical MicroSensors, Inc.	14 Pathogens (FLU A, FLU A subtype H1N1/2009, H1, and H3; FLU B; RSV A, B; PIV 1, 2, and 3; h-MPV; RV; ADV species B/E; ADV species C)	About 8 h	Multiplex microarray, competitive DNA hybridization	[Popowitch, E.B. et al. 2013]
FilmArray Pneumonia plus Panel	BioFireDiagnostics, LLC	27 Pathogens and 7 resistant genes (Semi-quantitative detection: *Acinetobacter calcoaceticus-baumannii complex*; *Enterobacter cloacae*; *Escherichia coli*; *Haemophilus influenzae*; *Klebsiella aerogenes*; *Klebsiella oxytoca*; *Klebsiella pneumoniae* group; *Moraxella catarrhalis*; *Proteus* spp.; *Pseudomonas aeruginosa*; *Serratia marcescens*; *Staphylococcus aureus*; *Streptococcus agalactiae*; *Streptococcus pneumoniae*; *Streptococcus pyogenes* Qualitative detection: *Legionella pneumophila*; *Mycoplasma pneumoniae*; *Chlamydia pneumoniae*; FLU A; FLU B; ADV; CoV; PIV; RSV; RV/Enterovirus; h-MPV; Middle East Respiratory Syndrome Coronavirus Resistance: ESBL: CTX-M; Carbapenemases: KPC, NDM, Oxa48-like, VIM, IMP; Methicilin Resistance: mecA/mecC and MREJ)	About 1 h	Nested multiplex RT-PCR	[Webber, D.M. et al. 2020, Lee, S.H. et al. 2019, Murphy, C.N. et al. 2020, Buchan, B.W. et al. 2020]

Assay	Company	Target	Time-to-Result	Type of Amplification	References
FilmArray Respiratory Panel (RP)	BioFireDiagnostics, LLC	20 Pathogens (ADV; CoV 229E, HKU1, OC43, NL63; h-MPV; RV/Enterovirus; FLU A, FLU A subtype H1N1/2009, H1, and H3; FLU B; PIV 1, 2, 3, and 4; RSV; *Bordetella pertussis*; *Chlamydophila pneumoniae*; *Mycoplasma pneumoniae*)	About 1 h	Nested multiplex RT-PCR	[Popowitch, E.B. et al. 2013]
NxTAG Respiratory Pathogen Panel	Luminex Molecular Diagnostics, Inc.	22 Pathogens (FLU A, FLU A subtype H1N1/2009, H1, and H3; FLU B; RSV A, B; CoV 229E, OC43, NL63, HKU1; PIV 1, 2, 3, and 4; h-MPV; ADV; h-BocaV; RV/Enterovirus; *Chlamydophila pneumoniae*; *Mycoplasma pneumoniae*; *Legionella pneumophyla*)	About 4 h	RT-PCR	[Couturier, M.R. et al. 2019, Cassidy, H. et al. 2021, Popowitch, E.B. et al. 2013]
xTAG Respiratory Viral Panel Fast (RVP FAST)	Luminex Molecular Diagnostics, Inc.	18 Pathogens (FLU A, FLU A subtype H1 and H3; FLU B; RSV A, B; CoV 229E, OC43, NL63, HKU1; PIV 1, 2, 3, and 4; h-MPV; ADV; h-BocaV; RV/Enterovirus)	About 4 h	RT-PCR	[Couturier, M.R. et al. 2019]
Verigene Respiratory Pathogens Flex NucleicAcid Test (RP Flex)	Nanosphere, Inc.	16 Pathogens (ADV; h-MPV; FLU A, FLU A subtype H1 and H3; FLU B; PIV 1, 2, 3, and 4; RV; RSV A, B; *Bordetella pertussis*; *Bordetella parapertussis/bronchiseptica*; *Bordetella holmesii*)	About 2 h	RT-PCR and microarray hybridization	[Couturier, M.R. et al. 2019, Cassidy, H. et al. 2021]
FilmArray Respiratory Panel 2.1 (RP 2.1)	BioFireDiagnostics, LLC	19 Pathogens (ADV; CoV 229E, HKU1, OC43, NL63; SARS-CoV-2; h-MPV; RV/Enterovirus; FLU A, FLU A subtype H1N1/2009, H1, and H3; FLU B; PIV; RSV; *Bordetella pertussis*; *Bordetella parapertussis*; *Chlamydophila pneumoniae*; *Mycoplasma pneumoniae*)	About 1 h	Nested multiplex RT-PCR	[Cassidy, H. et al. 2022, Tazi, S. et al. 2022]

Assay	Company	Target	Time-to-Result	Type of Amplification	References
FilmArray Respiratory Panel 2.1 plus (RP2PLUS)	BioFireDiagnostics, LLC	21 Pathogens (ADV; CoV 229E, HKU1, OC43, NL63; Middle East Respiratory Syndrome Coronavirus; SARS-CoV-2; h-MPV; RV/Enterovirus; FLU A, FLU A subtype H1N1/2009, H1, and H3; FLU B; PIV 1, 2, 3, and 4; RSV; *Bordetella pertussis; Bordetella parapertussis; Chlamydophila pneumoniae; Mycoplasma pneumoniae*)	About 45 min	Nested multiplex RT-PCR	[Tazi, S. et al. 2022]

Source: *Calderaro A, Buttrini M, Farina B, Montecchini S, De Conto F, Chezzi C. Respiratory Tract Infections and Laboratory Diagnostic Methods: A Review with A Focus on Syndromic Panel-Based Assays. Microorganisms. 2022; 10(9):1856. https://doi.org/10.3390/microorganisms10091856.*

4.3.2. Acute Bronchitis

4.3.2.1. Definition and Diagnosis

The hallmark of acute bronchitis is an abrupt inflammation of the bronchi, typically brought on by viral infections like the "common cold," rhinovirus, or influenza. In patients without underlying lung disease, it is typically clinically characterized by the presence of an acute, productive cough. In contrast, a viral infection is characterized by a low fever and milder symptoms in the early stages, whereas a bacterial infection typically causes a fever and occasionally chills as well as an acute, severe illness. In bacterial infections, sputum is purulent and abundant, while it is uncommon in viral infections.

4.3.2.2. Etiology

Most cases of acute bronchitis are caused by viral infections such as influenza virus, adenovirus, and rhinovirus. The incidence of bacterial infections playing a primary role is hard to determine. The involvement of *H. influenzae* and *Streptococcus pneumoniae* is uncertain, while the contributions of *Mycoplasma pneumoniae*, *Chlamydia pneumoniae*, and *B. pertussis* should not be overlooked.

4.3.2.3. Treatment

The majority of viral respiratory infections are benign, exhibiting no fever or purulent sputum production. Seven days after onset, symptoms start to lessen. In most cases, antibiotics are not advised. In chronic situations, or in cases of proven bacterial infection. Both macrolides and β-lactams have been employed.

4.3.3. Nosocomial Pneumonia

The virulence of the causative organism is the primary determinant of the disease process. However, there may be a predisposition to pneumonia caused by reduced host defenses, particularly suppression of the cough reflex, impairment of mucociliary clearance, the presence of a foreign body, or reduced systemic and local immunity. The microbiological etiology of pneumonia varies greatly depending on whether it is community-acquired or nosocomial.

4.3.3.1. Definition and Diagnosis

Individuals who contract nosocomial pneumonia frequently have compromised immune systems and a range of serious underlying conditions. They also receive a variety of medications and supportive care, which makes them more vulnerable to infectious complications. Pneumonia is particularly dangerous to develop after intubation. A sudden onset of malaise, fever, chills, increased sputum production, and leukocytosis are the hallmarks of the clinical signs and symptoms. An infiltrate can usually be identified on a chest X-ray.

4.3.3.2. Etiology

Along with the majority of bacteria responsible for community-acquired pneumonia, Gram-negative bacteria like K are also included in the spectrum of nosocomial pneumonia pathogens. Acinetobacter species, and *Escherichia coli*, *Staphylococcus aureus*, *P. aeruginosa* and related organisms, and occasionally fungi. However, the majority of pathogens are Gram-negative bacteria, with *H. influenza* and *Streptococcus pneumoniae* coming in second. Influenzae are usually not thought to be important. Of cases of nosocomial pneumonia, 10–30% have a polymicrobial etiology.

4.3.3.3. Treatment

Nosocomial pneumonia is the second most common hospital-acquired infection, leading to longer hospital stays and high mortality rates. Typically, parenteral drug administration is utilized, with the choice of antibiotic and dosage regimen dependent on various factors including the severity of the pneumonia, presence of other illnesses, prior therapy, and length of hospitalization. Second-generation cephalosporins are effective in cases without severe underlying conditions, while special risk groups may require combination therapy with aminoglycosides or third-generation cephalosporins. Macrolides like erythromycin are effective against certain pathogens but may cause gastrointestinal intolerance, while newer macrolides have fewer side effects. For patients with severe illnesses and respiratory issues, third-generation cephalosporins or carbapenems may be used alone or in combination with other antibiotics. Patients unable to take β-lactams may receive fluoroquinolones as an alternative therapy.

4.3.3.4. Fluoroquinolones

Research has demonstrated that when used as a monotherapy to treat severe nosocomial pneumonia, ciprofloxacin is just as effective as imipenem. Intravenous ciprofloxacin at high doses (400 mg every 8 h) produced significantly better rates of clinical cure or improvement than that achieved with imipenem (1 g every 8 h) and a significantly higher rate of bacteriologic eradication in a multicenter study of 189 patients with severe pneumonia that had been acquired in the community (16%) or in hospitals (84%). This was assumed to be the outcome of the ciprofloxacin group's considerably higher rate of Enterobacteriaceae bacteriologic eradication (93% versus 66%, p = 0.001). Peloquin et al. demonstrated that intravenous ciprofloxacin 200 mg twice a day was effective against Gram-negative pathogens in an open study involving 50 patients, Less than half of the patients had no trace of *P. aeruginosa*. According to Gentry et al, ofloxacin (400 mg b. I. d. was successful in treating nosocomial pneumonia; in 109 patients treated with ofloxacin 200 mg twice a day, Petermann reported an overall satisfactory response rate of 93%.

4.3.4. Community-Acquired Pneumonia

4.3.4.1. Definition and Diagnosis

The definition of pneumonia is an infectious agent-induced consolidation and inflammation of the lung tissue. Fever, chills, pleuritic chest pain, and a cough with purulent sputum are signs of pneumonia. It can be challenging to make a microbiological diagnosis, especially if the patient doesn't produce sputum.

4.3.4.2. Etiology

Most cases of community-acquired pneumonia (CAP) are caused by Streptococcus pneumoniae. Typically, complications arise from bloodstream invasion, leading to meningitis, septic arthritis, and bacteremia with shock. Another significant contributor is *H. influenzae* infection; common pathogens also include respiratory viruses and *Moraxella catarrhalis*. There is a connection between viral (influenza) infection and staphylococcal pneumonia. The majority of gram-negative pathogens are detected in immunosuppressive treatments or in high-risk patients, such as the elderly or those with multiple comorbidities. *Streptococcus pneumoniae* and *H. influenzae* may be the cause of two or more aerobic pathogens in as many as 10% of CAP cases. *Mycoplasma pneumoniae* is the most prevalent atypical pathogen, followed by *Chlamydia pneumoniae* and *L. pneumophila*, and when combined, they represent about 30–40% of cases. Reports on the prevalence of *Coxiella burnetii* vary.

4.3.4.3. Treatment

In most cases, including in the outpatient setting, the treatment strategy for community-acquired pneumonia (CAP) must be empirical, despite the fact that a Gram stain of bronchial secretions can aid in guiding therapy.

Table 4.5. *Tests for Community-Acquired Pneumonia*

(i) Outpatients with failure of antibiotic therapy: sputum culture, urinary antigen test for *Legionella pneumophila* and *Streptococcus pneumoniae.*
(ii) Hospitalized patients with positive urinary antigen test for pneumococcus: sputum and blood culture.
(iii) Severe obstructive lung disease: sputum culture.
(iv) Pleural effusion: sputum and blood culture, urinary antigen test for pneumococcus and *Legionella*, pleural fluid culture.
(v) Cavitary infiltrates: sputum culture (bacteria, fungi, and mycobacteria) and blood culture.
(vi) Active alcoholism: sputum and blood culture, urinary antigen test for *pneumococcus* and *Legionella.*
(vii) Severe CAP admitted to intensive care unit (ICU): sputum and blood culture, urinary antigen test for pneumococcus and *Legionella*, tracheal aspirate or bronchoalveolar lavage culture and viral studies also need to be performed.
(viii) Epidemiological factor or specific risk factors suggesting pathogen: urinary antigen test for *Legionella* (Legionnaires disease), influenza test during influenza season.

Source: Cilloniz C, Martin-Loeches I, Garcia-Vidal C, San Jose A, Torres A. Microbial Etiology of Pneumonia: Epidemiology, Diagnosis, and Resistance Patterns. International Journal of Molecular Sciences. 2016; 17(12):2120. https://doi.org/10.3390/ijms17122120.

As soon as possible after diagnosis, therapy must be started due to the possibility of severe morbidity, especially at the beginning. It is typically advised to use an antibiotic whose spectrum is tailored to the possible pathogens. There aren't any distinctive or particular clinical traits that match the etiologic diagnosis. It has been demonstrated that erythromycin and clarithromycin are effective against the majority of pathogens that cause illness, such as Mycoplasma, Chlamydia, and Legionella. In situations where it is believed that organisms other than atypical pathogens are the cause, aminopenicillins or oral cephalosporins may be employed.

Guidelines have been developed by several nations for the empirical treatment of CAP. Table 4.5 summarizes the recommendations from the American Thoracic Society, the British Thoracic Society, the Canadian Community-acquired Pneumonia Consensus Group, and the French guidelines. The fact that there are multiple guidelines with differing recommendations emphasizes the necessity of agreement in this therapeutic field.

4.3.4.4. Fluoroquinolones

The antibacterial spectrum of fluoroquinolones is tailored to most respiratory pathogens, and they exhibit fast bactericidal activity. They are effective against H and other Gram-negative bacilli. influenzae, Pseudomonas species, and Enterobacteriaceae. along with Acinetobacter spp. , and Gram-positive bacteria with varying degrees of activity against *Streptococcus pneumoniae*, such as some streptococci, coagulase-negative staphylococci, and *Staphylococcus aureus*.

Table 4.6. *State-of-the-Art in Treatments Against Pneumonia Caused by Gram-Positive Bacteria*

Strategies	Effect	Examples	
Antibiotics	Bacterial killing or growth inhibition	Fluoroquinolones	Levofloxacin
			Moxifloxacin
		β-lactams	Amoxicillin
			Ampicillin
			Amoxicillin-clavulanate
			Ampicillin-sulbactam
			Cefotaxime
			Ceftriaxone
			Oxacillin
			Flucloxacillin
			Ceftaroline fosamil
		Macrolides	Azithromycin
			Clarithromyxin
		Oxazolidinones	Linezolid
		Glucopeptides	Vancomycin
		Pleuromutilins	Lefamulin

Antibodies	Toxin neutralization		Ab pneumolysin
			Ab choline-binding PspA
		Monoclonal Ab	Human mAb IgG1 AR-301
			mAb MED14893
			2A3 and its variant LC10
			mAb LTM14
		Ab leukocidins	mAb ASN-1
			mAb ASN-2
Natural compounds	Toxin prevention	Flavonoids	Baicalin
			Morin hydrate
		Liposomes	
		Hydroxamate inhibitor	GI254023X
Antimicrobial peptides	Bacterial killing	AMPs	CATH-1
			CATH-2
			CRAMP
			LL-37
Immune modulators	Reduction inflammatory response	Toll-like	
		NOD-like	
Phages and phage proteins	Bacterial killing		Phages AB-SA01
			Pyophage
			Phage Sb-1
			Lysin Cpl-1
			Lysin Pal
			Lysin Cpl-7
			Lysin Cpl-711
			Lysin PL3
			Lysin ClyJ
			Lysin 23TH_48
			Lysin SA01_53
			Lysin SAL200

Source: *Fernández L, Cima-Cabal MD, Duarte AC, Rodríguez A, García-Suárez MdM, García P. Gram-Positive Pneumonia: Possibilities Offered by Phage Therapy. Antibiotics. 2021; 10(8):1000. https://doi.org/10.3390/antibiotics10081000.*

They are actively combating all pathogens that causes atypical pneumonia. Their range was restricted before ciprofloxacin was introduced because it did not include the majority of respiratory pathogens. Initially, it was thought that ciprofloxacin would offer a sufficient treatment for CAP. Nevertheless, issues with ciprofloxacin's weak antimicrobial activity. The presence of *Streptococcus pneumoniae* indicated that neither ciprofloxacin nor the fluoroquinolone class as a whole would be appropriate for treating pneumococcal pneumonia. With the advent of the more recent fluoroquinolones, which have better activity against these pathogens, especially *Streptococcus pneumoniae*, the situation is now shifting. (Table 4.6)

A lot of prescriptions for ciprofloxacin have been written down to treat LRTIs. But a series of anecdotal reports of ciprofloxacin's comparatively weak action against *Streptococcus pneumoniae* resulted in a change in the package labeling, which now advises against using the fluoroquinolones that are currently on the market to treat pneumococcal infections. The recommended intravenous ciprofloxacin dosage regimen was increased from 200 mg twice daily to 400 mg twice or three times daily, in part because of this.

Ofloxacin has been used to treat CAP, according to several studies. Nielsen et al. found that the combined cure/improvement rates for ofloxacin and erythromycin were 82% and 96%, respectively, in a study that compared the two drugs. According to Plouffe et al, ofloxacin had clinical success rates of 87% and 92%, respectively, and was just as effective as standard therapy (β-lactam plus a macrolide) for patients hospitalized for CAP. Petermann reported a 93% overall satisfactory response rate in 212 patients.

A study by Carbon et al. compared amoxicillin and temafloxacin in 246 hospitalized patients. Overall, the rates of bacterial eradication (98%, 96%) and clinical recovery (85%, 80%) did not show any discernible differences between temafloxacin and amoxicillin. When it came to treating pneumococcal infections, both worked just as well. The high frequency of serious adverse events led to the antibiotic's withdrawal from use in 1992, despite multiple additional studies demonstrating its effectiveness in treating CAP.

All common LRTI pathogens, including atypical organisms like *Chlamydia pneumoniae*, and *Mycoplasma pneumoniae* are susceptible to the action of sparfloxacin. However, because of the serious phototoxic reactions linked to its use, prescribing guidelines have been restricted. After an oral loading dose of 400 mg, 12 hours later, sparfloxacin showed rapid and high diffusion into respiratory tract tissues and fluids, with concentrations of 2.6 mg/L in bronchial mucosa, 9.8 mg/L in the epithelial lining fluid, and 61.3 mg/L in alveolar macrophages.

This antibiotic has been used in numerous CAP studies. The effectiveness of erythromycin (1000 mg twice daily), amoxicillin/clavulanic acid (500/125 mg three times daily), and sparfloxacin (200 mg once daily, after a 400-mg loading dose) was compared in two double-blind trials. When the findings from these studies were combined, they covered 1137 CAP episodes in hospitalized patients (560 of whom received sparfloxacin treatment and 577 of whom were randomly assigned to the comparator agents). The global efficacy rates of 88 and 84%, respectively, for sparfloxacin and the comparators were found to be comparable.

Another study examined the effects of a 10-day combination of amoxicillin 1 g three times a day and ofloxacin 200 mg twice a day against sparfloxacin 200 mg once daily. This double-blind, placebo-controlled trial was carried out on 211 elderly hospital patients or patients who had failed their initial round of antibiotics. In the groups treated with sparfloxacin and amoxicillin plus ofloxacin, the percentage of isolated pathogens that were identified as *Streptococcus pneumoniae* was 40% and 36%, respectively. At the conclusion of the treatment, the treatment groups receiving amoxicillin plus ofloxacin and sparfloxacin had respective overall efficacy rates of 92% and 82%, which are defined as successful clinical cure and resolution or improvement of signs or symptoms. Another controlled study of 304 patients found that oral treatment with sparfloxacin was superior to roxithromycin (82% success rate versus 72%) for CAP, which is caused by *Streptococcus pneumoniae* in 20% of cases.

The l-isomer of ofloxacin, levofloxacin, has a wide spectrum of activity against the majority of Gram-positive and Gram-negative bacteria, including atypical organisms. It is typically twice as potent as ofloxacin. Levofloxacin's oral bioavailability is almost 100%, similar to that of ofloxacin, allowing oral dosing for all but the most critically ill and incapacitated patients. Furthermore, following a 500 mg single dose, levofloxacin exhibits good penetration into lung tissue, bronchial mucosa, epithelial lining fluid, and alveolar macrophages. Oral levofloxacin (20 and 40 mg/kg) dramatically decreased the amount of viable *Streptococcus pneumoniae* organisms in the lungs in a mouse pneumonia model, while ciprofloxacin had no greater effect than no therapy at all.

Levofloxacin does not appear to significantly affect theophylline metabolism, in contrast to ciprofloxacin or enoxacin, according to recent pharmacokinetic studies conducted in humans and animals. Comparing levofloxacin to other fluoroquinolones like lomefloxacin, sparfloxacin, and enoxacin, it may also have a far lower potential for photosensitivity reactions.

It has been shown in two published studies that levofloxacin is effective in treating CAP. Intravenous or oral levofloxacin once daily was highly effective in treating mild-to-moderate and severe CAP in an open, non-comparative, multicenter trial involving 68 patients; 100% of the 60 clinically evaluable patients had a successful clinical response. Every pathogen identified in this investigation, such as *Streptococcus pneumoniae*, *H. influenzae*, *Chlamydia pneumoniae*, and *Staphylococcus aureus* were eliminated. In a randomized, open-label, active-control trial, patients with a primary diagnosis of CAP were compared between intravenous or oral levofloxacin (500 mg once daily) and parenteral ceftriaxone (1–2 g once or twice daily) and/or cefuroxime axetil (500 mg twice daily). For seven to 14 days, the patients were given the following study medications: 500 mg of levofloxacin once daily, either orally or as a one-hour infusion; 1 or 2 g of ceftriaxone once or twice daily; and 500 mg of oral cefuroxime axetil twice daily. A total of 456 patients (226 levofloxacin, 230 ceftriaxone cefuroxime) were eligible for efficacy evaluation. 96% of patients treated with ceftriaxone/cefuroxime and 96% of patients treated with levofloxacin had clinical success (defined as cure or improvement). Compared to 85% of patients treated with ceftriaxone/cefuroxime, 98% of levofloxacin patients had the pre-treatment pathogen completely eliminated. The two most prevalent pretreatment pathogens, *Streptococcus pneumoniae* and *H influenzae,* were completely eradicated in the group receiving levofloxacin treatment, as opposed to 94% and 79%, respectively, in the group receiving ceftriaxone/cefuroxime. Levofloxacin was well tolerated; the most frequent side effects were diarrhea (1%), and nausea (2%).

When it comes to trovafloxacin and ciprofloxacin are equally active. enhanced activity against group A streptococci and *Streptococcus pneumoniae*, as well as *H. influenzae* and *Moraxella catarrhalis.* Furthermore, it exhibits high activity against Legionella species. and Chlamydia pneumoniae, as well as being equally effective against pneumococci resistant to penicillin and those susceptible to it. Clinical trials are currently evaluating trovafloxacin's strong *in vitro* activity against pneumococci and other respiratory tract pathogens (Ray et al., 1993; Stroud and Friedman, 2001; Samuels M, Wieteska, 2011; Wald, 2014).

4.4. Viral Infections of the Lower Respiratory Tract

It is estimated that acute respiratory diseases claim the lives of 3 to 5 million children worldwide each year. In the US, between 75 and 80% of all acute morbidity is caused by respiratory disorders. The majority of the morbidity rate, or about 80% of respiratory illnesses, is caused by viral infections. Many of these infections cause minor, self-limiting upper respiratory tract symptoms. Most severe disease is caused by lower respiratory tract illness (LRI), especially when it manifests as parenchymal disease on a chest radiograph or as crackles or wheezes on physical examination. In the first year of life, LRI develops in one-third of children. In certain cases, it can be challenging to initially distinguish childhood asthma from lung respiratory illness (LRI); in fact, both conditions can coexist.

Even though viruses account for 60% or more of LRIs, it's frequently unclear whether bacterial infection is the main cause or a side effect of the viral infection. The most prevalent bacteria are by far *Streptococcus pneumoniae*, *Haemophilus influenzae*, and Staphylococcus aureus. A sudden onset or a change in symptoms over a few to several hours, toxicity, and radiographic findings of parenchymal consolidation, pleural effusions, or both are clinical features that point to these causes. White blood cell counts can be helpful, but higher neutrophil band counts (>1500 cells/mm^3) or extreme leukocytosis (>20,000 cells/mm^3) may indicate bacterial involvement.

Table 4.7. *Characteristics Between Short- and Long-Antibiotic-Course Treatment Groups and Appropriateness of Antibiotics. Significant p-value is <0.05*

	Indication (*n*, %)	**Duration of Antibiotic Use**			***p*-Value**
		≤5 Days *n* = 463	**6–7 Days *n* = 109**	**>8 Days *n* = 68**	
		***n* (%)**	***n* (%)**	***n* (%)**	
Appropriateness of antibiotics	CAP (262, 40.9%)	84 (18.1)	25 (22.9)	14 (20.6)	*0.02*
	HAP (119, 18.6%)	45 (9.7)	11 (10.1)	7 (10.3)	0.7
	VAP (6, 0.9%)	3 (0.6)	1 (0.9)	1 (1.5)	0.6
	COPD infective exacerbation (44, 6.9%)	17 (3.7)	5 (4.6)	1 (1.5)	0.6
	COVID-19 pneumonia (47, 7.3%)	8 (1.7)	1 (0.9)	1 (1.5)	0.4
	Unspecified (162, 25.3%)	7 (1.5)	2 (1.8)	0 (0)	*0.07*
	Overall (640, 100%)	164 (35.4)	45 (41.3)	24 (35.3)	0.5

CAP, community-acquired pneumonia; HAP, hospital-acquired pneumonia; VAP, ventilator-associated pneumonia; COPD, chronic obstructive pulmonary disease; COVID-19, coronavirus.

Source: Abdelsalam Elshenawy R, Umaru N, Aslanpour Z. Shorter and Longer Antibiotic Durations for Respiratory Infections: To Fight Antimicrobial Resistance—A Retrospective Cross-Sectional Study in a Secondary Care Setting in the UK. Pharmaceuticals. 2024; 17(3):339. https://doi.org/10.3390/ph17030339.

These results, however, are not conclusive since leukocytosis and varying shifts to the left can result from severe viral infections. On the other hand, severe bacterial pneumonia may manifest as concerning leukopenia. While some believe that the intensity of fever can help identify whether a bacterial infection is present, viral LRI can also cause high fevers that last for several days or longer. To date, serum levels of procalcitonin and C-reactive protein have demonstrated the greatest potential in differentiating between serious bacterial infections and viral diseases; however, these conclusions have not been applied to respiratory illnesses (Table 4.7).

Chlamydia trachomatis, Chlamydia pneumoniae, Mycoplasma pneumoniae, Mycobacterium tuberculosis, deep mycoses, and *Pneumocystis jirovecii* are some additional nonviral agents. The most common age group for trachomatis pneumonia in infants is between two weeks and six months. The infant is typically afebrile, the onset of respiratory symptoms is gradual over several days, and chest radiographs frequently show air trapping with interstitial infiltrates. M. Pneumoniae infections rarely cause pneumonia in children under the age of five, but they often do so in those between the ages of 5 and 19. *Chlamydia pneumoniae* infections seem to mimic the age- and clinical-specific patterns of M. pneumonia infections, but additional information is required before a definitive comparison can be made. When symptoms and abnormalities on radiographs slowly worsen over several days to weeks, it is advisable to consider tuberculosis and deep mycoses. Lastly, *P. jirovecii* infections are suggested in patients with alveolar infiltrates, congenital or acquired immunodeficiency, malignancy, and severe protein malnutrition, as well as progressive hypoxemia (often without significant hypercarbia).

A frequent clinical conundrum is the inability to consistently distinguish viral agents that might not respond to particular treatments from treatable causes, like bacteria. Almost all pediatric patients with acute lower respiratory infections (LRIs) are treated with antibiotics in the event that a bacterial agent is implicated. Such therapy has not been demonstrated to change the risk of bacterial superinfection and is ineffective in treating viral diseases. In addition, if secondary infection does occur, it may lead to the selection of more resistant organisms. The development of molecular diagnostic techniques has made it feasible to diagnose many viral LRIs quickly and precisely. Furthermore, for certain viral infections, specialized antiviral therapy is available and has the potential to lower rates of morbidity and mortality.

Viral infections continue to be the most frequent cause of pediatric LRIs, particularly in children under the age of five, despite the worry about bacterial coinfection. Most common among them are respiratory syncytial virus (RSV), human metapneumovirus (hMPV), influenza virus types A and B, parainfluenza virus types 1, 2, and 3, and adenoviruses. Though comparatively little is known about their role in lung respiratory illness (LRI), rhinoviruses, human coronaviruses (HCVs), influenza virus type C, and parainfluenza virus type 4 are known to play roles in upper respiratory disease. Occasionally, LRI has been linked to other viruses, including human herpesvirus-6 (HHV-6), cytomegalovirus (CMV), and Epstein-Barr virus (EBV), either as primary pathogens or as potential cofactors with other agents. In the context of immunocompromise, all three become more significant overall; this is particularly true for CMV. LRI has long been known to be significantly caused by the measles virus. Even though it appears that this virus can be eradicated, it still poses a serious threat to developing countries.

4.4.1. Respiratory Syncytial Virus

Respiratory syncytial virus (RSV) is the primary culprit behind lower respiratory infections in infants and young children, particularly those under the age of 2 who tend to experience more severe symptoms. RSV can lead to various illnesses such as croup, tracheobronchitis, bronchiolitis, pneumonia, or a combination of these conditions, and can also result in complications like progressive pulmonary failure, cor pulmonale, and an increased risk of bacterial superinfection. There is some evidence suggesting a potential link between severe RSV lower respiratory infections in infancy and the development of asthma or allergic airways disease in childhood.

4.4.2. Human Metapneumovirus

The infectious agent known as human metapneumovirus (hMPV) appears to have been around for a while, but it wasn't until 2001 that it was identified as a primary cause of lung respiratory illness (LRI). Since its initial description in patients with LRI in the Netherlands, hMPV has been found in both adult and pediatric LRI patients worldwide. hMPV shares a syncytial formation with RSV in cell culture and belongs to the same subfamily of Paramyxoviruses. Due to variations in the sensitivity of detection techniques, comparative prevalence studies can be challenging to assess; however, it is apparent that hMPV contributes significantly to LRI globally. 12% of nasopharyngeal samples from patients with LRI had hMPV prevalence in one prospective 25-year study, compared to 15% for RSV, 10% for parainfluenza virus, and five% for influenza virus. Typically, the infection happens in childhood, resulting in hMPV seropositivity in up to 52% of 24-month-old infants and 100% of 5-year-old children. Similar to RSV, hMPV exhibits a seasonal pattern, peaking during the winter. It seems that co-infection with hMPV and other respiratory viruses exacerbates the illness.

Table 4.8. *Diagnostic Strategies for RSV Detection*

Test	Turnaround Time	Sensitivity	Specificity	Note
Cell culture	Days	Low	Excellent	Traditional gold standard; long time for results
RT-PCR	Hours	Excellent	Excellent	New gold standard; expensive; needs expertise; positive results may not indicate active infection; possibility of multiplex tests
DFAs	<1 h	Low	Low	Needs expertise; rapid results
RADTs	Minutes	Low	Variable	Traditional tests depend on operator skills; newer platforms have better sensitivity/ specificity
Novel rapid molecular diagnostic assays	Minutes–few hours	Excellent	Good	Variability; not detection of RSV types; qualitative but not quantitative results

RT-PCR = reverse transcriptase polymerase chain reaction; DFAs = direct immunofluorescence assays; RADTs = rapid antigen detection tests.

Source: Bianchini S, Silvestri E, Argentiero A, Fainardi V, Pisi G, Esposito S. Role of Respiratory Syncytial Virus in Pediatric Pneumonia. Microorganisms. 2020; 8(12):2048. https://doi.org/10.3390/ microorganisms8122048.

Clinically speaking, hMPV infection resembles RSV disease in that it causes mild upper respiratory tract illness, croup, pneumonia, and, most frequently, bronchiolitis. It also mimics influenza-like symptoms, such as fever, myalgia, and vomiting. While most patients have less severe signs of respiratory distress, they typically present with symptoms that are commonly associated with RSV. Patients who are extremely old or have compromised immune systems, however, are more likely to experience more severe LRI. Similar hospital stays (6 to 7 days) are needed for patients hospitalized for hMPV-associated LRI as opposed to RSV patients. Studies have shown both beneficial and negative effects of hMPV, so the relationship between it and reactive airways disease and asthma is unclear (Table 4.8). hMPV is hard to diagnose because the virus does not grow well in standard cell cultures. These days, the preferred identification techniques are reverse transcription–polymerase chain reaction (RT-PCR) assays. Serologic testing (enzyme-linked immunosorbent assays [ELISAs] and immunofluorescence) is not widely accessible and is hampered by the nearly universal infection in childhood; to confirm a recent infection, there must be evidence of a ≥4-fold increase in antibody titers. Although research is ongoing to assess the effectiveness of ribavirin and intravenous immunoglobulin preparations, supportive care for hMPV infection is still in place. When wheezing is a part of a patient's symptom complex, bronchodilators like albuterol may help, but corticosteroids have no proven effect. The best course of action is still to prevent hMPV infection, however there have been no reported studies on hMPV vaccine products for humans.

4.4.3. Parainfluenza Viruses

The next most frequent cause of LRI in children under the age of five is parainfluenza viruses. Among this population, influenza virus type 3 is the most frequent cause of lung damage (LRI). Although they can occur at any time of year, these infections are most prevalent in the spring and summer. Autumn and early winter are often associated with isolated outbreaks of parainfluenza virus types 1 or 2, which cause bronchitis, croup, and upper respiratory illnesses. Type 4 parainfluenza virus is rarely found and is mostly linked to symptoms related to the upper respiratory tract.

Parainfluenza virus infection follows a similar clinical course to that of RSV, as shown in Figure 4.18. The primary symptoms include mild nasal stuffiness and coryza, which progress in different ways over the course of one to three days as the infection moves deeper into the respiratory tract and causes coughing as its main symptom. Children who are less than one-year-old are susceptible to bronchitis, pneumonia, and croup due to parainfluenza 3. Pneumonia linked to parainfluenza 3 can cause significant morbidity and mortality in patients with compromised immune systems. An acute illness typically lasts 7 to 10 days, though it can last up to 21 days. The fundamental management concepts for parainfluenza LRIs are the same as those previously discussed for RSV. An intravenous drip is typically required to give the patient enough fluids when eating and drinking become difficult for them. When hypoxemia is present, humidified oxygen is also administered; the usual starting concentration is between 30 and 40%. When conditions are severe, blood gas measurements are used to guide an increase in oxygen concentration. Mechanical ventilatory support and endotracheal intubation are necessary if there is clinical evidence of progressive respiratory failure.

Bronchodilators can also be tried, but they need to be used carefully and stopped if no obvious benefits are seen. There is no proof that corticosteroids help treat lower respiratory infections. Their function in upper respiratory infections is covered in another article. Ribavirin can be effective against parainfluenza types 1 and 3, but its application in treating these infections has not yet been supported by randomized clinical trials.

4.4.4. Influenza Viruses

It is widely known that influenza virus types A and B cause quickly changing outbreaks that typically happen in the winter months. Serious, fatal LRI in infants and children can result from both types. In contrast to RSV and parainfluenza viruses, the clinical course of this virus typically manifests as fever, malaise, and frequently myalgia that rapidly worsens over the course of 12 to 24 hours. Frequently, respiratory distress, coughing, and nasal congestion do not manifest for one or two days following the onset of systemic symptoms. While the acute illness's average duration of 3 to 7 days is slightly shorter than that of RSV or parainfluenza viruses, the convalescent phase typically lasts several weeks, and at any point during the illness' course, rapid deterioration due to bacterial superinfection can happen. In rare cases, patients may experience a severe viral pneumonia that progresses quickly and kills them two to three days after it first appears. In the last century, there have been three pandemics that have killed millions of people and caused exceptionally severe hemorrhagic pneumonia. The lack of neutralizing serum immunity against the pandemic strain, most likely as a result of antigenic drift of its hemagglutinin antigen, appears to be linked to the pathogenicity of these pandemics.

The basic management and diagnosis procedures are comparable to those outlined for parainfluenza and RSV viruses. Amantadine hydrochloride taken orally works ok to treat influenza A but not at all to treat influenza B. It may shorten the duration of fever and systemic symptoms and hasten the improvement of peripheral airway function if started within 24 to 48 hours of onset and continued for 5 to 7 days. During influenza A outbreaks, it is also used as prophylaxis in children who are considered high-risk. Rimantadine, a related medication, works similarly to amantadine and seems to have fewer side effects. It has been noted that viral resistance to amantadine and rimantadine develops quickly, especially when both drugs are used in households to treat symptomatic infections and prevent contacts at the same time.

If taken within 30 hours of the onset of the illness, the neuraminidase inhibitors zanamivir and oseltamivir can also greatly shorten the illness's duration and lessen its severity. Crucially, both medications work effectively against influenza A and B, are well tolerated, and don't always seem to be linked to viral resistance.

Every year, the influenza virus types A and B combination vaccines are assessed and adjusted as needed to better match the strains that are anticipated to be broadly distributed in the following year. Their effectiveness in providing protection varies annually, with ranges of 50% to 95% in immunologically normal adults over the age of six months. The influenza vaccine is not advised for individuals under the age of six months due to unknown efficacy; otherwise, individuals of all ages can receive the yearly immunization, which starts in the fall, with the exception of those who have previously had anaphylactic reactions to chickens or eggs. It is advised that children receiving the vaccine for the first time receive two doses spaced one month apart. For adults and children aged 5 to 49, there is also an intranasal live attenuated influenza vaccine available. This product offers an alternative to additional injections and is very effective and well-tolerated. For high-risk, immunocompromised patient populations, influenza vaccination is advised; otherwise, it is contraindicated (Table 4.9).

Table 4.9. *Antiviral Drugs Recommended For Use Against Influenza Viruses*

Drug Class	Active Substance	CID	Trade Name
NAI	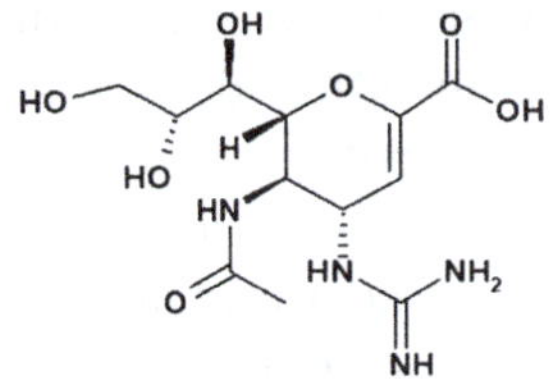 zanamivir	60855	Relenza® registered in EU, USA, and AsiaDectova® registered in EU
NAI	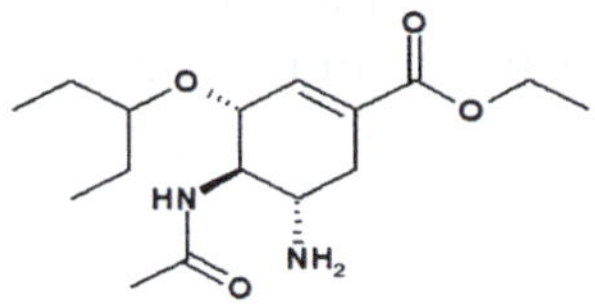 oseltamivir	65028	Tamiflu® registered in EU, USA, and Asia
NAI	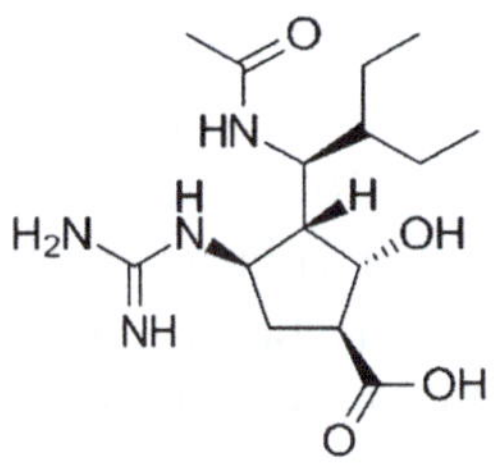 peramivir	154234	Rapivap® registered in USA and Asia
NAI	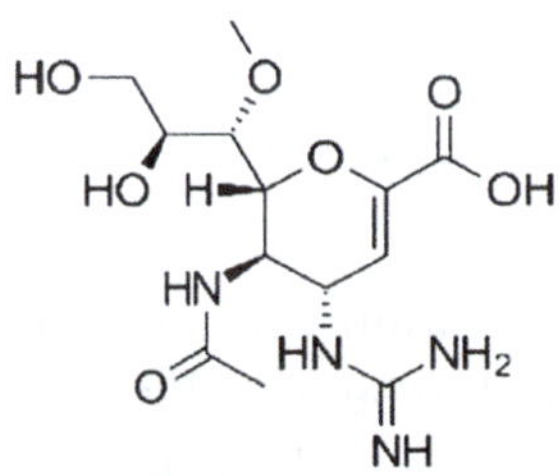 laninamivir	502272	Inavir® registered in Asia
CENI	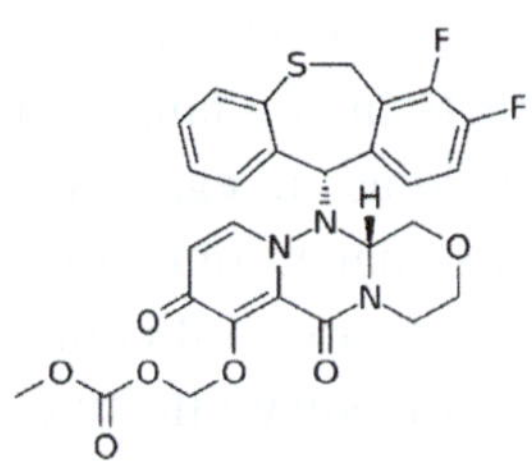 baloxavir marboxil	124081896	Xofluza® registered in EU, USA, and Asia

Source: Świerczyńska M, Mirowska-Guzel DM, Pindelska E. Antiviral Drugs in Influenza. International Journal of Environmental Research and Public Health. 2022; 19(5):3018. https://doi.org/10.3390/ijerph19053018.

Children with long-term salicylate therapy and those with chronic pulmonary, cardiac, hematologic, immunologic, and metabolic conditions should receive an annual influenza vaccination in particular. Furthermore, these high-risk children's household contacts and other caregivers (e.g., therapists, doctors, and nurses) ought to be the focus. If a yearly vaccination is not received and a serious exposure is later suspected (e.g,, when there is a confirmed outbreak), vaccination can offer "bridging" protection until there is a vaccine response if it is promptly followed by chemoprophylaxis with amantadine or rimantadine for two weeks following the vaccination schedule of one or two doses.

Outbreaks of feverish respiratory illnesses have been linked to influenza virus type C, particularly in pediatric clinic patients and children under three years old. Children aged 5 and under had a 64% prevalence of antibodies to this virus, according to a Los Angeles survey. Longitudinal studies, however, have not demonstrated that influenza virus type C plays a significant role in LRI, at least in children under three years old.

In Asian nations, avian influenza A (H5N1) has recently surfaced as a highly pathogenic source of poultry infection that can also occasionally infect humans. The clinical manifestations of influenza A (H5N1) infection in humans include fever, severe respiratory symptoms, lymphopenia, and an elevated risk of mortality. The majority of the at least 44 infected people who died in 2004 had direct contact with infected poultry. However, since few people will be immune to this strain, a probable case of person-to-person transmission raises concerns about the possibility of an impending pandemic. Although there seems to be some benefit to chemoprophylaxis using neuraminidase inhibitors, their use may be restricted due to concerns about emerging viral resistance. Therefore, it is essential to take preventive actions like developing vaccines and screening and culling chickens in advance. Regretfully, very few nations have prepared for an influenza pandemic, and even fewer have the financial and social means to work toward developing vaccines and accumulating antivirals. The financial reality of domestic poultry destruction in those countries hardest hit by this virus has perhaps had the biggest impact to date (Ray et al., 1993; Stroud and Friedman, 2001; Samuels M, Wieteska, 2011; Wald, 2014).

4.4.5. Adenoviruses

Young children's conjunctivitis, fevers, and upper respiratory infections are frequently brought on by adenoviruses. Thankfully, they only sporadically and infrequently generate LRI. The most common types of adenoviral pneumonia are types 3, 5, and 7. Adenoviral pneumonia initially progresses similarly to the pneumonia caused by RSV and parainfluenza viruses, but it can also be extremely severe and last for several weeks. Epidemics of LRI have been linked to Adenovirus types 3 and 7. Immunocompromise, congenital heart disease, and protein-calorie malnutrition are risk factors for serious, possibly fatal diseases. Chest radiographs during the acute phase frequently show extensive consolidation, especially in perihilar areas. These findings can make it challenging to distinguish these infections from bacterial illnesses, especially since high fevers, leukocytosis, and multisystem involvement are common. Hepatic dysfunction (including Reye's syndrome), encephalopathy, coagulopathies, measles-like exanthems, and diarrhea are other systemic manifestations that can occasionally appear.

When the virus is found in tissues, such as lung aspirates or biopsy specimens, the diagnosis is most reliably confirmed. Isolation of the virus from the throat must be considered as diagnostically supportive but not confirmatory, and isolation from stools or rectal swabs needs to be interpreted even more cautiously because asymptomatic shedding from the throat or gastrointestinal tract is common in young children. Confirming the diagnosis may also be aided by serologic analyses of paired acute and convalescent sera collected at least two weeks separated. Assays for immunoenzyme and immunofluorescence have been used for rapid detection. These techniques are typically very specific, with sensitivity ranging from 30 to 60%.

Right now, the only thing that can be provided is supportive management. These patients are at risk for bacterial superinfection for several weeks, so they need to be closely monitored. They may also develop chronic lung conditions such as bronchiectasis, recurrent wheezing, pulmonary fibrosis, and bronchiolitis obliterans. There have been reports of nutritional or immunologic deficiencies, as well as young age and a history of illness similar to the measles. It has been suggested that the causes are the enduring expression of adenovirus genes in the airway epithelium and the persistence of adenoviral antigens.

4.4.6. Human Coronaviruses

The part played by human coronaviruses (HCoV) in LRIs was unclear until recently. The two strains 229E and OC43 were most commonly linked to LRI. Adults with HCoV OC43 infections experience cough and nasal symptoms, while children have fever, sore throat, cough, and coryza. Acute wheezing episodes in children with asthma have also been linked to HCoV infections. ELISA found HCoV antigens in 30% of 108 acute respiratory episodes in a thought-provoking study of pediatric HCoV LRI, which involved 30 children under 6 years old with a history of at least 10 recurrent respiratory illnesses in the year prior. Furthermore, HCoV was linked to 29% of the 51 acute respiratory episodes that the patients' siblings had to deal with. It's interesting to note that while none of the siblings with HCoV had LRI findings, 30% of the HCoV infections found in the former group were linked to LRI symptoms, such as wheezy bronchitis. Peaks in infections happened in late fall, early winter, and early summer, with HCoV 229E being the primary cause. Increased levels of antibodies to HCoV strains OC43 and 229E are more common in the winter, according to family studies conducted in Seattle. Children were found to be infected three times more frequently than adults, and serologic evidence indicating reinfection was frequently observed over a three-year period.

4.4.7. Severe Acute Respiratory Syndrome

A new era of international scientific and medical cooperation was sparked by the 2002 outbreak of severe acute respiratory syndrome (SARS), which also resulted in the identification of a third coronavirus with human pathogenicity (SARS-CoV). The first SARS cases were reported in China in November 2002. Over the course of the following year, there were 8098 cases in 26 countries, resulting in 774 deaths. China has reported the detection of SARS-CoV-like viruses in raccoon dogs and Himalayan palm civets. These viruses have also been isolated from human samples, including nasal secretions, serum, feces, and bronchial washings. There is strong evidence that the main hosts of these viruses are bats. Given that SARS-CoV infection in humans has not been previously documented, it is plausible that the virus has migrated from animals to humans across the species barrier.

There is a 2–10 day incubation period for SARS, after which there is an influenza-like prodrome with symptoms like fever, headache, myalgias, and watery diarrhea. A dry, ineffective cough and mild dyspnea are the first respiratory symptoms to appear two to seven days after the prodrome. Lung high-resolution CT scans reveal ground-glass consolidations in these patients' lungs. Eight to 12 days later, there is still more progression that varies from a chronic intractable cough with a "mild cough variant" to the more common "moderate to severe variant" with dyspnea and hypoxia. 10 to 20% of hospitalized patients will need mechanical ventilation and intubation; these procedures are frequently preceded by gradual drops in oxygen saturation. About 14 to 18 days after the onset of symptoms, recovery starts.

Both RT-PCR and culture can be used to diagnose SARS-CoV, though RT-PCR has a higher sensitivity than culture. The highest yield is linked to specimens collected 10 days after the onset of symptoms, which is consistent with the time of peak viral load. As such, they should be used for paired acute and convalescent-phase serologic diagnosis. Serologic assays for SARS-CoV include immunofluorescent assays, ELISA, and Western blot assays; however, none is sensitive early in the disease course to be useful for rapid diagnosis.

The majority of SARS patients' care is still supportive, focused on preventing respiratory failure. Pneumothorax and pneumomediastinum are caused by barotrauma, which appears to be a common consequence of SARS-CoV infection in 20–34% of ventilated patients. For patients using mechanical ventilation, a "lung protective" ventilation approach is advised. The use of lopinavir-ritonavir, ribavirin, interferon a, and immunomodulatory treatments like corticosteroids, intravenous immunoglobulin, and plasma exchange have all been used as additional therapeutic approaches. But no controlled trial has shown that these lead to better outcomes or lower mortality. Even though SARS-CoV had a high death rate and a terrible effect in 2002, the story of its emergence describes a victory because public health measures implemented globally were successful in controlling the outbreak. Additionally, NL63, a fourth HCoV, has been discovered and proven to be a major contributor to acute respiratory illnesses in humans. After being first reported in the Netherlands, HCV NL63 has since been shown in Australia, Canada, Japan, Belgium, China, Switzerland, and the United States, among other countries. Currently known as HCoV-New Haven (NH) in the United States, this virus most likely belongs to the same or a closely related species as the NL63 that has been reported elsewhere. 88% of the 895 children under the age of five who had an acute respiratory illness tested negative for other common viral respiratory pathogens but positive for HCoV-NH. Apart from experiencing symptoms related to the upper respiratory tract, children infected with HCoV NL63 virus may also experience croup, asthma flare-ups, febrile seizures, and abnormalities in chest radiographs and tachypnea, which are signs of abnormal breathing sounds. HCoV NL63 may exhibit variable seasonality, with spring and summer in tropical regions and fall and winter in temperate zones.

The fifth HCoV, HKU1, has most recently been reported. The 71-year-old man who had returned to Hong Kong from an area of China where SARS was endemic was the first to exhibit the symptoms. A subsequent prospective study of nasopharyngeal aspirates from 418 patients suffering from pneumonia acquired in the community revealed that 10 (2.4%) of them tested positive for HCoV-HKU1. Nine of the 10 cases—all adult—had underlying respiratory tract diseases, and four of the cases happened in the spring and winter. Each person's symptoms were identical to those of other research participants who had pneumonia that they had acquired in the community. It is yet unknown how this new virus will affect the world.

Table 4.10. ***Comparative List of Nucleic Acid Amplification Tests for the Detection of SARS Cov-2, by Manufacturer, Origin of Specimen, Target Gene, Sensitivity, Specificity, Limit of Detection and The Time to Produce One Successful Run***

Nucleic Acid Amplification Tests (NAAT)									
Name of Test	Developer	Nature of Specimen	Target Gene	Sensitivity (PPA)	Specificity (NPA)	Limit of Detection (LoD)	Time to Result	Status	References
Non-Isothermal: RT-PCR									
Xpert ® Xpress SARS-CoV-2/Flu/RSV	Cepheid	NS, NPS, OPS, MTS, NA, NW	*E, N2*	97.9%	100%	131 GCE/mL	45 min run	EUA	[Loeffelholz, M.J. et al. 2020, Fung, B. et al. 2020, Cepheid. 2021]
Cobas ® SARS-CoV-2 & Influenza A/B: cobas Liat System	Roche Molecular Systems	NPS, NS	*Orf1ab, N*	100%	97.4%	0.012 $TCID_{50}$/mL	20 min run	EUA	[Hansen, G. et al. 2020, Roche Molecular Systems 2020]
Cobas ® SARS-CoV-2 Test	Roche Molecular Systems	NS, NPS, OPS	*Orf1ab, E*	100%	95.5%	0.007 $TCID_{50}$/mL	3.5 h run	EUA; CE-IVD	[Loeffelholz, M.J. et al. 2020, Craney, A.R. et al. 2020, Roche Molecular Systems.2021, Roche Molecular Systems.2021]
Accula ™ SARS-CoV-2 Test	Mesa Biotech	NS, MTS	*N*	95.8%	100%	150 copies/mL	30 min run	EUA	[Mesa Biotech. 2021]
BioFire ® Respiratory Panel 2.1-EZ	BioFire Diagnostics	NPS	*S, M*	98%	100%	6000 copies/mL	45 min run	EUA	[BioFire Diagnostics. 2020]
TaqPath ™ COVID-19 Pooling Kit	ThermoFisher Scientific, Inc.	NPS, NA, BAL	*Orf1ab, S, N*	100%	100%	10 GCE/reaction	4 h run	EUA; CE-IVD	[Bal, A. et al. 2021, Waltham, MA 2021, Yu, C.Y. et al. 2021]
Abbott RealTime ™ SARS-CoV-2	Abbott Molecular	NS, NPS, OPS, BAL	*RdRp, N*	100%	100%	100 copies/mL	6.8 h run	EUA	[Fung, B. et al, 2020, Abbott Diagnostics. 2021]
Non-Isothermal: RT-qSTAR Amplification									
PerkinElmer ® SARS-CoV-2 RT-qPCR Reagent Kit	Perkin Elmer Genomics	NPS, OPS, NA	*Orf1ab, N*	100%	100%	120 copies/mL	1 h run	CE-IVD; WHO-EUL	[Perkin Elmer Genomics. 2020]
LumiraDx ™ SARS-CoV-2 RNA STAR complete	LumiraDx UK, Ltd.	NPS, OPS, NA, MTS	*Orf1ab*	95%	100%	1875 copies/mL	20 min run	EUA	[Huang, Z. et al. 2020]
Isothermal: Transcription Mediated Amplification									
Aptima ® SARS-CoV-2 Assay	Hologic, Inc.	NPS, OPS, NS, NA	*Orf1ab*	100%	99.7%	0.026 $TCID_{50}$/mL	2.5 h run	EUA; CE-IVD	[Hologic. 2021]
Isothermal: RT-LAMP/NEAR									
Cue ™ COVID-19 Test for Home and OTC Use	Cue Health, Inc.	NS	*N*	97.4%	99.1%	2700 copies/mL	20 min run	EUA	[Cue Health, Inc. 2021]

AQ-TOP ™ COVID-19 Rapid Detection Test PLUS	Seasun Biomaterials, Inc.	NPS, OPS, NS, NA, MTS	*Orf1ab, N*	100%	100%	1 copy/μL	2 h run	EUA	[Seasun Biomaterials, Inc. 2021]
Pro-AmpRT SARS-CoV-2 Test	Pro-Lab Diagnostics	NPS, OPS, NS, NW, MTS	*Orf1ab*	96.6%	100%	125 copies/ swab	30 min run	EUA	[Pro-Lab Diagnostics. 2020]
ID Now ™ COVID-19 (NEAR)	Abbott Diagnostics	NPS, OPS, NS	*RdRp*	100%	100%	125 GCE/mL	13 min run	EUA; CE-IVD	[Rhoads, D.D. et al. 2020, Harrington, A. et al. 2020, Abbott Diagnostics. 2020]
Isothermal: RT-PCR/CRISPR									
Sherlock ™ CRISPR SARS-CoV-2 Kit	Sherlock Biosciences Inc.	NPS, OPS, NS, NPW, NA, BAL	*Orf1ab, N*	100%	100%	6750 copies/ mL	1h run	EUA	[Broughton, J.P. et al. 2020, Sherlock Biosciences. 2021]
SARS-CoV-2 DETECTR ™ Reagent Kit	Mammoth Biosciences, Inc.	NPS, OPS, MTS, NPA, NA	*N*	95%	100%	20,000 copies/mL	15 min run	EUA	[U.S. Food and Drug Administration. 2021]
Caspr Lyo-CRISPR SARS-CoV-2 Kit (FAM)	Caspr Biotech	NS, NPS, OPS	*Orf1ab, N*	99%	99%	25,000 copies/mL	1 h run	EUA	[Curti, L. et al. 2021]

Abbreviations: PPA, Positive Percentage Agreement; NPA, Negative Percentage Agreement; RT-PCR, Reverse Transcriptase-Polymerase Chain Reaction; RT-qSTAR, Reverse Transcriptase-Selective Temperature Amplification Reaction; RT-LAMP, Reverse Transcriptase-Loop Mediated Isothermal Amplification; NEAR, Nicking Enzyme Amplification Reaction; CRISPR, Clustered Regularly Interspersed Small Palindromic Repeats; NPS, Nasopharyngeal Swab; OPS, Oropharyngeal Swab; NS, Nasal Swab; NPA, Nasopharyngeal Aspirates; NA, Nasal Aspirates; NW, Nasal Wash; MTS, Mid-turbinate Nasal Swab; BAL, Bronchiolar Lavage; *E*, Envelope Protein; *N*, Nucleocapsid Protein; *S*, Spike Protein; *M*, Membrane Protein; $TCID_{50}$, tissue culture infectious dose infecting 50% of cells; GCE, Genomic copy equivalents; EUA, Emergency Use Authorization.

Source: Gitman MR, Shaban MV, Paniz-Mondolfi AE, Sordillo EM. Laboratory Diagnosis of SARS-CoV-2 Pneumonia. Diagnostics. *2021; 11(7):1270. https://doi.org/10.3390/diagnostics11071270.*

4.4.8. Rhinoviruses

The rhinovirus group, which consists of at least 115 distinct serotypes, is well recognized for being the causative agent of numerous upper respiratory ("common cold") symptoms in older children and adults. Although not at a rate that is appreciably different from children without respiratory illnesses, rhinoviruses have been isolated from newborns and kids who have been hospitalized with LRIs. Acute symptoms typically appear three to seven days after the typical two to three-day incubation period. In a retrospective analysis, bronchiolitis and pneumonia were identified in 44 children with respiratory symptoms who had positive rhinovirus cultures and were either hospitalized or seen in an emergency room; in some cases, both conditions were present (32 patients). Most of the patients were less than a year old. Even though they were rare, LRIs in kids with rhinovirus infections were identical to those brought on by RSV. Acute asthma episodes appear to be triggered by rhinoviruses. The standard method for diagnosing rhinovirus infections is through tissue culture, although a PCR assay is available that is more sensitive than culture. Challenges in identifying rhinoviruses in diagnostic samples may lead to an underestimation of their impact on lower respiratory infections. Treatment for rhinovirus infections primarily involves supportive care, as no antiviral medications are currently recommended. While there has been interest in using zinc and Echinacea as potential preventatives or treatments, controlled studies have not shown any clear benefits from either option so far.

4.4.9. Herpesviruses

All members of the herpesvirus family (herpes simplex virus [HSV] types I and II, varicella-zoster virus [VZV], CMV, EBV, HHV-6, HHV-7, and HHV-8) can cause lower respiratory infections (LRI) in immunocompromised patients, despite being uncommon as pulmonary pathogens in healthy children. These infections are typically hematogeneously spread as part of a systemic infection. Allogeneic bone marrow transplant recipients are primarily at risk for CMV; however, normal children who experience symptoms related to the lower respiratory tract may also test positive for the virus. Serologic research typically does not support a primary role for CMV in LRI in healthy children; however, reports of pneumonia in otherwise normal infants have been linked to acute, primary, systemic CMV infection.

Reactivation of latent virus is the most common cause of CMV pneumonitis in recipients of bone marrow transplants; transmission via blood products to seronegative patients is less common. Pneumonitis caused by CMV is significantly less common in recipients of autologous and syngeneic bone marrow transplants due to the substantial risk factor of graft-versus-host disease. Tachypnea, fever, and progressive pulmonary distress are the usual primary pulmonary process symptoms of CMV pneumonitis. On chest radiographs, diffuse, bilateral pulmonary infiltrates are typically visible. The virus can be cultured from lung tissue or bronchoalveolar lavage fluid to make the diagnosis, however nucleic acid detection techniques that show an elevated viral load in the context of lung radiation therapy are highly suggestive. The incidence of CMV during the first three months following bone marrow transplantation has significantly decreased since the introduction of prophylaxis with intravenous ganciclovir or oral valacyclovir in high-risk patients. When CMV pneumonitis is treated in patients after the disease manifests clinically, gangliovir is less effective.

Although it can spread during resuscitation efforts, herpes simplex pneumonitis is most frequently observed as a component of disseminated infections that are acquired during pregnancy. At all ages, immunocompromise of any kind increases the risk of developing HSV pneumonitis.

A potentially fatal consequence of primary VZV infection in newborns, immunocompromised individuals, and in rare cases, healthy children, is varicella pneumonitis. The first round of viral replication takes place in the lungs, and VZV is disseminated by aerosolized respiratory secretions. After that, there is a primary wave of viremia, which is followed by additional viral replication in lymphatic tissue. Following a secondary viremia, distinctive cutaneous lesions appear. Usually, varicella pneumonitis appears two to five days following a rash outbreak. The radiographic and clinical presentations differ. Miliary lung lesions that are asymptomatic (particularly in adult varicella) may eventually show up as calcified foci. In certain cases, mild interstitial pneumonia may be mistaken for a more serious bacterial pneumonia brought on by organisms like S or group A streptococci. aureus. These can be very challenging to treat and are frequently accompanied by effusions and empyemas. In immunocompromised individuals, varicella alone can result in fatal pneumonia that progresses over time. Neonates can contract VZV when their mothers develop chickenpox within 3 weeks of giving birth. If the mother becomes ill with varicella 5 days before delivery, minimal amounts of VZV-specific antibodies are transferred to the baby through the placenta. This increases the risk of systemic disease and pneumonitis in the neonate, with a case-fatality rate of 5%.

In healthy hosts, varicella is typically diagnosed through clinical observation. To rule out disseminated herpes simplex infections in immunocompromised hosts, vesicular lesions should be cultured or stained with immunofluorescence. Serologic antibody tests help determine one's level of immunity. If administered shortly after exposure, g-Globulin preparations with high titers of anti-VZV activity can effectively prevent varicella. This treatment is appropriate for immunocompromised children and newborns. When treating high-risk patients, acyclovir, and other related agents are the preferred medications because they lessen the severity of the illness when given within two days of the rash outbreak. Thankfully, primary varicella and its complications have significantly decreased as a result of the live VZV vaccine.

Similar to other herpesviruses, EBV can cause a range of clinical syndromes, including nasopharyngeal carcinoma, infectious mononucleosis, illnesses of the central nervous system, and malignant lymphoproliferative diseases. It can also cause lifelong infections. As a result of a primary EBV infection, pneumonia, pleural effusion, and pneumonia are rare but may go undiagnosed. Six of the 113 normal children in the group who had confirmed EBV-induced mononucleosis also had pneumonia during the illness; they were all younger than 4 years old. In every instance, pneumonia was self-limited. Clinical judgment combined with serologic testing for heterophil antibody or IgM anti-VCA antibody is used to diagnose primary EBV infection. It has been proposed that HHV-6, the common cause of roseola infantum, maybe the reason behind some cases of interstitial pneumonitis in recipients of bone marrow transplants. Approximately 90% of the population contracts this virus by the time they are 2 years old, making it one of the most common human viruses. Although HHV-6 detection by culture is not frequently available, evidence of serologic conversion can be used to diagnose primary infection. Since most healthy people have evidence of ongoing viral replication in their blood and salivary glands, reactivation is hard to prove. The more recently identified HHV-7 seems to share the pathogenicity and epidemiology of HHV-6, while HHV-8 is well known for its association with Kaposi sarcoma in patients who are immunocompromised and, in rare cases, immunocompetent. Patients who have received bone marrow transplants seem to develop interstitial pneumonitis from both HHV-7 and HHV-8. It is believed that HHV-6, HHV-7, and HHV-8 do not cause pneumonia in healthy individuals, and there is no known treatment for them (Ray et al., 1993; Stroud and Friedman, 2001; Samuels M, Wieteska, 2011; Wald, 2014).

4.4.10. Measles Virus

Pharyngitis and otitis media are common symptoms in the early stages of measles infection. While laryngitis can occasionally become severe, bronchitis is also common. The measles virus likely causes pneumonia in at least 50% of children. Most of the time, this is mild bronchopneumonia, identified only by hyperinflation on a chest radiograph and nonspecific lower respiratory symptoms. In other cases, the inflammation is more widespread, appearing on chest radiographs as diffuse infiltrates or even segmental or lobar consolidation.

In children with measles, secondary bacterial infections may be caused by *Streptococcus pneumoniae*, *Haemophilus influenzae*, *Streptococcus pyogenes*, and *Staphylococcus aureus*. This is especially critical in developing nations, where measles-related infections are a leading cause of mortality in young children. Measles may also adversely affect the development of tuberculosis in malnourished infants.

Within three weeks of exposure, immunocompromised children are at risk of developing a fatal infection that progresses slowly. Clinically, the illness presents as fever and possibly an unusual rash. For two to three days, nonspecific respiratory symptoms and signs develop. Air leaks are common, and chest radiographs typically reveal coarse nodular infiltrates.

Nasopharyngeal secretions or bronchoalveolar lavage fluid are typically used to diagnose measles through culture, though in rare cases, a lung biopsy may be required. The histopathologic findings often reveal giant cell pneumonia with inflammatory cell exudate and thickened alveolar walls containing inflammatory cells. Intracytoplasmic and intranuclear inclusions are seen in altered alveolar lining cells. Both serologic and immunofluorescence methods allow for rapid diagnosis.

Supportive measures and careful monitoring for signs of bacterial superinfection are key components of measles treatment. A live, attenuated vaccine is available for prevention, but it should not be administered to pregnant or immunocompromised individuals. Active community vaccination is a preventive measure against measles pneumonia in immunocompromised hosts. Immunoglobulin should be administered promptly to those exposed to the virus.

Partially immune hosts may contract modified measles, which presents as fever and an itchy maculopapular rash, especially around the wrists and ankles. This form of measles often involves respiratory symptoms, including dyspnea and diffuse crackles on auscultation. Chest radiographs show pleural effusion and nodular infiltrates, as well as hilar adenopathy.

4.4.11. Hantavirus

An outbreak of acute febrile illness that led to respiratory failure and shock was observed in the southwestern United States in 1993. This condition, known as hantavirus pulmonary syndrome, is characterized by severe noncardiogenic pulmonary edema in previously healthy individuals. Studies have identified three hantaviruses as the cause, which are typically carried by rodents. By November 2004, over 379 cases of hantavirus pulmonary syndrome had been reported in 31 U.S. states, with a mortality rate exceeding 50%. Cases have also been reported in Canada, Brazil, Argentina, and Paraguay. While rare in children under 16, the disease's severity and mortality rates are comparable to those seen in adults. Diagnosis can be made through serologic tests, PCR analysis of frozen tissues, immunochemistry, or examination of paraffin-embedded tissues. While there is no specific treatment, intravenous ribavirin has been suggested based on laboratory data and previous experiences with similar viruses.

4.4.12. Simultaneous Involvement by Multiple Pathogens

According to culture or antigen detection, 10.9% of previously healthy patients with RSV infection in the Tucson Children's Respiratory Study also had co-infection with another possible pathogen. This percentage increased when serologic results were also heavily utilized for diagnosis. Patients with RSV alone had the same clinical diagnosis and results as those who had previously been coinfected with other agents. When a primary pathogen, like RSV, is identified, routine searches for coinfecting agents are not advised for otherwise healthy infants and children. These types of diagnostic workup extensions are best saved for patients with known serious underlying medical conditions or whose clinical course deviates from what would be predicted for the pathogen found.

4.4.13. Prospects for Prevention and Treatment

The current understanding of the epidemiology, diagnosis, and primary causes of viral LRIs has advanced significantly. In the vital fields of molecular virology, antiviral therapy, and immunopathogenesis, exciting developments are currently being made. Future research will undoubtedly yield even more sensible prevention and treatment strategies, such as precisely crafted peptide vaccines that can more effectively enlist particular T-cell populations as partners in long-lasting defense. Other cutting-edge tactics include using cytokines to enhance the host's defenses and repurposing established ideas, like the use of particular antibodies for prophylaxis and therapy, in creative ways. Compared to the situation that Andrewes described more than 40 years ago when he proposed that doctors should consider these infections as "one of the stimulating risks of being mortal," there is a great deal of reason for hope (Ray et al., 1993; Stroud and Friedman, 2001; Samuels and Wieteska, 2011; Wald, 2014).

A Closer Look

Bronchi

Bronchi are the large air passages in the respiratory tract that branch off from the trachea (windpipe) and extend into the lungs. They play a crucial role in conducting air to and from the lungs during breathing.

The bronchi are divided into two main branches: the left bronchus and the right bronchus. The right bronchus is wider, shorter, and more vertical than the left bronchus, which makes it more susceptible to the aspiration of foreign objects. Each main bronchus enters its respective lung and further divides into smaller branches called bronchioles.

The primary function of the bronchi is to conduct air from the trachea into the lungs and vice versa. As air passes through the bronchi, it is humidified, warmed, and filtered to prepare it for gas exchange in the alveoli (air sacs) of the lungs.

The bronchi, along with their smaller branches (bronchioles), form what is known as the bronchial tree. This branching network extends deep into the lungs, with each successive branch becoming smaller in diameter. This branching pattern allows for the distribution of air to all parts of the lungs.

The inner lining of the bronchi is composed of a mucous membrane that contains goblet cells, which secrete mucus. The mucus helps to trap and remove dust, bacteria, and other foreign particles from the airways. Additionally, the bronchial walls are lined with cilia, tiny hair-like structures that beat in coordinated waves to move the mucus and trapped particles upward towards the throat, where they can be swallowed or expelled by coughing.

Various conditions can affect the bronchi, including bronchitis (inflammation of the bronchi), bronchiectasis (permanent dilation of the bronchi), and bronchial asthma (chronic inflammation and constriction of the bronchi). These conditions can cause symptoms such as coughing, wheezing, shortness of breath, and chest tightness. Treatment typically involves medications to alleviate symptoms and manage underlying inflammation, as well as lifestyle changes to reduce triggers and promote lung health.

Summary

- Upper and lower airway infections encompass a spectrum of respiratory tract illnesses caused by various pathogens, including viruses, bacteria, and fungi.
- Obstructive sleep apnea (OSA) is a condition wherein the upper airway undergoes partial or total collapse during inspiration, resulting in a significant (greater than 50%) decrease in airflow.
- Laryngostenosis is a congenital or acquired narrowing of the airway, often termed subglottic stenosis. Although it may be congenital, it most commonly occurs after endotracheal intubation.
- The junction of the underside of the true vocal cords and infraglottic larynx is less acute in infants and small children than it is in older children and adults; this results in a less prominent normal subglottic "shoulder" effect.
- Upper airway infections encompass a spectrum of respiratory illnesses affecting the structures above the vocal cords, including the larynx, trachea, and bronchi.
- Croup is viral laryngotracheitis although the term is often used to describe a range of pathologies including laryngotracheobronchitis and "spasmodic croup" characterized by nocturnal paroxysms of stridor without fever or inflammation.
- The thin cartilage of the epiglottis is covered on its anterior (superior) surface by stratified squamous epithelium.
- Acute infection of the uvula may occur at any age and is most commonly caused by Group A Streptococcus, although other infective organisms that have been implicated include Hib.
- Lower respiratory trace infections (LRTIs) are among the most common infections in humans, comprising approximately 45% and 25% of all community-acquired and nosocomial infections, respectively.

References

1. Armon, K., Stephenson, T., Gabriel, V., et al. (2001). Determining the common medical presenting problems to an accident and emergency department. *Archives of Disease in Childhood*, *84*, 390–392.
2. Berman, S., & McIntosh, D. (1985). Selective primary health care: Strategies for control of disease in the developing world. XXI. Acute respiratory infections. *Reviews of Infectious Diseases*, *7*, 674–691.
3. Bjornson, C., Russell, K., Vandermeer, B., et al. (2013). Nebulized epinephrine for croup in children. *Cochrane Database of Systematic Reviews*, *10*, CD006619.
4. Brook, I. (2004). Microbiology and management of peritonsillar, retropharyngeal, and parapharyngeal abscesses. *Journal of Oral and Maxillofacial Surgery*, *62*, 1545–1550.
5. Cantrell, R. W., Bell, R. A., & Morioka, W. T. (1978). Acute epiglottitis: Intubation versus tracheostomy. *Laryngoscope*, *88*, 994–1005.
6. Cherry, J. D. (2008). Clinical practice. Croup. *New England Journal of Medicine*, *358*, 384–391.

7. Cherry, J. D. (2014). Croup (laryngitis, laryngotracheitis, spasmodic croup, laryngotracheobronchitis, bacterial tracheitis, and laryngotracheobronchopneumonitis) and epiglottitis (supraglottitis). In J. D. Cherry, G. J. Harrison, S. L. Kaplan, et al. (Eds.), *Feigin and Cherry's Textbook of Pediatric Infectious Diseases* (7th ed., pp. 241–260). Philadelphia, PA: Elsevier Saunders.

8. Christian, M. D., Poutanen, S. M., & Loutfy, M. R. (2004). Severe acute respiratory syndrome. *Clinical Infectious Diseases, 38*, 1420–1427.

9. Eckel, H. E., Widemann, B., Damm, M., et al. (1993). Airway endoscopy in the diagnosis and treatment of bacterial tracheitis in children. *International Journal of Pediatric Otorhinolaryngology, 27*, 147–157.

10. Esper, F., Weibel, C., & Ferguson, D. (2005). Evidence of a novel human coronavirus that is associated with respiratory tract disease in infants and young children. *Journal of Infectious Diseases, 191*, 492–498.

11. Goldstein, N. A., & Hammerschlag, M. R. (2014). Peritonsillar, retropharyngeal, and parapharyngeal abscesses. In J. D. Cherry, G. J. Harrison, S. L. Kaplan, et al. (Eds.), *Feigin and Cherry's Textbook of Pediatric Infectious Diseases* (7th ed., pp. 167–174). Philadelphia, PA: Elsevier Saunders.

12. Graf, J., & Stein, F. (2006). Tracheitis in pediatric patients. *Seminars in Pediatric Infectious Diseases, 17*, 11–13.

13. Heath, P. T., Booy, R., Azzopardi, H. J., et al. (2000). Antibody concentration and clinical protection after conjugate vaccination in the United Kingdom. *JAMA, 284*, 2334–2340.

14. Jenkins, I. A., & Saunders, M. (2009). Infections of the airway. *Pediatric Anesthesia, 19*, 118–130.

15. Jones, R., Santos, J. I., & Overall, J. C., Jr. (1979). Bacterial tracheitis. *JAMA, 242*, 721–726.

16. Kobasa, D., Takada, A., & Shinya, K. (2004). Enhanced virulence of influenza A viruses with the haemagglutinin of the 1918 pandemic virus. *Nature, 431*, 703–707.

17. Kotloff, K. L., & Wald, E. R. (1983). Uvulitis in children. *Pediatric Infectious Disease, 2*, 392–393.

18. Midwinter, K. I., Hodgson, D., & Yardley, M. (1999). Paediatric epiglottitis: The influence of the Haemophilus influenzae b vaccine, a ten year review in the Sheffield region. *Clinical Otolaryngology, 24*, 447–448.

19. Perez, D. R., Sorrell, E. M., & Donis, R. O. (2005). Avian influenza: An omnipresent pandemic threat. *Pediatric Infectious Disease Journal, 24*(Suppl.), S208–S216.

20. Peters, C. J., & Khan, A. S. (2002). Hantavirus pulmonary syndrome: The new American hemorrhagic fever. *Clinical Infectious Diseases, 34*, 1224–1231.

21. Philpott, C. M., Selvadurai, D., & Banerjee, A. R. (2004). Paediatric retropharyngeal abscess. *Journal of Laryngology and Otology, 118*, 919–926.

22. Ray, C. G. (2004). Influenza, respiratory syncytial virus, adenovirus, and other respiratory viruses. In K. J. Ryan & C. G. Ray (Eds.), *Sherris Medical Microbiology: An Introduction to Infectious Diseases* (pp. 495–512). New York: McGraw-Hill.

23. Ray, C. G., Holberg, C. J., & Minnich, L. L. (1993). Acute lower respiratory illnesses during the first three years of life: Potential roles for various etiologic agents. *Pediatric Infectious Disease Journal, 12*, 10–14.

24. Rihkanen, H., Rönkkö, E., Nieminen, T., et al. (2008). Respiratory viruses in laryngeal croup of young children. *Journal of Pediatrics, 152*, 661–665.

25. Russell, K. F., Liang, Y., O'Gorman, K., et al. (2011). Glucocorticoids for croup. *Cochrane Database of Systematic Reviews, 1*, CD001955.

26. Sdralis, T., & Berkowitz, R. G. (1996). Early adenotonsillectomy for relief of acute upper airway obstruction due to acute tonsillitis in children. *International Journal of Pediatric Otorhinolaryngology, 35*, 25–29.

27. Shah, R. K., Roberson, D. W., & Jones, D. T. (2004). Epiglottitis in the Haemophilus influenzae type b vaccine era: Changing trends. *Laryngoscope, 114*, 557–560.

28. Stroud, R. H., & Friedman, N. R. (2001). An update on inflammatory disorders of the pediatric airway: Epiglottitis, croup, and tracheitis. *American Journal of Otolaryngology, 22*, 268–275.

29. Tebruegge, M., Pantazidou, A., Thorburn, K., et al. (2009). Bacterial tracheitis: A multi-centre perspective. *Scandinavian Journal of Infectious Diseases, 41*, 548–557.

30. The child with breathing difficulties. (2011). In M. Samuels & S. Wieteska (Eds.), *Advanced Pediatric Life Support: The Practical Approach* (5th ed., pp. 70–90). Oxford: Blackwell.

31. Ungkanont, K., Yellon, R. F., Weissman, J. L., et al. (1995). Head and neck space infections in infants and children. *Otolaryngology Head and Neck Surgery, 112*, 375–382.

32. Wald, E. R. (2014). Uvulitis. In J. D. Cherry, G. J. Harrison, S. L. Kaplan, et al. (Eds.), *Feigin and Cherry's Textbook of Pediatric Infectious Diseases* (7th ed., pp. 165–166). Philadelphia, PA: Elsevier Saunders.

33. Williams, J. V., Harris, P. A., & Tollefson, S. J. (2004). Human metapneumovirus and lower respiratory tract disease in otherwise healthy infants and children. *New England Journal of Medicine, 350*, 443–450.

34. Johns MW. A new method for measuring daytime sleepiness: The Epworth sleepiness scale. Sleep. 1991;14(6):540-5

35. Netzer NC, Stoohs RA, Netzer CM, Clark K, Strohl KP. Using the Berlin Questionnaire To Identify Patients at Risk for the Sleep Apnea Syndrome. Annals of Internal Medicine. 1999 Oct 5;131(7):485-91

36. Vasu TS, Doghramji K, Cavallazzi R, Grewal R, Hirani A, Leiby B, et al. Obstructive Sleep Apnea Syndrome and Postoperative Complications: Clinical Use of the STOP-BANG Questionnaire. Archives of Otolaryngology–Head & Neck Surgery. 2010 Oct 18;136(10):1020-4

37. Loeffelholz, M.J.; Alland, D.; Butler-Wu, S.M.; Pandey, U.; Perno, C.F.; Nava, A.; Carroll, K.C.; Mostafa, H.; Davies, E.; McEwan, A.; et al. Multicenter Evaluation of the Cepheid Xpert Xpress SARS-CoV-2 Test. J. Clin. Microbiol. 2020, 58.

38. Fung, B.; Gopez, A.; Servellita, V.; Arevalo, S.; Ho, C.; Deucher, A.; Thornborrow, E.; Chiu, C.; Miller, S. Direct Comparison of SARS-CoV-2 Analytical Limits of Detection across Seven Molecular Assays. J. Clin. Microbiol. 2020, 58.

39. Cepheid. Xpert Xpress SARS-CoV-2/Flu/RSV: Instructions for Use; Cepheid: Sunnyvale, CA, USA, 2021. Available online: https://www.fda.gov/media/142437/download (accessed on 21 June 2021).

40. Hansen, G.; Marino, J.; Wang, Z.-X.; Beavis, K.G.; Rodrigo, J.; Labog, K.; Westblade, L.F.; Jin, R.;

Love, N.; Ding, K.; et al. Clinical performance of the point-of-care cobas Liat for detection of SARS-CoV-2 in 20 minutes: A multicenter study. J. Clin. Microbiol. 2020, 59.

41. Roche Molecular Systems. cobas SARS-CoV-2 & Influenza A/B Nucleic Acid Test for Use on the cobas Liat System: Instructions for Use; Roche Molecular Systems: South Branchburg, NJ, USA, 2020. Available online: https://www.fda.gov/media/142193/download (accessed on 21 June 2021).
42. Craney, A.R.; Velu, P.D.; Satlin, M.J.; Fauntleroy, K.A.; Callan, K.; Robertson, A.; La Spina, M.; Lei, B.; Chen, A.; Alston, T.; et al. Comparison of Two High-Throughput Reverse Transcription-PCR Systems for the Detection of Severe Acute Respiratory Syndrome Coronavirus 2. J. Clin. Microbiol. 2020, 58.
43. Roche Molecular Systems. cobas® SARS-CoV-2 Qualitative Assay for Use on the cobas® 6800/8800 Systems; Roche Molecular Systems: South Branchburg, NJ, USA, 2021. Available online: https://www.fda.gov/media/136049/download (accessed on 21 June 2021).
44. Roche Molecular Systems. cobas SARS CoV-2 Test: Instructions for Use; Roche Molecular Systems: South Branchburg, NJ, USA, 2021. Available online: https://www.fda.gov/media/136049/download (accessed on 30 June 2021).
45. Mesa Biotech. Accula SARS-Cov-2 Test: Instructions for Use; Mesa Biotech: San Diego, CA, USA, 2021; Available online: https://www.mesabiotech.com/wp-content/uploads/2021/02/LBL-60061-Accula-SARS-CoV-2-IFU-03FEB2021).pdf (accessed on 1 July 2021).
46. BioFire Diagnostics. BioFire Respiratory Panel 2.1-E.Z. (RP2.1-E.Z.): Instructions for Use; BioFire Diagnostics: Salt Lake City, UT, USA, 2020; Available online: https://docs.biofiredx.com/wp-content/uploads/BFR0001-0044-BioFire-RP2.1-EZ-Instructions-for-Use-EUA-1.pdf (accessed on 21 June 2021).
47. Bal, A.; Destras, G.; Gaymard, A.; Stefic, K.; Marlet, J.; Eymieux, S.; Regue, H.; Semanas, Q.; D'Aubarede, C.; Billaud, G.; et al. Two-step strategy for the identification of SARS-CoV-2 variant of concern 202012/01 and other variants with spike deletion H69–V70, France, August to December 2020. Eurosurveillance 2021, 26, 2100008.
48. Thermo Fisher Scientific, Inc. TaqPath COVID-19 Combo Kit and TaqPath COVID-19 Combo Kit Advanced Instructions for Use; Thermo Fisher Scientific, Inc.: Waltham, MA, USA, 2021. Available online: https://www.fda.gov/media/136112/download (accessed on 21 June 2021).
49. Yu, C.Y.; Chan, K.G.; Yean, C.Y.; Ang, G.Y. Nucleic Acid-Based Diagnostic Tests for the Detection SARS-CoV-2: An Update. Diagnostics 2021, 11, 53.
50. Abbott Diagnostics. Abbott RealTime SARS-CoV-2: Instructions for Use; Abbott Molecular, Inc.: Des Plaines, IL, USA, 2020. Available online: https://www.fda.gov/media/136258/download (accessed on 1 July 2021).
51. Perkin Elmer Genomics. PerkinElmer SARS-CoV-2 RT-qPCR: Emergency Use Authorization Summary; Perkin Elmer Genomics: Pittsburg, PA, USA, 2020. Available online: https://www.fda.gov/media/147547/download (accessed on 1 July 2021).
52. Huang, Z.; Tian, D.; Liu, Y.; Lin, Z.; Lyon, C.J.; Lai, W.; Fusco, D.; Drouin, A.; Yin, X.; Hu, T.; et al. Ultra-sensitive and high-throughput CRISPR-powered COVID-19 diagnosis. Biosens. Bioelectron. 2020, 164, 112316.

53. Hologic. Aptima® SARS-CoV-2 Assay (Panther® System): Instructions for Use; Hologic: San Diego, CA, USA, 2021; Available online: https://www.hologic.com/sites/default/files/2021-06/AW-21492-001_007_01.pdf (accessed on 1 July 2021).

54. Cue Health, Inc. Cue COVID-19 Test for Home and Over-the-Counter (OTC) Use; Cue Health, Inc.: San Diego, CA, USA, 2021. Available online: https://www.fda.gov/media/146470/download (accessed on 1 July 2021).

55. Seasun Biomaterials, Inc. AQ-TOP COVID-19 Rapid Detection Kit PLUS: Instructions for Use; Seasun Biomaterials, Inc.: Seoul, Korea, 2021. Available online: https://www.fda.gov/media/142800/download (accessed on 21 June 2021).

56. Pro-Lab Diagnostics. Pro-AmpRT SARS-CoV-2 Test. Available online: https://www.fda.gov/media/141149/download (accessed on 2 November 2020).

57. Rhoads, D.D.; Cherian, S.S.; Roman, K.; Stempak, L.M.; Schmotzer, C.L.; Sadri, N. Comparison of Abbott ID Now, DiaSorin Simplexa, and CDC FDA Emergency Use Authorization Methods for the Detection of SARS-CoV-2 from Nasopharyngeal and Nasal Swabs from Individuals Diagnosed with COVID-19. J. Clin. Microbiol. 2020, 58.

58. Harrington, A.; Cox, B.; Snowdon, J.; Bakst, J.; Ley, E.; Grajales, P.; Maggiore, J.; Kahn, S. Comparison of Abbott ID Now and Abbott m2000 Methods for the Detection of SARS-CoV-2 from Nasopharyngeal and Nasal Swabs from Symptomatic Patients. J. Clin. Microbiol. 2020, 58.

59. Abbott Diagnostics. ID NOW COVID-19: Instructions for Use; Abbott Diagnostics: Scarborough, ME, USA, 2020. Available online: https://www.fda.gov/media/136525/download (accessed on 21 June 2021).

60. Broughton, J.P.; Deng, X.; Yu, G.; Fasching, C.L.; Servellita, V.; Singh, J.; Miao, X.; Streithorst, J.A.; Granados, A.; Sotomayor-Gonzalez, A.; et al. CRISPR–Cas12-based detection of SARS-CoV-2. Nat. Biotechnol. 2020, 38, 870–874.

61. Sherlock Biosciences. Sherlock CRISPR SARS-CoV-2 kit: Instructions for Use; Sherlock Biosciences: Boston, MA, USA, 2021. Available online: https://www.fda.gov/media/137746/download (accessed on 21 June 2021).

62. U.S. Food and Drug Administration. Available online: http://www.fda.gov/ (accessed on 21 June 2021).

63. Curti, L.; Primost, I.; Valla, S.; Alegre, D.I.; Perglione, C.O.; Repizo, G.; Lara, J.; Parcerisa, I.; Palacios, A.; Llases, M.; et al. Evaluation of a Lyophilized CRISPR-Cas12 Assay for a Sensitive, Specific, and Rapid Detection of SARS-CoV-2. Viruses 2021, 13, 420.

64. Webber, D.M.; Wallace, M.A.; Burnham, C.A.; Anderson, N.W. Evaluation of the BioFire FilmArray Pneumonia Panel for Detection of Viral and Bacterial Pathogens in Lower Respiratory Tract Specimens in the Setting of a Tertiary Care Academic Medical Center. J. Clin. Microbiol. 2020, 58, e00343-20.

65. Rytter, H.; Jamet, A.; Coureuil, M.; Charbit, A.; Ramond, E. Which Current and Novel Diagnostic Avenues for Bacterial Respiratory Diseases? Front. Microbiol. 2020, 11, 616971.

66. Leland, D.S.; Ginocchio, C.C. Role of Cell Culture for Virus Detection in the Age of Technology. Clin. Microbiol. Rev. 2007, 20, 49–78.

67. Couturier, M.R.; Bard, J.D. Direct-from-Specimen Pathogen Identification: Evolution of Syndromic Panels. Clin. Lab. Med. 2019, 39, 433–451.

68. WHO The Global Health Observatory. Global Health Estimates: Leading Causes of Death. Cause-Specific Mortality, 2000–2019. Available online: https://www.who.int/data/gho/data/themes/mortality-and-global-health-estimates/ghe-leading-causes-of-death (accessed on 29 July 2022).
69. WHO The Global Health Observatory. Global Health Estimates: Leading Causes of DALYs. Disease Burden, 2000–2019. Available online: https://www.who.int/data/gho/data/themes/mortality-and-global-health-estimates/global-health-estimates-leading-causes-of-dalys (accessed on 29 July 2022).
70. The World Bank World Bank Country and Lending Groups. Country Classification. Available online: https://datahelpdesk.worldbank.org/knowledgebase/articles/906519-world-bank-country-and-lending-groups (accessed on 29 July 2022).
71. Simoes, E.A.F.; Cherian, T.; Chow, J.; Shahid-Salles, S.A.; Laxminarayan, R.; John, T.J. Acute Respiratory Infections in Children; Jamison, D.T., Breman, J.G., Measham, A.R., Alleyne, G., Claeson, M., Evans, D.B., Jha, P., Mills, A., Musgrove, P., Eds.; The International Bank for Reconstruction and Development/The World Bank: Washington, DC, USA, 2006; ISBN 0-8213-6179-1.
72. WHO International Statistical Classification of Diseases and Related Health Problems (ICD). Available online: https://www.who.int/standards/classifications/classification-of-diseases (accessed on 29 July 2022).
73. Grief, S.N. Upper Respiratory Infections. Prim. Care 2013, 40, 757–770.
74. Miller, J.M.; Binnicker, M.J.; Campbell, S.; Carroll, K.C.; Chapin, K.C.; Gilligan, P.H.; Gonzalez, M.D.; Jerris, R.C.; Kehl, S.C.; Patel, R.; et al. A Guide to Utilization of the Microbiology Laboratory for Diagnosis of Infectious Diseases: 2018 Update by the Infectious Diseases Society of America and the American Society for Microbiology. Clin. Infect. Dis. Off. Publ. Infect. Dis. Soc. Am. 2018, 67, 813–816.
75. Flores, A.R.; Caserta, M.T. Pharyngitis. In Mandell, Douglas, and Bennett's Principles and Practice of Infectious Diseases; Elsevier: Amsterdam, The Netherlands, 2015; pp. 753–759.e2.
76. Arnold, J.C.; Nizet, V. Pharyngitis. In Principles and Practice of Pediatric Infectious Diseases; Elsevier: Amsterdam, The Netherlands, 2018; pp. 202–208.e2.
77. Mustafa, Z.; Ghaffari, M. Diagnostic Methods, Clinical Guidelines, and Antibiotic Treatment for Group A Streptococcal Pharyngitis: A Narrative Review. Front. Cell. Infect. Microbiol. 2020, 10, 563627.
78. Wolford, R.W.; Goyal, A.; Belgam Syed, S.Y.; Schaefer, T.J. Pharyngitis; StatPearls Publishing: Treasure Island, FL, USA, 2022.
79. Alcaide, M.L.; Bisno, A.L. Pharyngitis and Epiglottitis. Infect. Dis. Clin. N. Am. 2007, 21, 449–469.
80. Weber, R. Pharyngitis. Prim. Care 2014, 41, 91–98.
81. Anderson, J.; Paterek, E. Tonsillitis; StatPearls Publishing: Treasure Island, FL, USA, 2022.
82. Bartlett, A.; Bola, S.; Williams, R. Acute Tonsillitis and Its Complications: An Overview. J. R. Nav. Med. Serv. 2015, 101, 69–73.
83. Tristram, D. Laryngitis, Tracheitis, Epiglottitis, and Bronchiolitis: Sore Throat, Change in Voice, Feverora Wheezing Infant in Respiratory Distress. In Introduction to Clinical Infectious Diseases: A Problem-Based Approach; Springer: Cham, Switzerland, 2018; pp. 75–85.

84. Caserta, M.T. Acute Laryngitis. In Mandell, Douglas, and Bennett's Principles and Practice of Infectious Diseases; Elsevier: Amsterdam, The Netherlands, 2015; pp. 760–761.e1.

85. Blot, M.; Bonniaud-Blot, P.; Favrolt, N.; Bonniaud, P.; Chavanet, P.; Piroth, L. Update on Childhood and Adult Infectious Tracheitis. Med. Mal. Infect. 2017, 47, 443–452.

86. Bower, J.; McBride, J.T. Croup in Children (Acute Laryngotracheobronchitis). In Mandell, Douglas, and Bennett's Principles and Practice of Infectious Diseases; Elsevier: Amsterdam, The Netherlands, 2015; pp. 762–766.e1.

87. Woodfork, K. Bronchitis. In xPharm: The Comprehensive Pharmacology Reference; Elsevier: Amsterdam, The Netherlands, 2007; pp. 1–13.

88. Walsh, E.E. Acute Bronchitis. In Mandell, Douglas, and Bennett's Principles and Practice of Infectious Diseases; Elsevier: Amsterdam, The Netherlands, 2015; pp. 806–809.e1.

89. de Conto, F.; Conversano, F.; Medici, M.C.; Ferraglia, F.; Pinardi, F.; Arcangeletti, M.C.; Chezzi, C.; Calderaro, A. Epidemiology of Human Respiratory Viruses in Children with Acute Respiratory Tract Infection in a 3-Year Hospital-Based Survey in Northern Italy. Diagn. Microbiol. Infect. Dis. 2019, 94, 260–267.

90. Rossi, G.A.; Medici, M.C.; Merolla, R. Incidence of Respiratory Syncytial Virus Positivity in Young Italian Children Referred to the Emergency Departments for Lower Respiratory Tract Infection over Two Consecutive Epidemic Seasons. Infection 2005, 33, 18–24.

91. Segal, L.N.; Weiden, M.D.; Horowitz, H.W. Acute Exacerbations of Chronic Obstructive Pulmonary Disease. In Mandell, Douglas, and Bennett's Principles and Practice of Infectious Diseases; Elsevier: Amsterdam, The Netherlands, 2015; pp. 810–817.e3.

92. Medici, M.C.; Arcangeletti, M.C.; Merolla, R.; Chezzi, C. Incidence of Respiratory Syncytial Virus Infection in Infants and Young Children Referred to the Emergency Departments for Lower Respiratory Tract Diseases in Italy. Acta Biomed. 2004, 75, 26–33.

93. WHO Pneumonia. Available online: https://www.who.int/news-room/fact-sheets/detail/pneumonia (accessed on 29 July 2022).

94. Fauci, A.S. Harrison's Principles of Internal Medicine; McGraw-Hill Education: New York, NY, USA, 2015; ISBN 0071802134.

95. Lanks, C.W.; Musani, A.I.; Hsia, D.W. Community-Acquired Pneumonia and Hospital-Acquired Pneumonia. Med. Clin. N. Am. 2019, 103, 487–501.

96. Calderaro, A.; Buttrini, M.; Montecchini, S.; Piccolo, G.; Martinelli, M.; Dell'Anna, M.L.; di Maio, A.; Arcangeletti, M.C.; Maccari, C.; de Conto, F.; et al. Detection of SARS-CoV-2 and Other Infectious Agents in Lower Respiratory Tract Samples Belonging to Patients Admitted to Intensive Care Units of a Tertiary-Care Hospital, Located in an Epidemic Area, during the Italian Lockdown. Microorganisms 2021, 9, 185.

97. Weinberger, S.E.; Cockrill, B.A.; Mandel, J. Principles of Pulmonary Medicine E-Book; Elsevier Health Sciences: Amsterdam, The Netherlands, 2017; ISBN 0323523722.

98. Albano, D.; Bertagna, F.; Alongi, P.; Baldari, S.; Baldoncini, A.; Bartolomei, M.; Boccaletto, F.; Boero, M.; Borsatti, E.; Bruno, A.; et al. Prevalence of Interstitial Pneumonia Suggestive of COVID-19 at (18)F-FDG PET/CT in Oncological Asymptomatic Patients in a High Prevalence Country during Pandemic Period: A National Multi-Centric Retrospective Study. Eur. J. Nucl. Med. Mol. Imaging 2021, 48, 2871–2882.

99. Das, S.; Dunbar, S.; Tang, Y.-W. Laboratory Diagnosis of Respiratory Tract Infections in Children-the State of the Art. Front. Microbiol. 2018, 9, 2478.

100. Murdoch, D.R.; Werno, A.M.; Jennings, L.C. Microbiological Diagnosis of Respiratory Illness: Recent Advances. In Kendig's Disorders of the Respiratory Tract in Children; Elsevier: Amsterdam, The Netherlands, 2019; pp. 396–405.e3.

101. Campbell, S.; Forbes, B.A. The Clinical Microbiology Laboratory in the Diagnosis of Lower Respiratory Tract Infections. J. Clin. Microbiol. 2011, 49, S30–S33.

102. Ramanan, P.; Bryson, A.L.; Binnicker, M.J.; Pritt, B.S.; Patel, R. Syndromic Panel-Based Testing in Clinical Microbiology. Clin. Microbiol. Rev. 2018, 31, e00024-17.

103. Leber, A.L. Clinical Microbiology Procedures Handbook; John Wiley & Sons: New York, NY, USA, 2020; ISBN 1555818811.

104. Centers for Disease Control and Prevention. Specimen Collection Guidelines; Centers for Disease Control and Prevention: Atlanta, GA, USA, 2020.

105. Charalambous, B.M.; Batt, S.L.; Peek, A.C.; Mwerinde, H.; Sam, N.; Gillespie, S.H. Quantitative Validation of Media for Transportation and Storage of Streptococcus Pneumoniae. J. Clin. Microbiol. 2003, 41, 5551–5556.

106. Poulsen, C.S.; Kaas, R.S.; Aarestrup, F.M.; Pamp, S.J. Standard Sample Storage Conditions Have an Impact on Inferred Microbiome Composition and Antimicrobial Resistance Patterns. Microbiol. Spectr. 2021, 9, e0138721.

107. Skevaki, C.L.; Papadopoulos, N.G.; Tsakris, A.; Johnston, S.L. Microbiologic Diagnosis of Respiratory Illness: Practical Applications. In Kendig & Chernick's Disorders of the Respiratory Tract in Children; Elsevier: Amsterdam, The Netherlands, 2012; pp. 399–423.

108. Cooley, L.; Dendle, C.; Wolf, J.; Teh, B.W.; Chen, S.C.; Boutlis, C.; Thursky, K.A. Consensus Guidelines for Diagnosis, Prophylaxis and Management of P Neumocystis Jirovecii Pneumonia in Patients with Haematological and Solid Malignancies, 2014. Intern. Med. J. 2014, 44, 1350–1363.

109. Falsey, A.R.; Walsh, E.E. Novel Coronavirus and Severe Acute Respiratory Syndrome. Lancet 2003, 361, 1312–1313.

110. Ksiazek, T.G.; Erdman, D.; Goldsmith, C.S.; Zaki, S.R.; Peret, T.; Emery, S.; Tong, S.; Urbani, C.; Comer, J.A.; Lim, W.; et al. A Novel Coronavirus Associated with Severe Acute Respiratory Syndrome. N. Engl. J. Med. 2003, 348, 1953–1966.

111. Goldsmith, C.S.; Miller, S.E. Modern Uses of Electron Microscopy for Detection of Viruses. Clin. Microbiol. Rev. 2009, 22, 552–563.

112. Zhang, Y.; Hung, T.; Song, J.; He, J. Electron Microscopy: Essentials for Viral Structure, Morphogenesis and Rapid Diagnosis. Sci. China Life Sci. 2013, 56, 421–430.

113. LaSala, P.R.; Bufton, K.K.; Ismail, N.; Smith, M.B. Prospective Comparison of R-Mix Shell Vial System with Direct Antigen Tests and Conventional Cell Culture for Respiratory Virus Detection. J. Clin. Virol. Off. Publ. Pan Am. Soc. Clin. Virol. 2007, 38, 210–216.

114. Ginocchio, C.C. Detection of Respiratory Viruses Using Non-Molecular Based Methods. J. Clin. Virol. Off. Publ. Pan Am. Soc. Clin. Virol. 2007, 40 (Suppl. S1), S11–S14.

115. Hematian, A.; Sadeghifard, N.; Mohebi, R.; Taherikalani, M.; Nasrolahi, A.; Amraei, M.; Ghafourian,

S. Traditional and Modern Cell Culture in Virus Diagnosis. Osong Public Health Res. Perspect. 2016, 7, 77–82.

116. Slinger, R.; Milk, R.; Gaboury, I.; Diaz-Mitoma, F. Evaluation of the QuickLab RSV Test, a New Rapid Lateral-Flow Immunoassay for Detection of Respiratory Syncytial Virus Antigen. J. Clin. Microbiol. 2004, 42, 3731–3733.

117. Chartrand, C.; Tremblay, N.; Renaud, C.; Papenburg, J. Diagnostic Accuracy of Rapid Antigen Detection Tests for Respiratory Syncytial Virus Infection: Systematic Review and Meta-Analysis. J. Clin. Microbiol. 2015, 53, 3738–3749.

118. WHO. Antigen-Detection in the Diagnosis of SARS-CoV-2 Infection; WHO: Geneva, Switzerland, 2021.

119. Loens, K.; van Heirstraeten, L.; Malhotra-Kumar, S.; Goossens, H.; Ieven, M. Optimal Sampling Sites and Methods for Detection of Pathogens Possibly Causing Community-Acquired Lower Respiratory Tract Infections. J. Clin. Microbiol. 2009, 47, 21–31.

120. Chkhaidze, I.; Manjavidze, N.; Nemsadze, K. Serodiagnosis of Acute Respiratory Infections in Children in Georgia. Indian J. Pediatr. 2006, 73, 569–572.

121. Kuypers, J.; Wright, N.; Ferrenberg, J.; Huang, M.-L.; Cent, A.; Corey, L.; Morrow, R. Comparison of Real-Time PCR Assays with Fluorescent-Antibody Assays for Diagnosis of Respiratory Virus Infections in Children. J. Clin. Microbiol. 2006, 44, 2382–2388.

122. File, T.M.J.; Tan, J.S.; Plouffe, J.F. The Role of Atypical Pathogens: Mycoplasma Pneumoniae, Chlamydia Pneumoniae, and Legionella Pneumophila in Respiratory Infection. Infect. Dis. Clin. N. Am. 1998, 12, 569–592.

123. Saikku, P. Diagnosis of Chlamydia Pneumoniae. Clin. Microbiol. Infect. Off. Publ. Eur. Soc. Clin. Microbiol. Infect. Dis. 1998, 4 (Suppl. S4), S7–S13.

124. Graham, F.F.; Hales, S.; White, P.S.; Baker, M.G. Review Global Seroprevalence of Legionellosis—A Systematic Review and Meta-Analysis. Sci. Rep. 2020, 10, 7337.

125. WHO. Laboratory Manual for the Diagnosis of Wooping Cough Caused by Bordetella Pertussis/ Bordetella Parapertussis; WHO: Geneva, Switzerland, 2014.

126. Loeffelholz, M.; Chonmaitree, T. Advances in Diagnosis of Respiratory Virus Infections. Int. J. Microbiol. 2010, 2010, 126049.

127. WHO. Clinical Care for Severe Acute Respiratory Infection; WHO: Geneva, Switzerland, 2022.

128. Messacar, K.; Parker, S.K.; Todd, J.K.; Dominguez, S.R. Implementation of Rapid Molecular Infectious Disease Diagnostics: The Role of Diagnostic and Antimicrobial Stewardship. J. Clin. Microbiol. 2017, 55, 715–723.

129. Dien Bard, J.; McElvania, E. Panels and Syndromic Testing in Clinical Microbiology. Clin. Lab. Med. 2020, 40, 393–420.

130. Hanson, K.E.; Couturier, M.R. Multiplexed Molecular Diagnostics for Respiratory, Gastrointestinal, and Central Nervous System Infections. Clin. Infect. Dis. Off. Publ. Infect. Dis. Soc. Am. 2016, 63, 1361–1367.

131. Zanella, M.-C.; Meylan, P.; Kaiser, L. Syndromic Panels or "Panel Syndrome"? A Perspective through the Lens of Respiratory Tract Infections. Clin. Microbiol. Infect. Off. Publ. Eur. Soc. Clin. Microbiol. Infect. Dis. 2020, 26, 665–668.

132. Fox, A.S.; Rao, S.N. Syndromic Testing for the Diagnosis of Infectious Diseases: The Right Test If Used for the Right Patient. J. Antimicrob. Chemother. 2021, 76, iii2–iii3.

133. Cassidy, H.; van Genne, M.; Lizarazo-Forero, E.; Niesters, H.G.M.; Gard, L. Evaluation of the QIAstat-Dx RP2.0 and the BioFire FilmArray RP2.1 for the Rapid Detection of Respiratory Pathogens Including SARS-CoV-2. Front. Microbiol. 2022, 13, 854209.

134. Lebourgeois, S.; Storto, A.; Gout, B.; le Hingrat, Q.; Ardila Tjader, G.; del Carmen Cerdan, M.; English, A.; Pareja, J.; Love, J.; Houhou-Fidouh, N.; et al. Performance Evaluation of the QIAstat-Dx® Respiratory SARS-CoV-2 Panel. Int. J. Infect. Dis. 2021, 107, 179–181.

135. Yu, C.Y.; Chan, K.G.; Yean, C.Y.; Ang, G.Y. Nucleic Acid-Based Diagnostic Tests for the Detection SARS-CoV-2: An Update. Diagnostics 2021, 11, 53.

136. Cassidy, H.; van Genne, M.; Lizarazo-Forero, E.; Gard, L.; Niesters, H.G.M. A Discussion of Syndromic Molecular Testing for Clinical Care. J. Antimicrob. Chemother. 2021, 76, iii58–iii66.

137. Popowitch, E.B.; O'Neill, S.S.; Miller, M.B. Comparison of the Biofire FilmArray RP, Genmark ESensor RVP, Luminex XTAG RVPv1, and Luminex XTAG RVP Fast Multiplex Assays for Detection of Respiratory Viruses. J. Clin. Microbiol. 2013, 51, 1528–1533.

138. Lee, S.H.; Ruan, S.-Y.; Pan, S.-C.; Lee, T.-F.; Chien, J.-Y.; Hsueh, P.-R. Performance of a Multiplex PCR Pneumonia Panel for the Identification of Respiratory Pathogens and the Main Determinants of Resistance from the Lower Respiratory Tract Specimens of Adult Patients in Intensive Care Units. J. Microbiol. Immunol. Infect. 2019, 52, 920–928.

139. Murphy, C.N.; Fowler, R.; Balada-Llasat, J.M.; Carroll, A.; Stone, H.; Akerele, O.; Buchan, B.; Windham, S.; Hopp, A.; Ronen, S.; et al. Multicenter Evaluation of the BioFire FilmArray Pneumonia/Pneumonia Plus Panel for Detection and Quantification of Agents of Lower Respiratory Tract Infection. J. Clin. Microbiol. 2020, 58, e00128-20.

140. Buchan, B.W.; Windham, S.; Balada-Llasat, J.-M.; Leber, A.; Harrington, A.; Relich, R.; Murphy, C.; Dien Bard, J.; Naccache, S.; Ronen, S.; et al. Practical Comparison of the BioFire FilmArray Pneumonia Panel to Routine Diagnostic Methods and Potential Impact on Antimicrobial Stewardship in Adult Hospitalized Patients with Lower Respiratory Tract Infections. J. Clin. Microbiol. 2020, 58, e00135-20.

141. Tazi, S.; Kabbaj, H.; Zirar, J.; Zouaki, A.; el Amin, G.; el Himeur, O.; Seffar, M. Comparative Performance Evaluation of FilmArray BioFire RP2.1 and MAScIR 2.0 Assays for SARS-CoV-2 Detection. Adv. Virol. 2022, 2022, 4510900.

Chapter 5

PEDIATRIC ASTHMA

Contents

Introduction

Edema, bronchospasm, and increased mucus production cause recurrent episodes of airflow obstruction in asthma, a chronic inflammatory disease of the airways. Often linked to eczema (atopic dermatitis) and seasonal allergies (allergic rhinitis), these three disorders together make up the atopic triad.

Asthma patients may have a variety of respiratory symptoms, including coughing, chest tightness, wheezing, and shortness of breath. The frequency and intensity of symptoms can vary greatly, but untreated asthma and severe flare-ups can result in fatal respiratory failure.

Information on the natural history, risk factors, and patterns of disease occurrence—as well as how therapy affects the course of the illness—is necessary for the prevention and management of asthma. A significant portion of this data is gathered via epidemiological research. The scientific techniques used to investigate the prevalence of disease in human populations are known as epidemiology. While it has proven challenging to define this field precisely, epidemiology differs from traditional clinical research in that it focuses on human populations rather than patient groups. It is possible to think of epidemiology as having two separate parts: the identification of risk factors for disease and the description of disease occurrence, usually by person, place, or time. Health services research and the evaluation of therapeutic modalities are two more uses for experimental study designs, such as the controlled clinical trial. A population's disease occurrence is described by its incidence, mortality, and prevalence rates. The ratio of new cases to the population at risk is known as the incidence rate for a given time period. Since it is hard to find new cases of asthma, incidence data are not easily accessible. Similar ratios apply to mortality, where the numerator is the total number of deaths. Cause-specific mortality, including mortality specific to asthma, is monitored closely in the majority of countries. The most popular measure of the occurrence of asthma is prevalence, which can be found through questionnaires in surveys. Prevalence represents the natural history of a disease since it is based on both the incidence rate and the length of the illness. Conditions like asthma that last longer but have a lower case-fatality rate are more common.

Disease prevalence is determined by cross-sectional surveys, such as the International Study of Asthma and Allergy in Children (ISAAC). Epidemiologists use case-control and cohort research to find risk factors for disease. In a case-control design, a suitable control group and a case series, such as individuals with asthma, are identified. Then, the proportions of cases and controls exposed to the relevant risk factor(s) are compared. Cohort design involves tracking study participants over time and making observations about natural history or risk factors for disease. For instance, tracking individuals with and without atopy and identifying any new cases of asthma in the two groups could be part of a cohort study on atopy and asthma. One famous example of a prospective cohort study is the respiratory health study conducted in Tucson, Arizona, on children. In this study, a cohort of infants was enrolled from birth, and the incidence of respiratory illnesses and potential asthma risk factors were prospectively recorded. Important information about the prevalence, causes, and natural history of childhood asthma has been made available by these epidemiological methods. The clinical series data, which are typically based on sick or receiving medical care children, are supplemented by the epidemiological data. This chapter examines the epidemiology of childhood asthma and highlights the growing body of research on the disorder's natural history and risk factors.

Orientation and Directional Terms

Term	Definition	Illustration
Chest tightness	Chest tightness is a common symptom of asthma in children, and can be present with or without other symptoms.	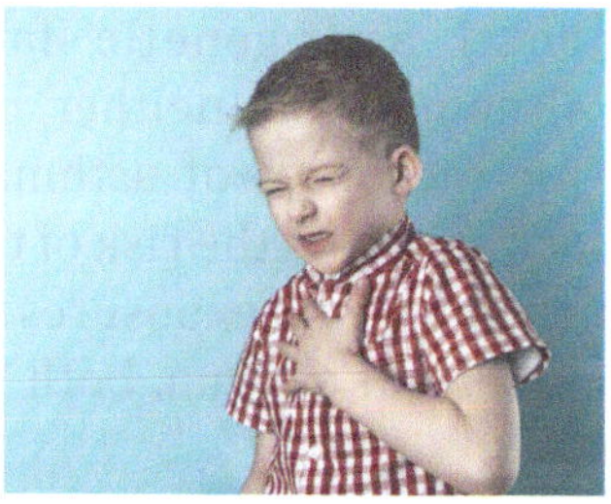
Childhood Asthma	Childhood asthma is a chronic lung disease that causes a child's airways to become inflamed and narrow when exposed to triggers.	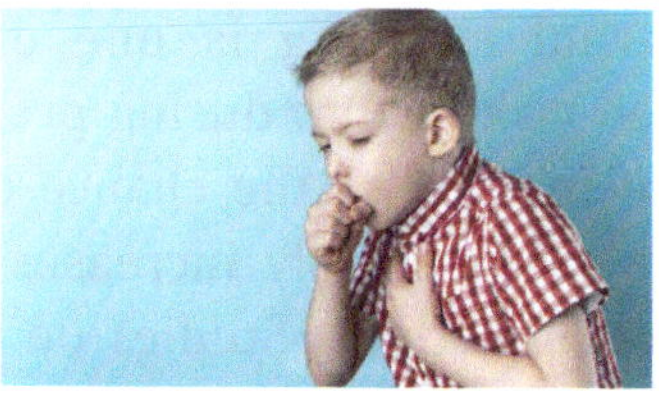
Coughing	Coughing is a common symptom of asthma in children, and is usually dry and hacking. It's often most noticeable at night, in the early morning, or after exercise, but can also be triggered by cold air, excitement, or laughing.	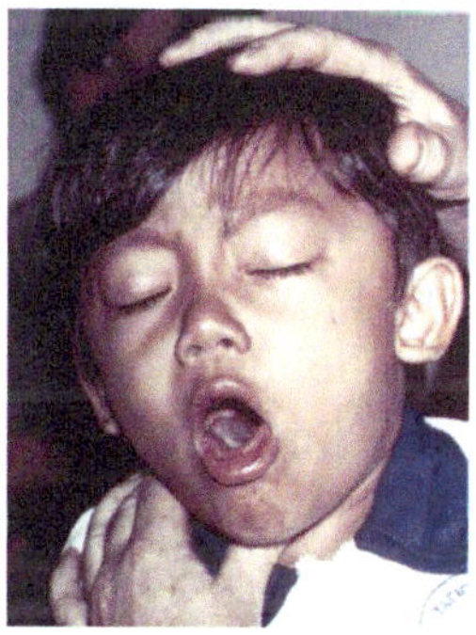
Shortness of breath	Shortness of breath is a classic symptom of pediatric asthma, which causes the airways to swell and narrow.	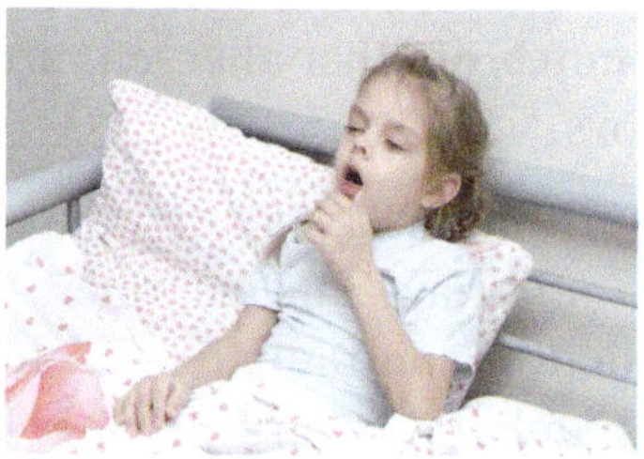
Wheezing	Wheezing is a common symptom of asthma in children under five years old. It can sound like a whistling or wheezing when breathing out.	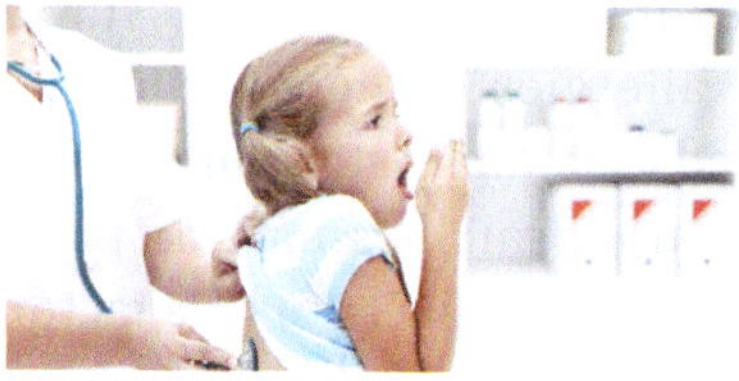

5.1. Etiology of Asthma

Asthma's precise etiology is still unknown and seems to be complex. It appears that environmental and genetic factors work together. Although it is neither required nor sufficient for the onset of asthma, a positive family history increases the risk of the condition. Multiple environmental exposures are linked to the development of asthma, both in utero and in children.

Maternal smoking is one of the well-researched risk factors during pregnancy, and it does seem to raise the chance of wheezing as a child and probably increases the chance of developing asthma. Studies on these other suggested prenatal risk factors have yielded less conclusive results. These include maternal diet and nutrition, stress, use of antibiotics, and cesarean delivery.

Numerous exposures during childhood have also been the focus of study. Exposure to tobacco smoke is known to aggravate asthma in those who already have a diagnosis and appears to raise the chance of developing the condition. Air pollution and other allergens such as mold, animals, mites, or other allergens are additional risk factors.

Many other risk factors that have been proposed still have unclear roles, and studies are frequently contradictory or inconclusive. There is debate regarding the benefits of breastfeeding and the need to stay away from dietary allergies while nursing. It has been suggested that family structure and size are risk factors; larger families may be protective, but birth order is less likely to be a factor. Although there is disagreement over the increased prevalence, there is a correlation between low socioeconomic status and higher morbidity. Antibiotic use and viral lower respiratory infections have been linked to wheezing in early childhood, but it is unclear how they contribute to persistent asthma. Asthma and the respiratory syncytial virus (RSV) have a specific correlation, but not a direct one. It is known that viral respiratory tract infections can exacerbate pre-existing asthma.

5.2. Problems in the Epidemiological Investigation of Childhood Asthma

In the framework of an epidemiological investigation, asthma in study participants can be identified using clinical, physiological, and questionnaire approaches. Regardless of the method used to diagnose the condition, the study of childhood asthma has been hampered by the difficulty of operationally defining the illness. Although individual authors and expert groups have produced definitions, none of them have produced precise, practical standards for separating children with asthma from those who do not. Indeed, participants in the Ciba Study Group on the Identification of Asthma in 1971 concluded that the information available at the time was insufficient to define asthma in a way that would satisfy people; newer data does not change this conclusion. We are still a long way from having definition-based criteria for clinical or research purposes, despite the fact that the definition of asthma has changed to include modern concepts of pathogenesis. Furthermore, any boundary along this spectrum is arbitrary because the asthma syndrome ranges in severity from intermittent and mild to continuous and severe.

Asthma and other major diseases linked to airflow obstruction are currently referred to using terminology developed in 1959 by attendees of a Ciba symposium. This group defined asthma by emphasizing different physiological dysfunction and addressed diseases that affect adults, such as emphysema, chronic airflow obstruction, asthma, and chronic bronchitis (Table 5.1). More recent definitions have included inflammation as the hallmark of pathogenesis and have added hyperresponsiveness of the airways as a fundamental abnormality. These definitions are conceptually appropriate for children, even though they were not created especially for childhood asthma, and they are used in research. However, the lack of useful, non-invasive markers of inflammation and the difficulty in assessing ventilatory function and airway responsiveness in younger children make their application challenging.

Table 5.1. *Asthma Definitions*

Asthma is defined as severe if it was treated with:
Asthma which requires treatment with guidelines suggested medications for GINA steps 4–5 asthma (high dose ICS# and LABA or leukotriene modifier/theophylline) for the previous year or systemic CS for ≥50% of the previous year to prevent it from becoming "uncontrolled" or which remains "uncontrolled" despite this therapy
Asthma is defined as uncontrolled when it has the following signs and symptoms: a) Poor symptom control: ACQ consistently ≥ 1.5, ACT <20 (or "not well-controlled" by NAEPP/GINA guidelines) b) Frequent severe exacerbations: Two or more bursts of systemic CS (≥3 days each) in the previous year c) Serious exacerbations: At least one hospitalization, ICU stay or mechanical ventilation in the previous year d) Airflow limitation: After appropriate bronchodilator withhold FEV1 <80% predicted (despite reduced FEV1/FVC, defined as less than the lower limit of normal)
#The definition of high dose inhaled corticosteroids (ICS) is age-specific.
GINA, Global Initiative for Asthma; LABA, long-acting β2-agonists; CS, corticosteroids; ACQ, Asthma Control Questionnaire; ACT, Asthma Control Test; ICU, Intensive Care unit; NAEPP, National Asthma Education and Prevention Program; FEV1, forced expiratory volume in 1 s.

Source: Ragnoli B, Pochetti P, Raie A and Malerba M (2021) Interrelationship Between Obstructive Sleep Apnea Syndrome and Severe Asthma: From Endo-Phenotype to Clinical Aspects. Front. Med. 8:640636. doi: 10.3389/fmed.2021.640636.

5.2.1. Questionnaires

In epidemiological studies of childhood asthma, questionnaires are the most common method of classifying subjects as affected because children may not cooperate well enough for physiological testing. This is due to practical concerns. Numerous instruments, some specifically designed for children, have been developed. The American Thoracic Society created one of the first standardized questionnaires for children's respiratory symptoms. While some of the questions are related to asthma, the questionnaire does not fully cover the symptoms of this condition. It does contain questions on common respiratory ailments and symptoms. More tailored instruments have been created specifically for childhood asthma. For the ISAAC study, a quick, uniform tool was created. The main symptoms of asthma and other allergy disorders are covered in this questionnaire. The three main questions about asthma are about wheezing, nocturnal coughing, and asthma reports. Additionally, a video version was created and verified using the traditional instrument.

Epidemiologists have regarded a parent's report of asthma, with or without a medical professional's diagnosis, as affirmative evidence in numerous questionnaire-based studies. The choice of diagnostic labels made by individual doctors and patterns of medical care utilization have an impact on this kind of estimate of the occurrence of the disease. Clinicians and epidemiologists may not use the same terminology when referring to children; this may have been especially true in the past when there was a widespread reluctance to use the term "asthma." In the late 1970s, Taussig et al. asked doctors in Tucson, Arizona, about the criteria they used to diagnose children with chronic bronchitis. The majority of the doctors placed a high value on allergies and wheezing, and they routinely treated children with chronic bronchitis with bronchodilator therapy. The authors concluded that there is a significant overlap between childhood asthma and chronic bronchitis diagnoses. In England, around the same period, Speight et al. found children who had a history of wheezing episodes, and then used bronchial challenge testing with histamine, school absenteeism, and treatment responses to confirm the wheezing's clinical significance. Just a small percentage of the wheezing children had received an asthma diagnosis, despite the fact that the majority had been examined by a doctor. However, many developed nations have likely moved past these outdated labeling practices.

The way that questionnaire-based prevalence estimates are worded may have an impact on asthma prevalence estimates. Physician-diagnosed asthma is less common than wheezing for people of all ages, and approximately half of those with a diagnosis have active asthma.

Table 5.2. *Epidemiological Definition of Asthma, Allergic Rhinitis (AR) and Atopic Dermatitis (AD)*

Allergic Conditions	
Wheezing ever-in-a-lifetime	Has your child ever had wheezing in his life?
Current asthma *	Has your child had wheezing during the last 12 months in the absence of a cold?
Self-reported diagnosed asthma	Has your child ever had asthma?
AR symptoms ever-in-a-lifetime	Has your child ever had a runny nose in the absence of a cold?
Current AR *	Has your child had a runny nose without a cold during last 12 months?
Self-reported diagnosed AR	Has your child ever had allergic rhinitis?
AD symptoms ever-in-a-lifetime	Has your child ever had an itchy rash which was coming and going for at least six months?
Current AD *	Has your child had an itchy rash which was coming and going during last 12 months?
Self-reported diagnosed AD	Has your child ever had atopic dermatitis?

* Current symptoms represent the self-reported prevalence of the disease. AR—allergic rhinitis, AD—atopic dermatitis.

Source: Topalušić I, Stipić Marković A, Artuković M, Dodig S, Bucić L, Lugović Mihić L. Divergent Trends in the Prevalence of Children's Asthma, Rhinitis, and Atopic Dermatitis and Environmental Influences in the Urban Setting of Zagreb, Croatia. Children. 2022; 9(12):1788. https://doi.org/10.3390/children9121788.

The prevalence estimates vary by age as well; in contrast to the pattern at older ages, the youngest age group reports fewer doctor-diagnosed diseases concerning nonspecific wheezing.

Patients who wheeze when prompted by a respiratory infection in infants and early children have been referred to as having "wheezy bronchitis" or "asthmatic bronchitis," but these labels do not distinguish these patients from those who have been diagnosed with asthma. Williams and McNicol, for instance, demonstrated that children with asthma and wheezy bronchitis had similar natural histories of their conditions. As a result, to fully evaluate the prevalence of asthma, a questionnaire needs to contain all labels that doctors may use locally. However, due to the imperfect sensitivity of questionnaires, some false-positive cases must be expected. Even a comprehensive questionnaire may not detect all cases of asthma.

5.3. Epidemiology of Childhood Asthma

There is still much to learn about the etiology of asthma, which is reflected in the lack of a consensus definition that can be used to analyze the disease's epidemiology in children. In clinical practice, the definition of asthma is widely used. It is defined as an obstructive lung disease with hyper-reactivity of the airways to a variety of stimuli and a high degree of reversibility of the obstructive process, either spontaneously or as a result of treatment. However, there isn't always a direct correlation between the clinical manifestation of the illness (measured by the frequency and severity of asthma symptoms) and the lung cellular and biochemical characteristics of asthma (as determined, for example, by bronchoalveolar lavage). Furthermore, the variety of clinical manifestations of asthma, including frequent wheezing, dyspnea during exercise, and persistent nocturnal cough, has led to uncertainty regarding the best way to describe the asthma phenotype. While all of these clinical characteristics are thought to be suggestive of the existence of asthma, they could also represent various phenotypic manifestations of this complex syndrome in childhood, each of which could have a unique set of underlying disease mechanisms. Furthermore, the fact that recurrent wheezing may exhibit distinct cellular, physiological, and clinical traits at various ages suggests that this illness is developmental in nature.

Epidemiological studies give rise to additional methodological issues. The most popular way to determine whether a population sample has asthma is to use questionnaires. Currently, children can choose between two primary standardized respiratory symptom questionnaires: the International Study of Asthma and Allergies in Childhood (ISAAC) (2) and the American Thoracic Society (1). When evaluating a parent's report of asthma as proof of the prevalence of the disease, it is important to keep in mind that parental responses are influenced by medical care patterns and the diagnosis labels that specific doctors choose to use. Language barriers may have an impact on estimates based on wheeze reports from parents. For instance, wheeze has no term in certain languages. Surveys that only consider a doctor's diagnosis of asthma have the potential to select participants who are sicker than average, which could distort the characteristics of the illness as reported. On the other hand, due to the low specificity of wheezing symptoms for asthma, studies that use the presence of the disease as an indicator may overestimate the prevalence of the illness.

5.3.1. Methods

The majority of data on the prevalence of asthma is gathered from cross-sectional surveys, which have been conducted widely across the globe. Prevalence estimates from nationwide probability samples are obtained in the United States through periodic surveys carried out by the National Center for Health Statistics. Only a small number of cohort studies offer incidence rates, in contrast to the wealth of information on prevalence. Hospitalization and death rates may provide more information about the prevalence of asthma. These metrics, however, incorporate differences in severity, diagnosis, and treatment protocols, and classification in addition to disease frequency.

5.3.2. Prevalence of Asthma

Many populations have had their asthma prevalence documented, and several developed nations—including the United States—have monitored it over time. Through the use of questionnaires, spirometry, and assessments of airway hyperresponsiveness, the prevalence of asthma has been estimated from surveys. Periodic prevalence estimates are provided by the National Center for Health Statistics' National Health Interview Survey (NHIS) and National Health and Nutrition Surveys (NHANES), which are conducted on random samples of the entire US population. Data from these surveys, which span 40 years, are currently available.

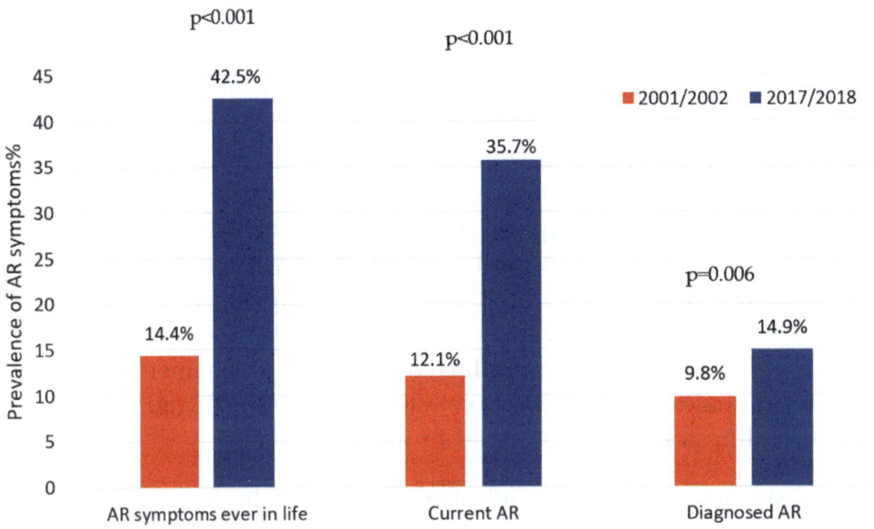

Figure 5.1. *Significant rise in the self-reported prevalence of AR symptoms and diagnoses, 2002–2018.*

Source: Topalušić I, Stipić Marković A, Artuković M, Dodig S, Bucić L, Lugović Mihić L. Divergent Trends in the Prevalence of Children's Asthma, Rhinitis, and Atopic Dermatitis and Environmental Influences in the Urban Setting of Zagreb, Croatia. Children. 2022; 9(12):1788. https://doi.org/10.3390/children9121788.

The NHIS is a survey that interviews households across the United States to gather longitudinal data on asthma prevalence. According to the latest available data from 1995, 5.6% of US residents, or 14.6 million people, have asthma. The survey asked participants if they had asthma in the past 12 months, with results showing that asthma is most common in younger age groups. In fact, 6.9% of children under 18 years old have asthma, making it the most common chronic illness of childhood in the US. Asthma prevalence rates were highest in the West and Northeast (5.9%), slightly lower in the South (5.5%), and even lower in the Midwest (5.2%). Analysis of NHIS data dating back to 1982 indicates a steady rise in asthma prevalence across all age and racial demographics. Rates differ between racial and ethnic groups, likely due to genetic, environmental, social, and cultural factors. Figure 5.1 illustrates the escalating prevalence of asthma in individuals aged 5–34 years old, with a 52% increase overall for black and white populations combined, from 34.6 to 52.6 per 1000.

Asthma is a global issue that is believed to be more prevalent in wealthier, developed countries compared to poorer, developing nations. The prevalence of asthma in children can range from 0% to 30%, with data for this age group being more reliable due to chronic obstructive pulmonary disease, which can be mistaken for asthma in older individuals, not affecting children.

Around the world, there are significant differences in the prevalence rates for children and young adults. The most comprehensive data on global variations in asthma prevalence can be found in the ISAAC study. The ISAAC Steering Committee published results for 463,801 children in 1998, who were between the ages of 13 and 14 and came from 155 partner centers spread across 56 nations. The prevalence figures for a positive response to the question, "Have you had wheezing or whistling in the chest in the last 12 months?" ranged across the countries by about 20 times, with more developed nations typically having higher rates. Similar patterns were seen for other allergic diseases (Figure 5.2).

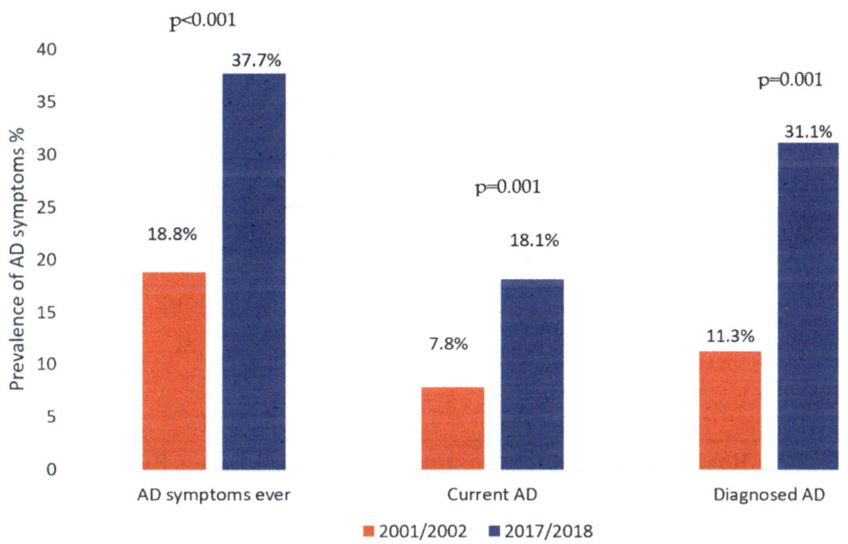

Figure 5.2. *Significant rise in the self-reported prevalence of AD symptoms and diagnoses, 2002–2018.*

Source: Topalušić I, Stipić Marković A, Artuković M, Dodig S, Bucić L, Lugović Mihić L. Divergent Trends in the Prevalence of Children's Asthma, Rhinitis, and Atopic Dermatitis and Environmental Influences in the Urban Setting of Zagreb, Croatia. Children. 2022; 9(12):1788. https://doi.org/10.3390/children9121788.

Apart from the significant differences between nations, global data also indicate an increase in prevalence. The methods of assessment differ significantly, and there is no discernible pattern of variation by economic status (Table 5.3). **Comparing countries within the same region, however, shows that prevalence has increased recently, including in the US. Between**

1971 and 1981, the prevalence of asthma among 18-year-old military conscripts in Sweden rose by 47%. The examining physician's interview and the patient's medical history were used to diagnose asthma. A study conducted on Finnish military conscripts revealed a five-fold rise in the prevalence of asthma between 1966 and 1989. There has also been a rise in asthma cases over the previous 20 years, according to data from Tahiti, France, Australia, New Zealand, and England (Table 5.3). The study conducted on schoolchildren in Melbourne produced significantly high prevalence rates; the outcome measure, any history of wheezing or asthma, is probably going to give an upwardly biased estimate of the incidence of asthma. However, over a 26-year period, there was a significant increase in prevalence using this potentially biased method.

Asthma prevalence has also increased in the Far East. Asthma cases are lower in other parts of the world and in Asia's less developed regions. As the richest nation in the Pacific region, Japan defies the trend by having a comparatively low prevalence of asthma.

Table 5.3. *The Prevalence of Asthma-Related Respiratory Symptoms*

Has Your Child Ever Had Wheezing or Whistling in the Chest at Any Time in the Past?		
Yes	834	21.7%
No	3002	78.3%
Has Your Child Had Wheezing or Whistling in the Chest in the Past 12 Months?		
Yes	356	9.3%
No	3480	90.7%
How Many Attacks of Wheezing Has Your Child Had in the Past 12 Months?		
none	3598	93.8%
1–3	183	4.8%
4–12	42	1.1%
≥ 12	13	0.3%
In the Past 12 Months, How Often, on Average, Has Your Child's Sleep Been Disturbed Due to Wheezing?		
Never woken with wheezing	3588	93.5%
Less than one night per week	162	4.2%
One or more nights per week	86	2.3%
In the Past 12 Months, Has Wheezing Ever Been Severe Enough to Limit Your Child's Speech to Only One or Two Words at a Time between Breaths?		
Yes	41	1.1%
No	3795	98.9%
Has Your Child Ever Had Asthma?		
Yes	290	7.6%
No	3546	92.4%
In the Past 12 Months, Has Your Child's Chest Sounded Wheezy during or after Exercise? (Physical Education, Running, Walking on Stairs)		

Has Your Child Ever Had Wheezing or Whistling in the Chest at Any Time in the Past?		
Yes	227	5.9%
No	3609	94.1%
In the Past 12 Months, Has Your Child Had a Dry Cough at Night Apart from a Cough Associated with a Cold or Chest Infection?		
Yes	422	11%
No	3414	89%
Has Your Child Had Asthma Diagnosed by a Physician?		
Yes	248	6.5%
No	3588	93.5%

Source: Molnár D, Gálffy G, Horváth A, Tomisa G, Katona G, Hirschberg A, Mezei G, Sultész M. Prevalence of Asthma and Its Associating Environmental Factors among 6–12-Year-Old Schoolchildren in a Metropolitan Environment—A Cross-Sectional, Questionnaire-Based Study. International Journal of Environmental Research and Public Health. 2021; 18(24):13403. https://doi.org/10.3390/ijerph182413403.

It may be possible to determine the frequency of asthma objectively by measuring airway responsiveness. Communities have measured air traffic responsiveness, and standardized procedures are available to determine it. Data on the prevalence of increased airway responsiveness in children across several nations used cold air, exercise, histamine, or methacholine to cause bronchial hyperresponsiveness (BHR). The prevalence rates of BHR were not consistently higher nor lower than those for asthma diagnosed by a physician, but they did differ, as the table shows. However, many individuals with BHR never have asthma attacks or symptoms; it's important to remember that BHR is just one aspect of the asthma phenotype. However, it remains a crucial element and useful in objective estimates of asthma prevalence. For instance, in the study of Chinese teenagers, 93% of those with severe to moderate BHR also had an asthma diagnosis from their doctor at the time of the study, and 73% had one from earlier. Just 0.5% of those with normal airway responsiveness had a prior diagnosis, and none of them had a diagnosis from a doctor as of yet. It is possible that there is uncertainty regarding the diagnosis and disease status at this level of pulmonary reactivity because 56% of individuals with mild BHR had a current doctor's diagnosis and 38% had a previous one (Table 5.4).

Table 5.4. *The Frequency of Asthma Symptoms Indicates the Severity in the CA Group*

Severity Indicator	Frequency/ Severity Response	*n* in CA	% in CA
In the past 12 months, how often, on average, has your child's sleep been disturbed due to wheezing?	Never woken with wheezing	292	60.33%
	Less than one night per week	119	24.59%
	One or more nights per week	73	15.01%

Severity Indicator	Frequency/ Severity Response	*n* in CA	% in CA
In the past 12 months, has wheezing ever been severe enough to limit your child's speech to only one or two words at a time between breaths?	Yes	37	7.64%
	No	447	92.36%
In the past 12 months, has your child's chest sounded wheezy during or after exercise? (physical education, running, walking on stairs)	Yes	149	30.79%
	No	335	69.21%

Source: *Molnár D, Gálffy G, Horváth A, Tomisa G, Katona G, Hirschberg A, Mezei G, Sultész M. Prevalence of Asthma and Its Associating Environmental Factors among 6–12-Year-Old Schoolchildren in a Metropolitan Environment—A Cross-Sectional, Questionnaire-Based Study. International Journal of Environmental Research and Public Health. 2021; 18(24):13403. https://doi.org/10.3390/ijerph182413403.*

5.3.3. Incidence of Childhood Asthma

Data on the incidence of asthma are available from a few studies conducted abroad as well as from a number of cohort studies conducted in the United States. For Rochester, Minnesota, home of the Mayo Clinic, some of the most complete data are available for the years 1964–1983 (Figure 5.3). Nearly every incident case of asthma in the Rochester population has been documented thanks to the extensive Mayo Clinic records. As predicted by prevalence statistics, boys, and the youngest age groups have the highest incidence rates of asthma. Little new asthma is discovered in adolescence and early adulthood. Even though early childhood has the highest incidence rates of asthma, the classification of wheezing during infections as asthma may have an upward bias on these rates. Martinez et al. observed children from birth until age six, and discovered that a significant percentage of kids who had wheezing in the first three years of life had stopped by the time they were six years old (Table 5.5).

Table 5.5. *The Association Between CA Asthma and Other Manifestations of Atopy*

QID	Atopic Condition: Has Your Child Ever Had...?	Yes/No	*n* (%) in CA	*p*-Values	OR	CI
A1	Any allergic diseases	Yes (*n* = 1206)	331 (27.45)	<0.0001	6.12	4.99–7.55
		No (*n* = 2630)	153 (5.82)			
A2	Eczema	Yes (*n* = 491)	86 (17.52)	0.0005	1.57	1.21–2.02
		No (*n* = 3345)	398 (11.90)			
A3	food allergy	Yes (*n* = 242)	61 (25.21)	<0.0001	2.53	1.85–3.42
		No (*n* = 3595)	423 (11.77)			

A4	allergic rhinitis	Yes (n = 357)	124 (34.73)	<0.0001	4.61	3.61–5.88
		No (n = 3479)	360 (10.35)			
A5	Has your child been diagnosed with allergic rhinitis by a physician?	Yes (n = 373)	149 (39.95)	<0.0001	6.21	4.90–7.86
		No (n = 3463)	335 (9.67)			

QID: question ID, OR: odds ratio, CI: confidence interval.

Source: *Molnár D, Gálffy G, Horváth A, Tomisa G, Katona G, Hirschberg A, Mezei G, Sultész M. Prevalence of Asthma and Its Associating Environmental Factors among 6–12-Year-Old Schoolchildren in a Metropolitan Environment—A Cross-Sectional, Questionnaire-Based Study. International Journal of Environmental Research and Public Health. 2021; 18(24):13403. https://doi.org/10.3390/ijerph182413403.*

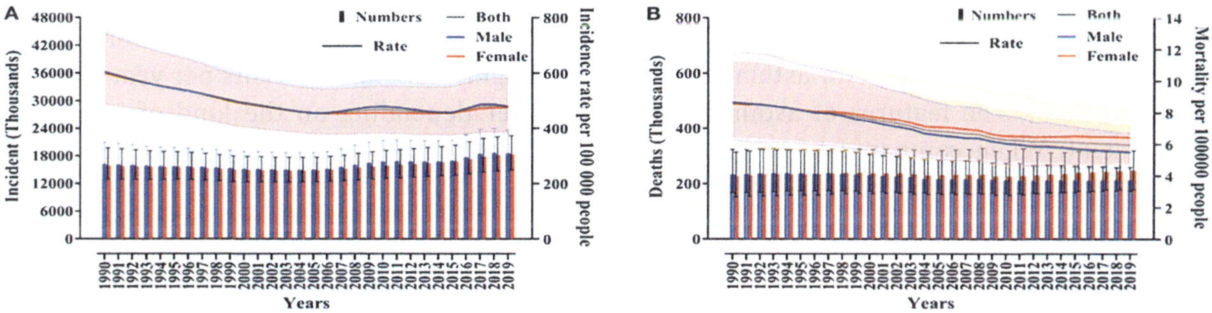

Figure 5.3. *Global asthma incidents, incidence **(A)**, deaths, and mortality **(B)** from 1990 to 2019.*

Source: Cao Y, Chen S, Chen X, Zou W, Liu Z, Wu Y and Hu S (2022) Global trends in the incidence and mortality of asthma from 1990 to 2019: An age-period-cohort analysis using the global burden of disease study 2019. Front. Public Health 10:1036674. doi: 10.3389/fpubh.2022.1036674.

5.3.4. Morbidity/Hospitalization Data

Measures of the use of medical services, such as hospital stays, prescription drug use, and quality of life, are indicators of morbidity. Based on hospital records of inpatients discharged from short-stay (less than 30 days) non-federal hospitals, data on asthma hospitalizations from the National Hospital Discharge Survey (NHDS) paints a picture of asthma prevalence and severity. In the US, asthma caused 198,000 hospital admissions in individuals under 25 in 1993. Furthermore, there was a 28% rise in hospitalizations in this age group between 1980 and 1993. The majority of this increase could be explained by admissions of children under the age of five. Furthermore, according to the report, hospitalization rates for asthma were consistently higher among Blacks, who had a 3.5 advantage over Whites in this regard (Figure 5.4).

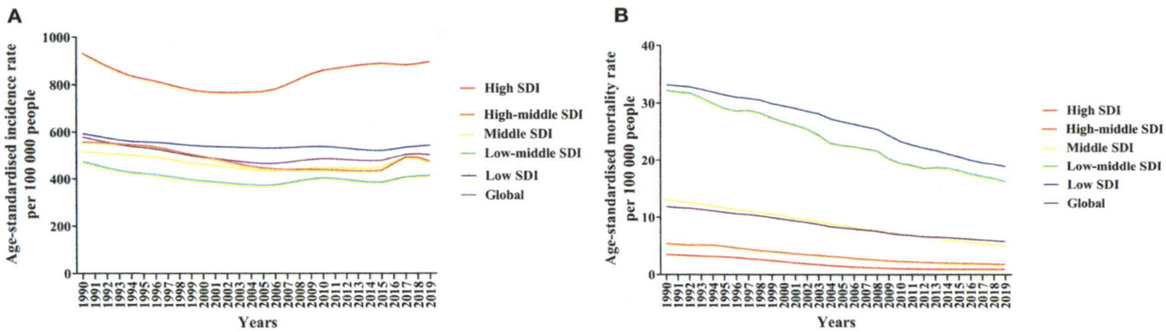

Figure 5.4. *Global age-standardized incidence rate* ***(A)*** *and age-standardized mortality rate* ***(B)*** *of asthma by SDI regions, 1990 to 2019.*

Source: Cao Y, Chen S, Chen X, Zou W, Liu Z, Wu Y and Hu S (2022) Global trends in the incidence and mortality of asthma from 1990 to 2019: An age-period-cohort analysis using the global burden of disease study 2019. Front. Public Health 10:1036674. doi: 10.3389/fpubh.2022.1036674.

Asthma-related ambulatory care visit counts provide an extra measure of asthma morbidity. In the US, the primary diagnosis for asthma was made in roughly 13.7 million visits per year between 1993 and 1994. The features of asthmatic patients differ depending on the kind of healthcare environment. When compared to patients who see doctors in offices, patients who depend on emergency rooms may have different conditions, require different care, and experience different results. Data from the National Ambulatory Medical Care Survey (NAMCS), a nationwide survey of visits to office-based physicians in the US, and the National Hospital Ambulatory Medical Care Survey (NHAMCS), a nationwide survey of visits to hospital emergency and outpatient departments in the US, were analyzed for the years 1993–1994 to characterize visits for asthma in the US.

Doctor's appointments made up the highest percentage of visits for asthma at 80.5%, with emergency room visits at 12% and outpatient department visits at 7.5%. Age was found to play a significant role in the type of provider sought, with individuals aged 15–24 having the lowest rate of doctor's appointments and the highest rate of emergency room visits.

Race was found to have a strong connection with the type of healthcare setting visited, as black individuals were more inclined to utilize emergency rooms and hospital outpatient departments instead of physicians' offices compared to white individuals. This suggests that black individuals may lack effective preventive asthma management, which could be due to potential obstacles in accessing proper medical treatment in these settings.

Vollmer and colleagues conducted a study in Portland, Oregon using Kaiser Permanente health care databases to analyze trends in asthma over a 20-year period. The study demonstrated an increase in asthma cases among the population, which grew from 86,200 in 1966 to 310,800 in 1987. The research presented a methodology for defining asthma episodes in order to address potential biases in asthma morbidity estimates resulting from changes in health care utilization and administration practices. For example, the study highlighted how economic incentives to reduce hospital stays in health maintenance organizations could lead to inaccurate conclusions about asthma morbidity based on hospital admission rates.

In addition, asthma hospitalizations account for only a small portion of total acute asthma healthcare usage. Instances of asthma were defined to encompass severe asthma events, including hospitalizations, visits to the emergency room, and utilization of hospital-based urgent care clinics. For boys and girls aged 0–14, the rise in asthma episodes was most noticeable in boys, but there was also a statistically significant trend in girls. Within this age group, boys aged 0–4 experienced the sharpest increase from 285 per 100,000 in 1965–1967 to 2025 per 100,000 in 1985–1987. Among age groups older than 14, there was no clear pattern of change in asthma episodes (Figure 5.5).

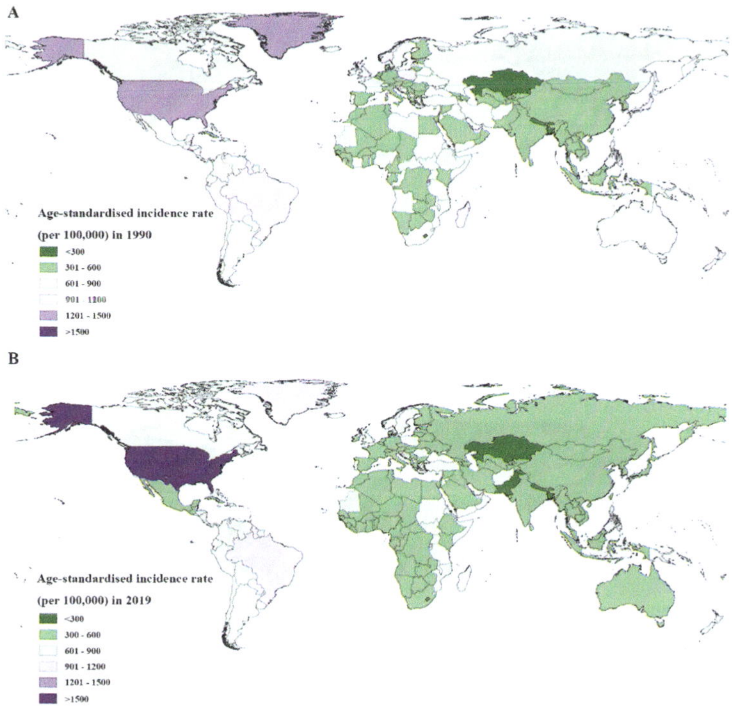

Figure 5.5. *The age-standardized incidence rate in 1990* ***(A)*** *and 2019* ***(B)*** *for asthma in 204 countries and territories worldwide.*

Source: Cao Y, Chen S, Chen X, Zou W, Liu Z, Wu Y and Hu S (2022) Global trends in the incidence and mortality of asthma from 1990 to 2019: An age-period-cohort analysis using the global burden of disease study 2019. Front. Public Health 10:1036674. doi: 10.3389/fpubh.2022.1036674.

5.3.5. Asthma Mortality

While death from asthma is not common, monitoring mortality rates is important for understanding the disease's impact on the population and the effectiveness of its management. There have been significant spikes in asthma-related deaths in recent years, leading to extensive investigations into the causes of these so-called asthma epidemics.

Asthma deaths are recorded using the International Classification of Disease (ICD), which is updated approximately every decade. Changes in coding between revisions can impact mortality rates, leading to observed increases or decreases. In the United States, the switch from the eighth to the ninth revision in 1979 is believed to have caused a 35% rise in overall asthma deaths, but for those under 45 years old, the increase was less than 5%. This coding change is thought to be due to how asthma-related bronchitis was classified in the different revisions. The upcoming tenth revision will also categorize bronchitis and asthma together under "asthma." Research into the accuracy of death certificates in listing asthma as the cause of death has mainly focused on adults, as there is a risk of misdiagnosis with chronic obstructive pulmonary disease (COPD).

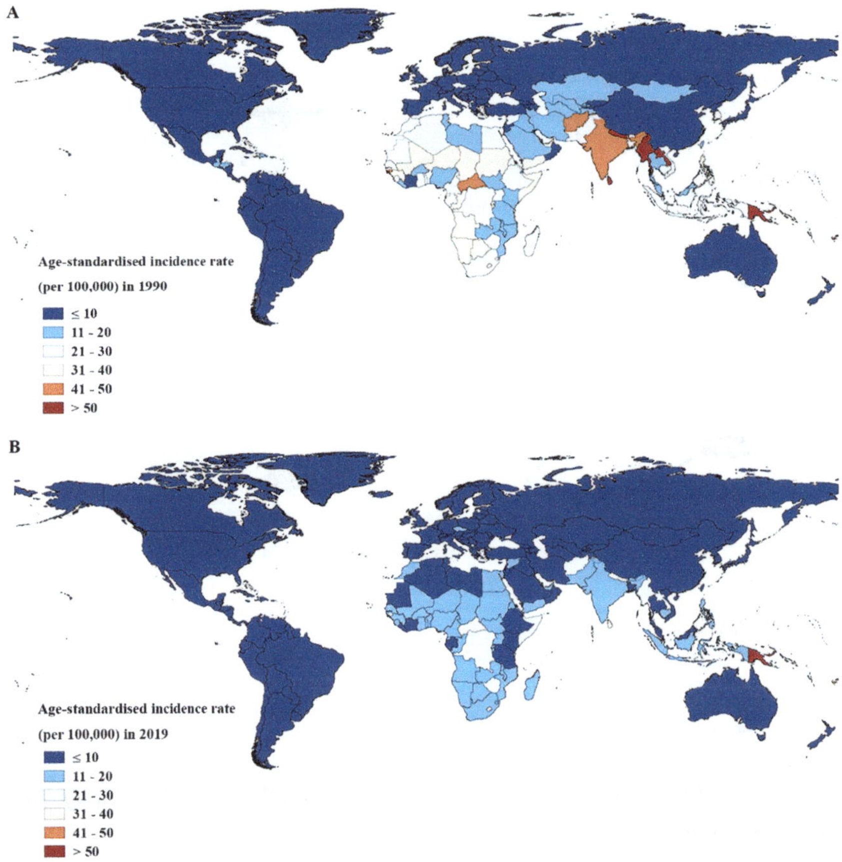

Figure 5.6. *The age-standardized mortality rate in 1990 (A) and 2019 (B) for asthma in 204 countries and territories worldwide.*

Source: Cao Y, Chen S, Chen X, Zou W, Liu Z, Wu Y and Hu S (2022) Global trends in the incidence and mortality of asthma from 1990 to 2019: An age-period-cohort analysis using the global burden of disease study 2019. Front. Public Health 10:1036674. doi: 10.3389/fpubh.2022.1036674.

A study on long-term trends in the US from 1941 to 1989 identified three separate eras of asthma mortality in individuals aged 5 to 34. The patterns were consistent across the ages of 5–14 and 15–34. There was a gradual increase in mortality rates from 1941 to 1964, followed by a noticeable decline from 1965 to 1977. However, there was a significant increase in asthma mortality from 1978 to 1989, almost doubling during that period. It is important to consider changes in ICD codes when interpreting these trends, but there is a consensus that the recent rise in childhood asthma mortality is not solely due to changes in coding practices (Figure 5.6).

Another trend analysis examined the rise in asthma mortality rates among US residents under 25 years old from 1980 to 1993. Blacks had consistently higher rates than Whites during this time period in every age group, with the 15–24 age group within each race having the highest rates for each year observed. Blacks were four times more likely than Whites to die from asthma in 1993, and blacks aged 5 to 14 were six times more likely than Whites to die from asthma in 1993 (Figure 5.7).

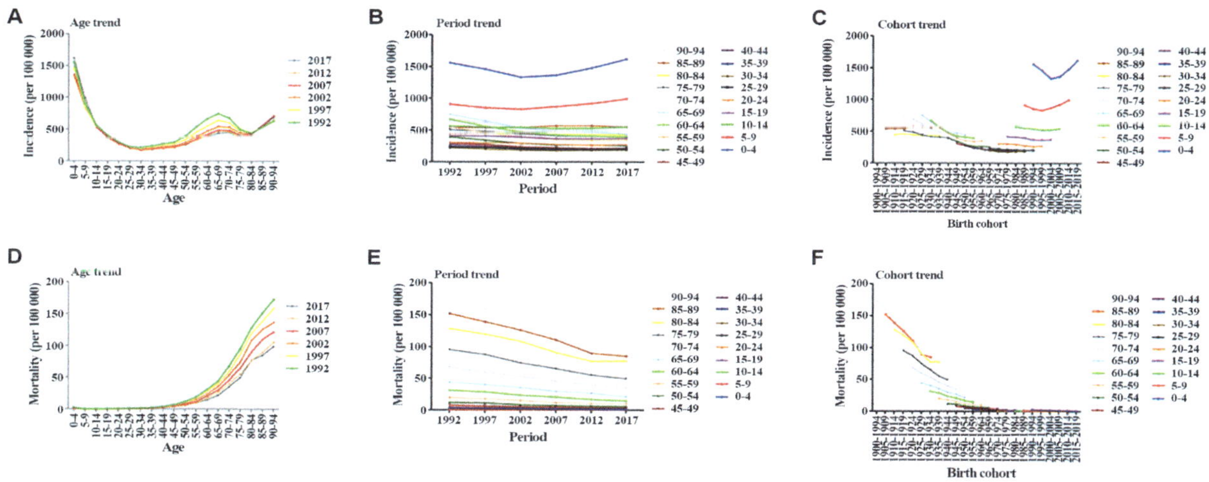

Figure 5.7. *Global trends in asthma incidence and mortality. (A) Global trends in asthma incidence by age. (B) Global trends in asthma incidence by period. (C) Global trends in asthma incidence by birth cohort. (D) Global trends in asthma mortality by age. (E) Global trends in asthma mortality by period. (F) Global trends in asthma mortality by birth cohort.*

Source: Cao Y, Chen S, Chen X, Zou W, Liu Z, Wu Y and Hu S (2022) Global trends in the incidence and mortality of asthma from 1990 to 2019: An age-period-cohort analysis using the global burden of disease study 2019. Front. Public Health 10:1036674. doi: 10.3389/fpubh.2022.1036674.

These national data demonstrate how the patterns of asthma mortality vary significantly amongst ethnic groups. Cook County, Illinois, and New York City had disproportionately high mortality rates from asthma, according to a study conducted to identify target populations of children and young adults in the US who were at high risk of passing away from the condition. In the city of New York, Carr et al. showed wide variations in asthma mortality, with the poorest neighborhoods having the highest rates. Also, it was shown that the death rates for Hispanics and Blacks were three to five times higher than those for Whites. In Cook County, Chicago, Targonski et al. looked at patterns in the mortality from asthma in people aged 5 to 34 between 1968 and 1991. Blacks had a higher death rate and a faster rate of increase than Whites during this period, and they also discovered an inverse relationship between income and asthma mortality. Similar results were seen in Philadelphia for individuals between the ages of 5 and 34, where asthma mortality rates exceeded Pennsylvania's average. Findings from the Rochester, Minnesota cohort study on asthma indicate that the rising mortality rates seen could potentially be linked to the increasing number of asthma cases. There was a noticeable increase in annual incidence rates from 1964 to 1983 among all age groups under 15 years old, with the exception of infants under 1 year old who had steady rates. Incidence rates also went up to a lesser extent in the 15–29, 30–49, and 50+ age groups. The study suggests that the rise in asthma-related deaths is more likely due to the rising prevalence of asthma rather than poor management of the disease.

It can be challenging to interpret straight comparisons of asthma mortality between nations due to variations in certification and diagnosis procedures. Also, many countries do not have readily available asthma mortality rates, especially the less developed ones. In contrast to other developed nations, the US, Canada, Hong Kong, and the Netherlands have comparatively low rates across all age groups, according to global estimates (Figure 5.8).

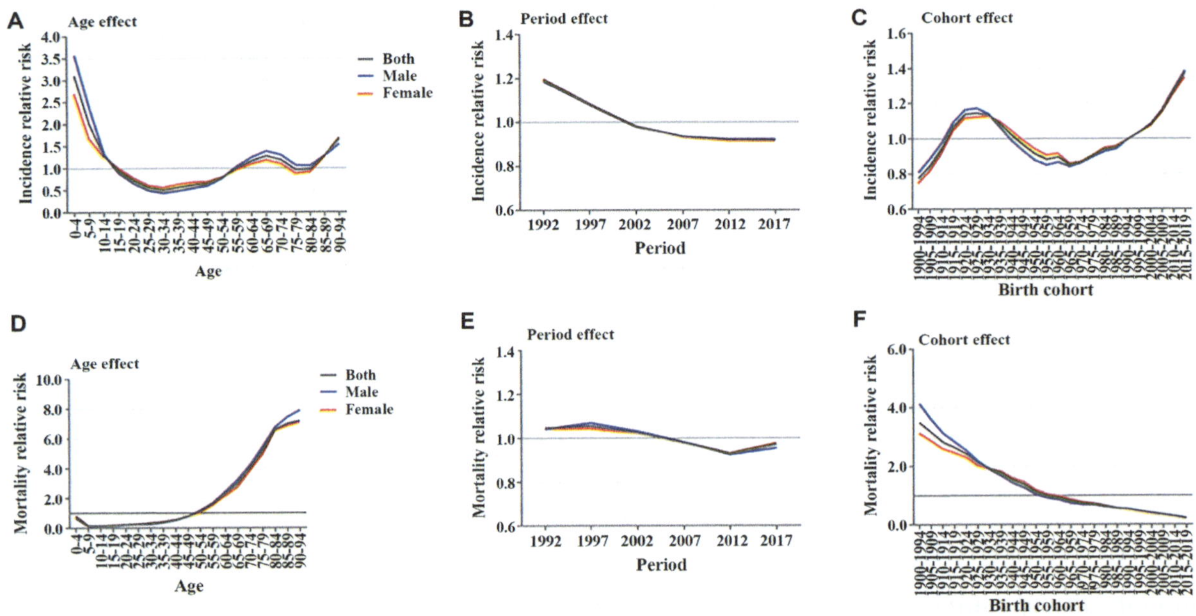

Figure 5.8. *Relative risk of asthma incidence and mortality. (A) Relative risk of asthma incidence due to age effect. (B) Relative risk of asthma incidence due to period effect. (C) Relative risk of asthma incidence due to birth cohort effect. (D) Relative risk of asthma mortality due to age effect. (E) Relative risk of asthma mortality due to period effect. (F) Relative risk of asthma mortality due to birth cohort effect.*

Source: Cao Y, Chen S, Chen X, Zou W, Liu Z, Wu Y and Hu S (2022) Global trends in the incidence and mortality of asthma from 1990 to 2019: An age-period-cohort analysis using the global burden of disease study 2019. Front. Public Health 10:1036674. doi: 10.3389/fpubh.2022.1036674.

Recent trend analyses show rising rates of asthma-related mortality. The sharp increase in asthma-related deaths that occurred in New Zealand between 1976 and 1980—including deaths of younger people—and the persistently high rates that were reported until 1989 are noteworthy.

Following a formal investigation, it was determined that this epidemic didn't seem to be the product of incorrect death certificates or classification changes. Instead, it appeared to be real. It was discovered that a number of factors, including the patient's, families, and physician's lack of understanding of the severity and mortality risk, were linked to fatal asthma. The adoption of self-management techniques resulted in the subsequent decline in the mortality rate from asthma that was seen after 1980. However, neither the total increase in asthma deaths nor any indication that any of these management factors had gotten worse during this time were consistent with these findings. Some New Zealand researchers believed that the primary cause of the epidemic was the beta-agonist fenoterol, which was introduced in 1976 and rose to a 30% market share in New Zealand during the same five-year period that mortality increased threefold. Following the drug's subsequent withdrawal in 1989, the mortality rate from asthma fell by two-thirds over the course of a year, and the mortality rate returned to levels comparable with those in other nations. This conclusion regarding fenoterol and asthma deaths is still up for debate, though (Figure 5.9).

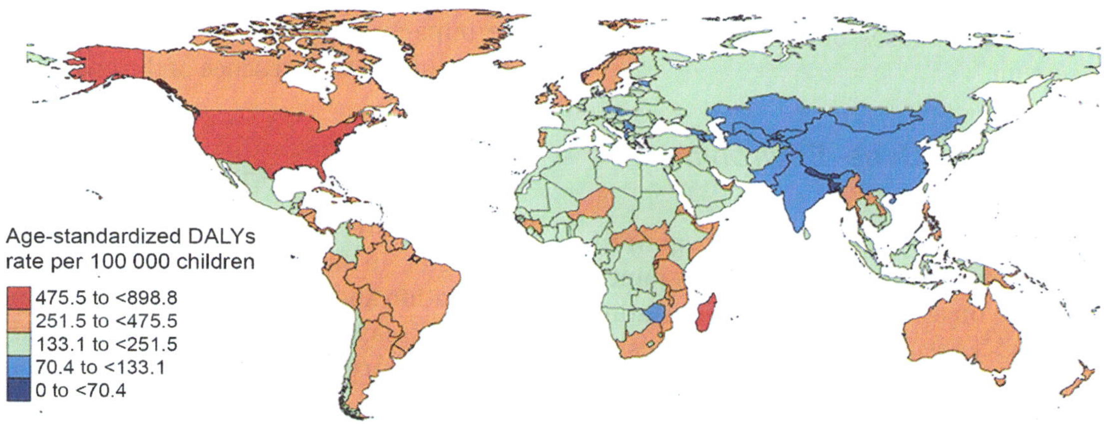

Figure 5.9. *Age-standardized DALYs due to childhood asthma per 100,000 children by country, both sexes, 2019. DALYs, disability adjusted life years.*

Source: Zhang D and Zheng J (2022) The Burden of Childhood Asthma by Age Group, 1990–2019: A Systematic Analysis of Global Burden of Disease 2019 Data. Front. Pediatr. 10:823399. doi: 10.3389/fped.2022.823399.

The data collected up until the mid-1990s reveal a shifting picture of asthma incidence. Both the prevalence and mortality rates are trending slightly higher. The frequency of the disease varies significantly between countries and regions. There has been significant public health concern over the rising prevalence; theories have been put forth but not fully tested. It seems that methodologic advancements are not the only cause of the increasing prevalence. A possible contributing factor has been identified as indoor air pollution, with a focus on bioallergens. It is still highly debatable how pharmacologic agents affect mortality trends.

5.3.6. Risk Factors for Childhood Asthma

Risk factors are traits, either inherited or learned, that can raise an individual's chance of developing a disease. Clinicians can identify people who are likely to develop a disease and counsel patients based on information about risk factors. Preventative measures also stem from an awareness of risk factors. Numerous epidemiologic studies on the etiology of asthma have identified several risk factors, including male sex, family history, early life respiratory infections, indoor, and outdoor allergens, and exposure to tobacco smoke. The majority of the data is cross-sectional in nature, and it lacks the necessary longitudinal perspective to adequately explain why asthma rates are rising at the moment. There are many theories explaining the increased prevalence of asthma, some of which include altered patterns of respiratory infections, indoor air pollution, sedentary lifestyles, and changes in diet. We'll go over the main causes of childhood asthma in this section.

5.3.6.1. Role of Gene–Environment Interactions

It has long been believed that genetic susceptibility and environmental factors jointly determine the onset and clinical manifestation of asthma. As a result of the recent explosion in knowledge about the human genome, genetic components are now extensively used in asthma research and will probably soon have a bearing on the treatment of asthmatic patients. According to current theories of asthma pathogenesis, a person must be both genetically predisposed to asthma and exposed to the right environmental stimulus for the disease to manifest. This means that the disease's onset and clinical trajectory are influenced by interactions between genes and the environment. The relative contributions of genes and environmental factors likely vary among the population's asthmatics.

Studies can evaluate gene-environment interactions in various ways, including case-control and cohort studies, as well as family-based genetic studies. The underlying idea is that individuals with different genetic predispositions for asthma may react differently to environmental triggers. Khoury et al. proposed different scenarios for gene-environment interactions. These include a situation where both a specific asthma susceptibility gene and exposure to a certain environmental factor are needed to increase the risk of the disease. Another scenario is when an environmental factor elevates the risk for everyone, but more so for individuals with the susceptible genotype. A third possibility is that the environmental factor alone may not raise the risk, but in combination with the susceptible genotype, it significantly increases the risk of asthma. A fourth scenario involves both genotype and environmental exposure contributing to higher risk. Ultimately, the impact of a particular genotype may vary depending on the presence of the environmental factor.

5.3.6.2. Genetic/Familial Factors

Clinicians are well aware that asthma tends to cluster in families, which has long led to speculation about a possible genetic component to the disease. Consequently, this theory has been supported by data from twin, familial aggregation, linkage, and association studies.

Studies on family aggregation compare the prevalence of illness among various family members. Increased aggregation between spouses implies that environment is more important, while the presence of disease aggregation between siblings and between parents and children supports a hereditary component. Aggregation among related individuals, however, might indicate a shared home environment or a set of genes. Numerous family-based studies have shown evidence of a hereditary component to asthma. Furthermore, studies based on population data have indicated a higher incidence of asthma in first-degree relatives of index cases. In twin studies, the frequency of disease varies between monozygotic (MZ) twins, who share all of their genes, and dizygotic (DZ) twins, who share half of their genes on average. This is an additional technique to ascertain the proportionate influence of genetic and environmental elements. Since both types of twins are thought to share similar environmental factors, a higher occurrence of disease in MZ twins than in DZ twins is evidence that the disease has a genetic component. Some small studies have found significantly higher concordance rates in MZ twins. Larger twin registry studies also point to a strong hereditary component for asthma. Edfors-Lubs discovered that 3.8% of 6996 twin pairs from the Swedish twin registry had an asthmatic. The fact that MZ pairs have a higher concordance of asthma (19.8%) than DZ pairs (4.8%) suggests that genetic factors play a role in asthma. Similarly, in a total of 2902 Australian pairs, Duffy, and colleagues found that 30% of MZ twins and 12% of DZ twins had concordance.

Another technique for determining the chromosomal locations of disease susceptibility genes and clarifying underlying genetic mechanisms is genetic linkage analysis. Numerous chromosomal regions, including 5q, 6p, 11q, 12q, 13q, and 14q, have been linked to the genetic control of asthma. These chromosomal regions were shown to be important in a recent multi-center US study that screened the entire human genome for asthma; additional regions (2q, 5p, 11p, 17p, 19q, and 21q) were also suggested to be important. The identification of underlying major and minor asthma susceptibility genes is anticipated through further fine mapping of these regions. A variety of association studies, such as linkage disequilibrium studies, can be employed to evaluate the significance of particular candidate genes as asthma risk factors. Initial findings from association and linkage analyses indicate the potential involvement of multiple genes, such as the IgE receptor, T-cell antigen receptor, HLA class II antigens, and the β_2-adrenergic receptor, in asthma and asthma-related phenotypes. To determine these candidate genes' role in the pathophysiology of asthma, more research is required as their causal involvement has not yet been established.

5.3.6.3. Male Sex

Data from epidemiologic studies consistently show that a child's gender is a risk factor for asthma. It has been demonstrated that boys are up to twice as likely as girls to have asthma before the age of 14. Nonetheless, the gender gap becomes less pronounced as people age.

A possible explanation for the higher prevalence of asthma observed in boys is that their airways differ in geometry. Research has indicated that boys have smaller airways than girls for a given lung size. Boys between the ages of 4 and 6 years old had higher airway resistance and lower flow rates. Boys may be more susceptible to lower respiratory tract infections and wheezing due to this variation in the structure of their airways. It has been demonstrated that lower respiratory tract infections are more common in boys.

Martinez et al. additionally proposed that a major factor contributing to wheezing in both boys and girls was decreased lung function. In the Tucson study, 124 healthy newborns had their lung function assessed a few weeks after birth. For the next six years of life, boys with high respiratory resistance and girls with low functional residual capacity had higher incidences of wheezing illness.

5.3.6.4. Atopy

The majority of children with asthma also have respiratory allergies, particularly to indoor allergens. Asthma and atopy are closely connected, with atopy referring to the allergic response to environmental allergens mediated by IgE. Allergy plays a significant role in childhood asthma, and there is a suggestion that sensitization in the womb could influence future immune responses. Atopy is evaluated in different ways in epidemiological studies, such as through total serum IgE levels, specific IgE for allergens, positive skin-test reactions, or questionnaires assessing conditions associated with atopy like eczema and allergic rhinitis. The relationship between atopy and asthma is briefly discussed.

Multiple studies have consistently found a connection between atopy and asthma, though the strength of this association can vary depending on the specific measurement used and the demographics of the study population. One study conducted by Burrows et al. in Tucson, Arizona, used skin tests with local antigens to assess atopic status in a random sample of children aged 3–14. They found that atopy was significantly linked to wheezing and difficulty breathing, regardless of an official asthma diagnosis. Further research in Tucson indicated that total serum IgE levels were more closely tied to asthma prevalence. In a separate study in western Pennsylvania, self-reported hay fever diagnoses revealed a higher incidence of atopy among asthmatic children compared to non-asthmatic children. Additional studies have shown that parental atopy and asthma can also increase the risk of asthma in their children, with a complex interplay between these factors and the child's gender. Asthma and atopy are undoubtedly related conditions, and it appears that their causal relationships are intricate. Furthermore, further research is needed to fully understand the elusive causal mechanistic pathways. Atopy does, however, raise the risk of asthma in both parents and children, and it can be utilized as an empirical predictor of the likelihood of developing asthma.

5.3.6.5. Environmental Factors

While a child's susceptibility to asthma may be influenced by genetic factors, asthma may not develop until environmental triggers are encountered. The main environmental factors that have been studied as asthma risk factors are tobacco smoke in the surrounding environment, outdoor or ambient air pollution, respiratory tract infections, and aeroallergens.

5.3.6.5.1. Aeroallergens

Although allergens are well-known to exacerbate asthma attacks, their part in the onset of asthma has only recently been investigated. An extensive analysis of the contribution of indoor allergens to asthma is given in a recent report published by the Institute of Medicine in the United States. Numerous epidemiologic studies have examined the possible impact of aeroallergens, specifically indoor allergens; however, the majority of these investigations have been cross-sectional in nature, providing limited insight into the role of allergens in initiating new cases.

Brunekreef et al. used parents' reports of mold and moisture in the house as a proxy for allergen exposure. discovered that there were relative risks of 1.42 (95% confidence interval 1.04–1.94) and 1.27 (95% confidence interval 0.93–1.74) for asthma diagnosed by a doctor, respectively, among a cohort of 4625 children aged 8 to 12 who lived in six US cities. Sporik et al. looked at the function of allergens more directly and collected baseline measurements of house-dust mite antigen in the homes of 93 infants whose parents had asthma or hay fever. When 67 kids were reassessed after 11 years, 17 of them had asthma. For children who tested positive for house dust mites on a skin test, the relative risk of developing asthma was 19 points, while for children who were exposed to high concentrations of the mite antigen during infancy, it was 4 points. These findings, along with the Institute of Medicine review, point to allergen exposure as a potentially significant risk factor for the onset of childhood asthma.

5.3.6.5.2. Respiratory Tract Infections

Lower respiratory tract viral infections are common in childhood and have been shown to cause wheezing in both asthmatic and non-asthmatic children. The part played by viruses or other respiratory infections in the genesis of asthma is, however, less clear. T-helper lymphocytes, which can be categorized into Th1 or Th2 subgroups according to the cytokines they produce when activated, mediate the inflammatory response of the airways. It has been demonstrated that viral antigens increase the cytokines linked to Th1 lymphocyte production. Studies on asthmatic patients' airways, however, reveal the presence of cytokines linked to the Th2 profile rather than the Th1 profile. It is thought that respiratory infections influence the balance between Th1 and Th2 immune responses as well as the immunological response phenotype. While the Th1 response is self-limiting and only produces low-level IgE, the Th2 response results in IgE production, eosinophilia, and airway responsiveness.

According to the "hygiene hypothesis," a decrease in early exposure to infectious pathogens causes the Th2 phenotype to mature more slowly than the Th1 phenotype, which in turn causes a shift towards the T2 phenotype and an increased risk of developing asthma. One effect of a downward trend in infections could have been a change in lung immunophenotype linked to an increased risk of asthma. Despite receiving a lot of attention, this hypothesis has not yet been put to the test.

Childhood lower respiratory tract infections are common and can be brought on by respiratory syncytial virus, parainfluenza viruses, or other pathogens. According to a community-based study conducted in Tecumseh, Michigan, children typically get 1.5 lower respiratory infections between the ages of 1 and 2 years old and 2.1 lower respiratory infections in their first year of life. Utilizing a surveillance system akin to Tecumseh, another cohort study of respiratory illnesses in Albuquerque, New Mexico, from birth to 18 months of age, discovered remarkably similar incidence rates from 1988 to 1992. In a different study, the prevalence of severe viral respiratory infection episodes was monitored through a pediatric group practice. According to this study, 25% of children were impacted in their first year of life, 12% had recurring episodes by the time they were 5 years old, and 8% of children in their 6–8-year-old age group had recurring episodes of infection.

According to follow-up studies, respiratory infections may put children at risk for developing asthma if they have previously been hospitalized for them. According to multiple studies, children who had previously been hospitalized tended to have abnormal lung function, such as reduced spirometric flow rates, hyperinflation, and increased respiratory resistance, all of which were signs of airflow obstruction. Elevated airway reactivity has also been observed in children who have previously been hospitalized following evaluation through physical activity, cold air inhalation, or methacholine or histamine inhalation challenge. These findings, however, only pertain to the more serious infections because the majority of children with lower respiratory tract diseases do not end up in hospitals. Even so, a population-based study conducted on kids in East Boston, Massachusetts, discovered that a history of croup or bronchiolitis was associated with heightened airway responsiveness.

The most pertinent data over a follow-up period spanning from birth to adolescence can be found in the Tucson Children's Respiratory Study. The first three years of the participants' lives were monitored for respiratory ailments that required medical attention, and later on, respiratory symptoms and lung function were monitored over time. Stein et al. looked at respiratory syncytial virus infection as a predictor of lung function and subsequent wheezing. Wheezing was found to be predicted by viral infection up to the age of 10, but not at age 13. Although another cohort study indicates that children with atopy may have higher rates of more severe respiratory illnesses, infection did not predict atopic status. Additionally, individuals with a history of respiratory syncytial virus also had significantly reduced lung function.

There are theories explaining the possible connection between viral respiratory infections and the ensuing onset of asthma. One theory that is currently being floated is that viral infections can intensify airway inflammation, which is a feature of the asthma phenotype. The idea that respiratory syncytial virus infection could increase allergic sensitization has also been put forth in the past, but there is little evidence to support this theory, and the most recent report from the Tucson study finds no connection between atopy and respiratory syncytial virus infection. Welliver and colleagues demonstrated several decades ago that certain respiratory viruses can elicit an IgE-specific response in a study of 79 children with respiratory syncytial virus infection. Furthermore, the degree of airway obstruction in lower airway disease was correlated with the intensity of this response as well as the levels of histamine and leukotriene C4 in nasal secretions. Furthermore, only 20% of the 38 infants with respiratory syncytial virus (RSV) infection who had undetectable RSV-specific IgE titers experienced wheezing episodes over the course of a 48-month follow-up, compared to 70% of those who had high RSV IgE antibodies. This research revealed that a person's genetic susceptibility to developing bronchial hyper-responsiveness may be identified by their capacity to produce an IgE response specific to a virus. It is unknown, nevertheless, if virus-specific IgE production is a sign or the root cause of subsequent asthma. According to a different, related mechanistic theory, viral respiratory infections heighten the pattern of the airway's response to inhaled allergens and consequently cause hyperresponsiveness of the airways. Eight out of 10 subjects experienced airway obstruction 4–8 hours after antigen inhalation (late-phase reaction) during rhinovirus infection, whereas only one subject had a late-phase reaction before infection, according to results from a small group that were examined before and after the virus infection. Furthermore, four weeks after the rhinovirus inoculation, five of the seven that were tested still showed signs of airway obstruction. These findings imply that elements involved in the pathophysiology of asthma may be impacted further by viral respiratory infections. The "hygiene hypothesis" suggests that viral respiratory antigens may have an indirect role in the genesis of asthma, but this is still up for debate.

5.3.6.5.3. Outdoor Air Pollution

It is possible to categorize outdoor air pollutants as either naturally occurring or man-made. Particulate matter, including bioaerosols, volatile organic compounds, and ozone, is one type of naturally occurring air pollution. The main sources of pollution caused by humans are the combustion of fossil fuels in automobiles, power plants, heating appliances, and industrial point sources. Chemical emissions from manufacturing plants, storage tanks, and unintentional releases also contribute to this problem. Air pollutants in the United States are classified as either air toxins or "criteria pollutants," which include lead, nitrogen dioxide, sulfur dioxide, particulate matter, ozone, and carbon monoxide, and are regulated under the Clean Air Act. The latter were designated as a specific list of 189 chemicals under the Clean Air Act Amendments of 1990, some of which were of concern as possible asthma triggers. The same kinds of pollutants are typically a cause for concern in all of the polluted cities and regions of the world. In-depth analyses of the data on exposures and health effects should be conducted using the recently published comprehensive reviews of these pollutant effects on health.

The main belief is that outdoor air pollution aggravates asthma rather than being the cause of it. Nonetheless, there are several air pollutants that have been connected to the onset of asthma. These agents have been recognized by the occurrence of asthmatic clusters. Soybeans and castor beans have been examples of responsible agents.

At the current concentrations, there is no correlation between the onset of asthma and the pollutants related to widespread combustion. Numerous studies have shown a connection between outdoor air pollution and asthma flare-ups. According to experimental research, ozone, and nitrogen dioxide are oxidant pollutants that may exacerbate the effects of allergens by permeabilizing airways.

5.3.6.5.4. Indoor Air Pollution

Children and adults inhale a variety of pollutants in the home and other indoor environments that may increase their risk of developing asthma. These pollutants include volatile and semi-volatile organic compounds released from household products, furnishings, and other sources; combustion-source emissions from cooking stoves and ovens, gas or kerosene-fueled space heaters, wood-burning stoves and fireplaces, and tobacco smoking; and allergens from insects and mites, rodents, pets, and other sources. It's unclear if these exposures by themselves, in the absence of underlying genetic susceptibility, can trigger asthma. However, there is growing evidence that the incidence of wheezing and asthma is influenced by allergen exposure levels and that maternal smoking is linked to an increased risk of both asthma exacerbation and asthma onset. As a matter of fact, the Scientific Committee on Tobacco in the United Kingdom and the Environmental Protection Agency of the State of California have determined a connection between tobacco smoke exposure and the prevalence of asthma.

However, research on the relationship between indoor air pollution and asthma incidence for variables other than passive tobacco smoke exposure has been scant to date. Numerous studies have examined the prevalence of asthma and exposure to nitrogen oxides from cooking stoves as combustion sources other than cigarette smoking. Nitrogen dioxide levels in homes with cooking stoves powered by natural gas or propane are typically significantly higher than those in homes with electric stoves. Some studies show that homes with gas stoves have a higher risk of respiratory symptoms, such as wheezing; however, the results are contradictory and do not support the idea that nitrogen oxides increase the incidence of asthma. It has not been determined whether the numerous exposures to volatile and semi-volatile organic compounds that can happen in homes and other locations are risk factors for childhood asthma.

Research on indoor allergens has mostly concentrated on how children's asthma status relates to allergen levels, rather than how allergen levels predict asthma. According to a prospective cohort study conducted in the UK and published by Sporik and colleagues, a child's exposure to house dust mites during their early years may have an impact on their chance of developing asthma. 93 children who were at high risk for asthma due to having a parent with hay fever or asthma were enrolled in this prospective study. Children who had higher levels of house dust mite antigen in their homes tended to wheeze at a younger age, and the presence of house dust mites in the home was predictive of the later development of asthma. Reducing early childhood allergen exposure has been shown in a preventive trial to delay the onset of allergic diseases, including asthma. There are currently more prevention trials underway.

Infante-Rivard's case-control study on asthma looked at many risk factors, such as family history and environmental exposures, for the onset of the condition. In this study, the features of kids who came to the ER with recently developed asthma were contrasted with those of suitable controls. As predicted by the exacerbation data, there was an increased risk associated with family history, as well as with exposure to cigarette smoke, specific indoor heating systems, and other factors.

5.3.6.5.5. Environmental Tobacco Smoke

The mixture of mainstream smoke exhaled back into the atmosphere by the smoker and side stream smoke released by the burning cigarette is known as environmental tobacco smoke (ETS), and it is exposed to the nonsmoking child. One of the main sources of fine particles in the air of US homes is smoking, which also adds gases and respirable particles to indoor air. Through the use of biomarkers, which show the amounts of tobacco smoke constituents that have actually been absorbed into the body, as well as personal exposure measurements, the exposure of children to the particles and gases in tobacco smoke has been documented. A significant metabolite of nicotine, cotinine, has been studied in children with parental smoking in great detail. Children who live with smokers typically have significantly higher levels of cotinine than children who live in non-smoking homes.

In addition to exacerbating the condition of children who already have asthma, environmental tobacco smoke exposure may also be a contributing factor in the development of asthma. The risk of more severe lower respiratory tract infections in the first few years of life may be increased by passive smoking, which may then have an impact on the risk of developing asthma. Second, it's possible that ETS directly causes toxicity, which would then cause and sustain the elevated nonspecific airway responsiveness that asthmatic kids experience. Third, a sizable percentage of kids are exposed to ETS both before and after birth. As a long-term result of the higher incidence of lower respiratory infections in early childhood or through other pathophysiological mechanisms, such as inflammation of the respiratory epithelium, exposure to ETS may cause asthma. When the responsiveness of the airways is measured soon after birth, it is observed that babies whose mothers smoked during their pregnancies have more responsive airways than babies whose mothers do not smoke. Pregnancy-related maternal smoking also decreased the ventilatory function assessed soon after delivery. These findings imply that lung development may be impacted by maternal smoking exposures during pregnancy, possibly leading to a reduction in the relative size of the airways. Research points to the possibility that prenatal exposure to tobacco smoke constituents may have an impact on postpartum airway responsiveness. Young et al. evaluated nonspecific airway responsiveness with 63 healthy infants at a mean age of 4 weeks and a histamine challenge. Parental smoking and a family history of asthma were linked, even at this young age, to heightened airway responsiveness. Hanrahan and colleagues discovered that children whose mothers smoked during pregnancy had reduced airway function shortly after birth in a similar prospective study.

The link between childhood asthma and passive smoking has been well-documented. An early case report detailed a baby whose asthma was hard to control until they were kept away from any tobacco smoke exposure. There is inconsistent evidence supporting the claim that children who are exposed to smoke from smoking at home experience wheezing more frequently. The Environmental Protection Agency examined the data regarding ETS as a cause and aggravating factor for asthma in its 1992 risk assessment of the substance. It concluded that there was enough data to link parental smoking to a higher risk of exacerbating a child's asthma symptoms. For instance, it has been observed that children whose parents smoke have more responsive airways and seek medical attention for their asthma more frequently. Although there was some evidence that suggested passive smoking may also contribute to asthma, it was not thought to be strong enough to establish a causal link.

In another study, the California Environmental Protection Agency examined data from 37 relevant investigations conducted up to 1996. Through meta-analysis, it was found that there was a 50% increased risk of clinically diagnosed asthma and other wheezing syndromes in children exposed to parental smoking. Cook and Strachan also found a significant link between childhood asthma and exposure to environmental tobacco smoke (ETS), particularly if both parents or the mother smoke. This growing body of evidence suggests a strong causal association between childhood asthma and ETS exposure.

Research also suggests that smoking when involuntarily quits aggravates asthma symptoms. As early as 1950, a case report titled "Bronchial asthma due to allergy to tobacco smoke in an infant" discussed the possibility that ETS negatively impacts children who have asthma. Murray and Morrison assessed asthmatic kids who were being watched in a clinic more recently. Maternal smoking had a negative impact on lung function level, frequency of symptoms, and response to inhaled histamines. Studies on populations have also demonstrated that children with asthma who have been exposed to ETS have more responsive airways. It is expected that exposure to ETS will increase airway responsiveness, which will exacerbate asthma symptoms. In this sense, it has been demonstrated that children with asthma visit the ER more frequently when exposed to smoking in the home. The finding that children with asthma who have mothers who smoke have a higher likelihood of using asthma medications supports the clinically significant effects of ephedrine therapy (ETS) on asthmatic children. All asthma management guidelines recommend minimizing exposure to allergens at home.

5.4. The Natural History of Asthma

Researchers, clinicians treating the children, and parents of affected children have long been concerned about the natural history of childhood asthma. When parents and children with asthma inquire about whether their child will outgrow their asthma, clinicians must be able to respond. Researchers have looked for factors influencing prognosis and descriptively described the natural history of asthma. The former child asthmatic may be exposed to environmental factors, such as cigarette smoke, in their adult years that could negatively impact their respiratory health; the hypothesis that childhood asthma increases the risk of negative effects is still being researched.

Most studies on the natural history of asthma have used cohort or prospective designs, following up on asthmatic participants. Surveys and cross-sectional studies have been used to characterize asthma prevalence and risk factors, but they don't provide useful information about natural history. Cohort studies can be broadly classified based on the types of participants they include: children enrolled in particular medical facilities, individuals gathered through school or population surveys as participants in epidemiological studies, or birth cohort studies.

The studies' methodologies differ significantly from one another, especially in how they characterize the existence of asthma. The majority of studies have employed a clinical diagnosis or data gathered through questionnaires on self- or parent-reported histories of asthma, illnesses related to wheezing, or other conditions that resemble asthma. Furthermore, the studies have been carried out over the course of a century, and during this time, asthma diagnosis methods and classification have changed.

5.4.1. Natural History of Asthma in Childhood

Cohort studies of kids who visited clinics or practices provided the majority of the first data on the natural history of childhood asthma. These studies, some of which go back to the 1930s, served as the main source of information about the natural history of asthma until the 1960s when population-based studies of the disease were started. These earlier studies showed that a significant percentage of children with asthma experienced a decline in clinical symptoms over time. Still, the vast majority of kids continued to exhibit symptoms. The lack of certainty regarding the representativeness of children receiving care at a specific facility and the variety of methods used limit how these data can be interpreted. Participants in these studies were recruited from practices and clinics, where presumably more severe cases of asthma were represented. However, they offer proof that the prognosis for certain kids with asthma can be positive (Table 5.6).

Table 5.6. *Comparison of Childhood and Adult Asthma*

Feature	Childhood asthma	Adult asthma
Variable Phenotypes	Yes	Yes
Symptoms	Age 0–6 years: Cough, wheezing, acute episodes of dyspnea and increased work of breathing Age 6–11 years: cough, wheezing, dyspnea or cough with exertion Age 11–18 years: cough, wheezing, dyspnea, dyspnea on exertion, chest tightness, chest pain	Shortness of breath, wheeze, chest tightness and cough. *Allergic bronchopulmonary aspergillosis:* Above symptoms plus sputum production. *Aspirin exacerbated respiratory disease:* Above symptoms plus nasal polyps and sensitivity to aspirin.
Sex predominance	Males < 10 years	Females
Remission	Common	Rare
Factors associated with severity	Asthma duration, medication use, lung function, neutrophilic phenotype, low socioeconomic status, racial/ethnic minorities	IgE, FeNO, eosinophilia, obesity, smoking, low socioeconomic status
Mortality	Rare	Uncommon

Source: Trivedi M and Denton E (2019) Asthma in Children and Adults—What Are the Differences and What Can They Tell us About Asthma? Front. Pediatr. 7:256. doi: 10.3389/fped.2019.00256.

The physiological effects of childhood asthma have been better-understood thanks to more recent epidemiological research, which has also suggested that children with asthma may already have more responsive airways from birth. Through birth cohort studies that include measures of ventilatory function and airway responsiveness during the first few weeks of life, we are now starting to look into the early stages of asthma. Infants who are already at risk for asthma due to a parental history of atopy and asthma already frequently respond more strongly to challenges. The early natural history of wheezing has also been made clearer by the Tucson study. Martinez et al. provided an account of the natural history of wheezing that starts before the age of three years old in a birth cohort study. It is possible that the early wheezing did indicate asthma because children who wheezed until they were six years old were more likely to have mothers who had a history of asthma and to have an elevated serum IgE level.

Wheezing children who did not continue to wheeze had early airway dysfunction but were not more likely to have mothers with asthma or high IgE levels. These findings suggest that physicians should exercise caution when classifying all early childhood illnesses accompanied by wheezing as asthma because some kids are more likely to wheeze during the critical period of respiratory infections due to impaired airway function.

A growing body of data from prospective cohort studies that have tracked age- and population-based child groups over time is now available to us. The majority of these studies have participants selected from defined populations, so selection bias resulting from a specific healthcare facility that treats children with asthma is less likely. Several studies only offer data up to childhood. Park and Kim gathered data on a national cohort of 11,465 children in the United Kingdom at birth, as well as at the ages of five and 10. Wheezing was determined in retrospect by giving the parents questionnaires. Just 20% of the kids who experienced a wheezing fit before turning five had one or more by the time they were nine years old. The number of wheezing episodes before age five was a highly reliable indicator of the prognosis at age 10. By the time they were 10 years old, half of the kids who had been diagnosed with asthma at age five had recovered. Sporik and associates examined 67 kids who had a family history of asthma. While children who started wheezing later in life tended to have more persistent wheezing and higher bronchial hyperresponsiveness (BHR), early wheezing children did not tend to continue wheezing and had normal bronchial hyperreactivity at age 11 (Table 5.7).

Table 5.7. *Asthma Presentations Across the Lifecourse*

Age	Presentation/Phenotype	Description
Child	Asthma diagnosis	Physician's diagnosis of asthma at least once per lifetime or recurrent diagnoses of spastic, obstructive, or asthmatic bronchitis as reported by the parents at age 6 years
	Frequent wheeze	Wheeze on a monthly basis for at least 1 year between age 1 and 6 years

	Unremitting wheeze	Having symptoms between wheezing episodes or having wheeze without a cold at least once between age 1 and 6 years
	Recurrent unremitting wheeze	Having symptoms between wheezing episodes or wheeze without a cold for 2 or more years between age 1 and 6 years
	Multi-Trigger wheeze	Having at least 2 common asthma triggers leading to wheeze between ages 3 and 6 years
	Episodic wheeze	Wheezing episodes associated only with viral upper respiratory infection between age 1 and 6 years.
	Severe asthma Difficult to control asthma Therapy resistant asthma	Asthma which is poorly controlled based on frequent symptoms and significant morbidity Often due to incorrect diagnosis, poor adherence to therapy, incorrect inhaler/spacer technique, uncontrolled comorbidities (allergic rhinitis) Poorly controlled asthma after ruling out "Difficult to control asthma"
	Eosinophilic predominant asthma	Allergic asthma
	Neutrophilic predominant asthma	Non-allergic asthma
	Recurrent croup Middle lobe syndrome	Repeated episodes of croup Repeated episodes of middle lobe infiltrate or atelectasis
	Recurrent pneumonia	Repeated episodes of lung infection
Adult	Late onset eosinophilic asthma	Later onset, predominately female, and elevated sputum and serum eosinophils, associated with sinusitis
	Obesity related asthma	Associated with increased levels of TNFa, IL-6, leptins, less eosinophils, FeNO, and corticosteroid responsiveness
	Neutrophilic asthma	Difficult to characterize, often severely obstructed with only partial reversibility and a high healthcare utilization
	Aspirin- associated asthma	Subset of late-onset eosinophilic asthma, associated with sinusitis, nasal polyps, and sensitivity to cyclooxygenase-1 inhibitors
	Allergic bronchopulmonary aspergillosis	Lower airway allergic sensitization to *Aspergillus fumigatus* causing asthma exacerbations, pulmonary function deterioration, mucous plugging, central bronchiectasis, and transient pulmonary infiltrate

Source: Trivedi M and Denton E (2019) Asthma in Children and Adults—What Are the Differences and What Can They Tell us About Asthma? Front. Pediatr. 7:256. doi: 10.3389/fped.2019.00256.

Many studies have produced data that covers the years from childhood to early adulthood. One of the earliest investigations using this design was carried out in Australia, first by McNicol and associates. The sample's age at enrollment in 1964 was 7 years old; follow-up has now been completed for a maximum of 21 years, or 28 years old. Wheezing tended to follow over time, but only 32% of people still wheezed at least once a week at age 28 and 43% had stopped by then. On spirometry, those with more severe wheezing at age 28 tended to have lower lung function levels and higher airway responsiveness during a methacholine challenge. Some got better with time, but about the same amount got worse.

The United Kingdom's 1958 birth cohort has now been followed up to age 33 years in another extensive, long-term study. Participants' parents were questioned when they were 7, 11, and 16 years old, and the participants themselves were questioned when they were 23 and 33 years old. Over time, asthma symptoms tend to subside. Among children who were diagnosed with asthma or wheezy bronchitis before turning 7, only 10% reported experiencing wheezing in the previous year at age 23, a percentage that rose to 27% at age 33. A sample of 1060 participants with a history of wheezy bronchitis or asthma and 275 controls had their lung function assessed. Lung function was only marginally lower in those who did not report wheezing at age 33 when compared to the controls. Wheezing patients had a FEV 1 that was about 10% lower than that of the control group.

Several smaller studies have produced similar results. Of the adult population with a history of childhood asthma, about half no longer had symptoms. In these studies, adult status was predicted by childhood history. Specifically, childhood atopy predicted adult status, and childhood airway responsiveness predicted adult airway responsiveness, which was greater in those with persistent symptoms but did not tend to wane over time.

5.4.2. Determinants of the Natural History of Childhood Asthma

5.4.2.1. Gender

Boys are more likely than girls to have asthma, but the disease does not seem to progress differently based on a person's gender. The clinical course was similar in males and females over 20-year follow-up intervals in the early studies by Rackenmann, Edwards, and Blair. According to the results of the Australian cohort study, which McNicol and Williams started, women may have an easier time in their early adult life. Men were much more likely than women to have transitioned to a more severely symptomatic group between the ages of 21 and 28.

5.4.2.2. Age and Severity of Onset

Regarding the age at which asthma attacks begin and how long they last in children, the early clinic-based research gave contradictory results. More recent prospective cohort studies have demonstrated that wheezing during early childhood and infancy does not always indicate asthma and has a different natural history from wheezing with a later onset. In the follow-up study of the United Kingdom's 1958 birth cohort, individuals who reported wheezing for the first time before the age of 7 years old tended to be less symptomatic at age 33. The initial severity of childhood asthma may be a useful clinical marker, even though the age of onset may not be a reliable indicator of how the condition will develop.

5.4.2.3. Atopic Status

Numerous studies have linked atopy indicators to a worse prognosis. Children who tested positive for asthma on skin tests and had eczema had more severe asthma in the early Buffum and Settipane study. The continuation of asthma has also been linked to the persistence of eczema. The 1958 United Kingdom birth cohort follow-up yielded similar results. When it came to people who had asthma or wheezy bronchitis by the age of 16, those who reported having hay fever, allergic rhinitis, or eczema in the previous year were about twice as likely to have wheezed in the same time period. In Sporik and colleagues' cohort study of infants at high risk for allergic diseases, atopy was also linked to persistent wheezing.

5.4.2.4. Family History

Numerous studies have demonstrated that a child's risk for a chronic illness is increased when there is a family history of asthma. Further insightful studies of genotype and prognosis will surely come after these scant data.

5.4.2.5. Smoking

There has been a correlation found between smoking during adolescence and early adulthood and a higher chance of symptom persistence. The United Kingdom's 1958 birth cohort study found that current smokers were more likely to relapse at age 33. In a 25-year follow-up study, smoking was linked to a higher risk of wheezing and other symptoms in kids who were initially enrolled in an Aberdeen school survey.

5.4.2.6. Treatment

While treatment has been demonstrated to significantly improve the condition of children with asthma, there is no evidence that early intervention or intensive therapy changes the disease's natural course. The Australian study found no correlation between the intensity of therapy reported at previous evaluations and the severity of asthma at age 21. The National Heart, Lung, and Blood Institute-funded Childhood Asthma Management Program (CAMP) is a randomized trial that is currently investigating the hypothesis that frequent and intensive treatment may have a positive impact on the natural course of childhood asthma.

A Closer Look

Natural History of Asthma in Adulthood

Asthma in adults is a more diverse condition than in children. In addition to the inherent problem of defining asthma, the reversible airway obstruction of asthma may become irreversible to a degree in some adults, and separating such individuals from those with cigarette smoke-induced chronic obstructive pulmonary disease (COPD) may be difficult. The presence of atopy is not a useful criterion, as atopy is present in about 35% of the adult population, and adults with COPD may have increased airway responsiveness with inhalation challenge testing.

Asthma in adults is a mixture of the disease that has started in childhood and is following its natural course and asthma developing de novo during the adult years. This mixed composition of asthma in adults makes studies of adult asthma relevant to childhood asthma. Difficulties arise in evaluating natural history because the effects of asthma on the lung must be separated from effects of factors that vary with the calendar period (e.g., changing environmental factors) and aging of the lung itself.

The problem of defining asthma has plagued the adult studies as it has those of childhood. Most investigators have used the response to a self-administered questionnaire to identify the presence of asthma. This approach appears to have satisfactory validity in general. Enarson and colleagues have shown that a positive response to the question Have you ever had bronchial asthma? is closely correlated with BHR. Almind and co-workers have also used reversibility of FEV 1 or diurnal variation of peak expiratory flow rates (PEFR), as possible diagnostic criteria for asthma. Patients' knowledge of their own diagnosis may underestimate the prevalence of asthma in some settings; consequently some researchers have asked about wheeze and followed this symptom prospectively in addition to the self-reported diagnosis of asthma. Most of the studies have evaluated subjects at only two points in time with no data on the intervening years. Peat and co-workers have provided the longest study to date, with four observations made over 18 years in Busselton, West Australia. Busselton had a population study every 3 years. In 1981, every fourth attender was assigned to the asthma study, in which 922 subjects had lung function and bronchial responsiveness measured. A total of 484 of these subjects were restudied in 1984. The final sample consisted of 92 asthmatics and 186 controls, with four measurements taken between 1966 and 1984. This study has provided the first description of FEV 1 decline in asthmatics and normals drawn from the general population.

The natural history of asthma in adults has been evaluated in terms of (1) effect of asthma on rate of decline of pulmonary function, (2) clinical course, (3) the development of irreversible airway obstruction, and (4) mortality.

Summary

- Asthma is a chronic inflammatory disease of the airways, characterized by recurrent episodes of airflow obstruction resulting from edema, bronchospasm, and increased mucus production. Commonly associated with seasonal allergies (allergic rhinitis) and eczema (atopic dermatitis), these three conditions form what is known as the atopic triad.
- The exact etiology of asthma remains unclear and appears to be multifactorial. Both genetic and environmental factors seem to contribute. Positive family history is a risk factor for asthma but is neither necessary nor sufficient for the development of the disease. Multiple environmental exposures, both prenatal and during childhood, are associated with the development of asthma.
- Epidemiologic data have provided substantial insights into the patterns of occurrence of pediatric asthma and the factors that determine risks for the disease. Incidence has been described and its natural history has been evaluated. Striking variation in the frequency of childhood asthma has been demonstrated, comparing urban, inner-city areas and suburban and rural areas in the United States, and across countries. The prevalence of pediatric asthma has been convincingly shown to be rising in a number of developed countries. Methodologic differences in the techniques used to identify persons as having asthma do not appear to be the sole explanation. Mortality from asthma has again risen in a number of countries.
- The rising prevalence of asthma has sparked speculation about changes in risk factors for asthma, particularly related to indoor air pollution and respiratory infections. However, definitive research has not yet been conducted to test these hypotheses; neither have the periodic fluctuations of asthma mortality been fully explained. The epidemic asthma mortality of the 1960s was attributed to the use of specific, potent bronchodilators, and similar concerns about therapeutic agents have been raised in relation to the more recent rise in asthma mortality. Epidemiologic studies have provided an indication that drug therapy could be playing a role, although observational data have inherent limitations for isolating the effects of therapy, since the more severe asthmatics tend to be treated more aggressively.
- A number of risk factors have been identified for the development of asthma. For some—indoor allergens and tobacco smoke exposure— the evidence is sufficient to warrant programs of intervention. Current concepts of the pathogenesis of asthma emphasize gene–environment interaction; we do not yet know; however, how genes and environmental factors act together to determine asthma risks. Future research, incorporating genetic marks of susceptibility, will ultimately be informative for clinicians and for those concerned with preventing asthma.

References

1. Ball, T. M., Castro-Rodriguez, J. A., Griffith, K. A., et al. (2000). Siblings, day-care attendance, and the risk of asthma and wheezing during childhood. *New England Journal of Medicine, 348*, 538–543.
2. Bont, L., Heijnen, C. J., Kavelaars, A., et al. (2000). Monocyte IL-10 production during respiratory syncytial virus bronchiolitis is associated with recurrent wheezing in a one-year follow-up study. *American Journal of Respiratory and Critical Care Medicine, 161*, 1518–1523.
3. Castro-Rodriguez, J. A., Holberg, C. J., Morgan, W. J., et al. (2000). Increased incidence of asthma-like symptoms in girls who become overweight or obese during the school years. *American Journal of Respiratory and Critical Care Medicine, in press.*
4. Collins, A., Ennis, S., Tapper, W., et al. (2000). Mapping oligogenes for atopy and asthma by meta-analysis. *Genetics and Molecular Biology, 23*, 1–10.
5. Cookson, W. O. C., & Moffatt, M. F. (2000). Genetics of asthma and allergic disease. *Human Molecular Genetics, 9*, 2359–2364.
6. Ernst, P., & Cormier, Y. (2000). Relative scarcity of asthma and atopy among rural adolescents raised on a farm. *American Journal of Respiratory and Critical Care Medicine, 161*, 1563–1566.
7. Gereda, J. E., Leung, D. Y. M., Thatayatikon, A., et al. (2000). Relation between house-dust endotoxin exposure, type 1 T-cell development, and allergen sensitization in infants at high risk of asthma. *Lancet, 355*, 1680–1683.
8. Gordis, L. (2000). *Epidemiology* (2nd ed.). Philadelphia: W. B. Saunders.
9. Matricardi, P. M., Rosmini, F., Riondino, S., et al. (2000). Exposure to foodborne and orofecal microbes versus airborne viruses in relation to atopy and allergic asthma: Epidemiological study. *BMJ, 320*, 412–417.
10. O'Donnell, A. R., Hayden, C. M., Laing, I. A., et al. (2000). Association study of CC16 and CD14 polymorphisms in an unselected population assessed at age 8 and 25. *American Journal of Respiratory and Critical Care Medicine, 161*, A928.
11. Ober, C., & Moffatt, M. F. (2000). The pathobiology of asthma: Implications for treatment. *Clinical Chest Medicine, 21*, 1–18.
12. Riedler, J., Eder, W., Oberfeld, G., et al. (2000). Austrian children living on a farm have less hay fever, asthma and allergic sensitization. *Clinical and Experimental Allergy, 30*, 194–200.
13. Sampogna, F., Demenais, F., Hochez, J., et al. (2000). Segregation analysis of IgE levels in 335 French families (EGEA) using different strategies to correct for the ascertainment through a correlated trait (asthma). *Genetic Epidemiology, 18*, 128–142.
14. Tulic, M. K., Wale, J. L., Holt, P. G., et al. (2000). Modification of the inflammatory response to allergen challenge after exposure to bacterial lipopolysaccharide. *American Journal of Respiratory Cell and Molecular Biology, 22*, 604–612.
15. Von Ehrenstein, O. S., von Mutius, E., Illi, S., et al. (2000). Reduced risk of hay fever and asthma among children of farmers. *Clinical and Experimental Allergy, 30*, 187–193.
16. Wang, T. N., Ko, Y. C., Wang, T. H., et al. (2000). Segregation analysis of asthma: Recessive major gene component for asthma in relation to history of atopic diseases. *American Journal of Medical Genetics, 93*, 373–380.

17. Welliver, R. C. (2000). Immunology of respiratory syncytial virus infection: Eosinophils, cytokines, chemokines and asthma. *Pediatric Infectious Disease Journal, 19*, 780–783.

18. Wright, A. L., Holberg, C. J., Taussig, L. M., et al. (2000). Maternal asthma status alters the relation of infant feeding to asthma and recurrent wheeze in childhood. *Thorax, in press.*

19. Young, S., Arnott, J., O'Keeffe, P. T., et al. (2000). The association between early life lung function and wheezing during the first 2 years of life. *European Respiratory Journal, 15*, 151–157.

Chapter 6

NONINFECTIOUS PULMONARY DISORDERS

Contents

Introduction

Noninfectious pulmonary disorders encompass a broad spectrum of conditions affecting the respiratory system that are not caused by infectious agents. These disorders can arise from various factors including environmental exposures, genetic predispositions, autoimmune reactions, and lifestyle choices. Chronic obstructive pulmonary disease (COPD) stands out as a leading cause of morbidity and mortality worldwide, primarily driven by smoking and environmental pollutants. Characterized by progressive airflow limitation, COPD encompasses conditions such as emphysema and chronic bronchitis, leading to symptoms like coughing, wheezing, and dyspnea. Asthma, another prevalent disorder, involves airway inflammation and hyperresponsiveness, often triggered by allergens or irritants, resulting in recurrent episodes of wheezing, chest tightness, and coughing. Occupational lung diseases, induced by exposure to harmful substances in the workplace, encompass conditions like pneumoconiosis (e.g., coal workers' pneumoconiosis) and occupational asthma. Interstitial lung diseases (ILDs) comprise a diverse group of disorders affecting the interstitium of the lungs, including idiopathic pulmonary fibrosis (IPF), sarcoidosis, and connective tissue disease-associated ILDs. IPF, in particular, is characterized by progressive scarring of lung tissue with an unknown cause and poor prognosis. Other noninfectious pulmonary disorders include pulmonary hypertension, pulmonary embolism, and lung cancer, each with its distinct etiology, pathophysiology, and clinical manifestations. While treatment approaches vary depending on the specific disorder, management often involves a combination of pharmacotherapy, pulmonary rehabilitation, oxygen therapy, and, in some cases, surgical interventions such as lung transplantation. Overall, noninfectious pulmonary disorders pose significant challenges in healthcare due to their diverse nature, chronicity, and impact on patients' quality of life, necessitating comprehensive approaches to diagnosis, treatment, and prevention.

Orientation and Directional Terms

Term	Definition	Illustration
Chronic obstructive pulmonary disease (COPD)	Chronic obstructive pulmonary disease, or COPD, refers to a group of diseases that cause airflow blockage and breathing-related problems. It includes emphysema and chronic bronchitis. COPD makes breathing difficult for the 16 million Americans who have this disease.	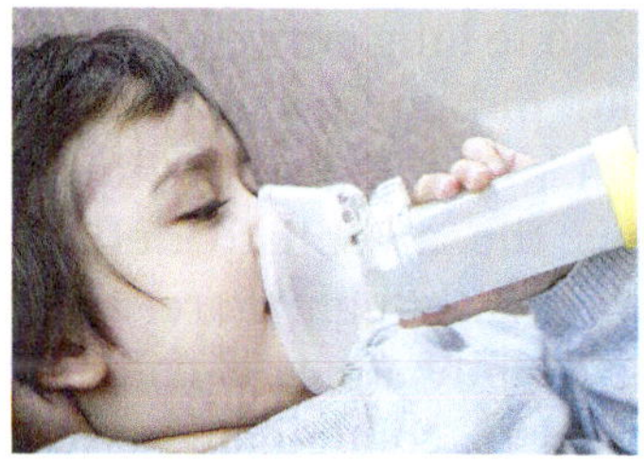
Interstitial lung diseases (ILDs)	Interstitial lung diseases (ILDs) are a group of several disorders that can cause scarring in your lungs. The scar tissue in your lungs affects your lungs' ability to carry oxygen and can make it harder for you to breathe normally.	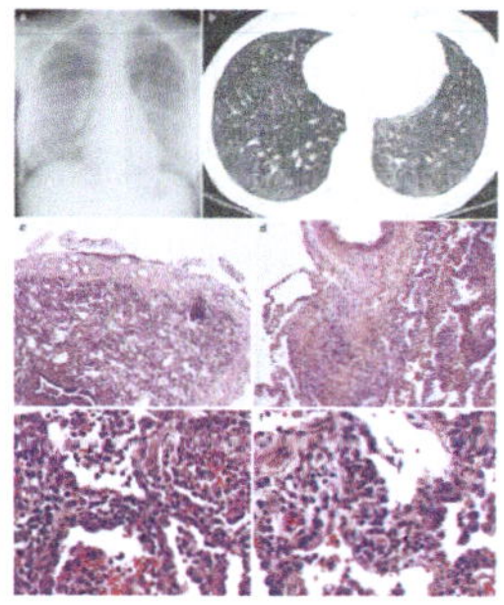
Atelectasis	Atelectasis is the collapse of a lung or part of a lung, also known as a lobe. It happens when tiny air sacs within the lung, called alveoli, lose air. Atelectasis is one of the most common breathing complications after surgery.	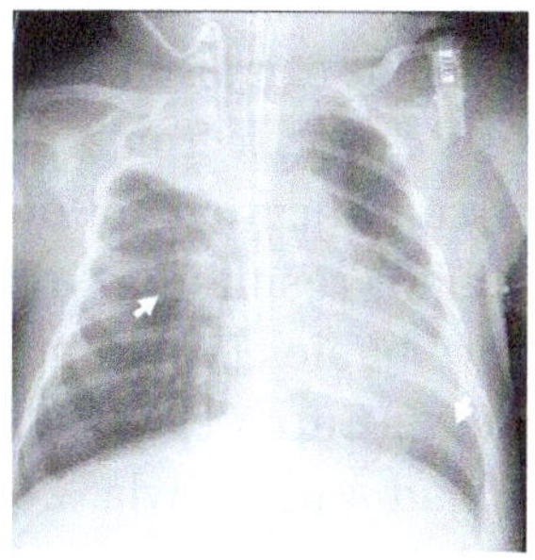
Rheumatoid arthritis (RA)	Rheumatoid arthritis can cause pain, swelling, and deformity. As the tissue that lines your joints (synovial membrane) becomes inflamed and thickened, fluid builds up and joints erode and degrade. Rheumatoid arthritis is a chronic inflammatory disorder that can affect more than just your joints.	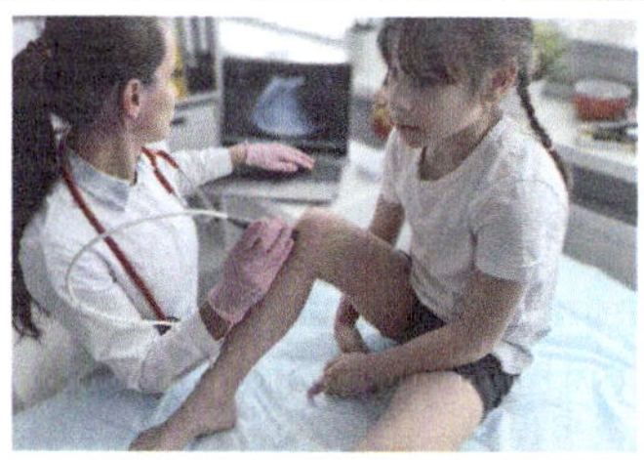
Idiopathic pulmonary fibrosis (IPF)	Idiopathic pulmonary fibrosis (IPF) is the most common type of pulmonary fibrosis. It is a disease that causes scarring (fibrosis) of the lungs. The word "idiopathic" means it has no known cause. Scarring causes stiffness in the lungs and makes it difficult to breathe.	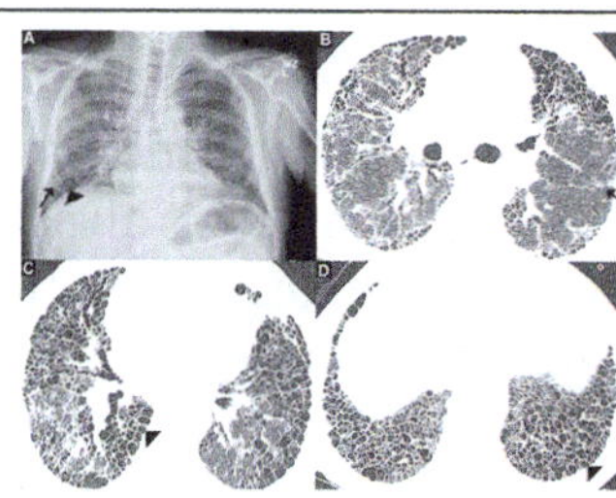

6.1. Atelectasis

Athelectasis is a partial lung collapse or closure that leaves little to no gas exchange. Usually, it affects one lung entirely or partially unilaterally. Unlike pulmonary consolidation, when the alveoli are filled with liquid, this condition causes the alveoli to deflate to little or no volume. Although more accurately it usually involves only a partial collapse, it is commonly referred to colloquially as a "collapsed lung." However, that ambiguous term is also used colloquially for a fully collapsed lung caused by a pneumothorax.

It can be caused by a number of medical conditions or by normal exhalation, and it is a very common finding in chest X-rays and other radiological studies. While atelectasis is often defined as a collapse of lung tissue, it should not be confused with pneumothorax, a more specific condition that can also cause atelectasis. Acute atelectasis can arise from a surfactant deficiency or as a complication following surgery. This causes infant respiratory distress syndrome in premature babies (Wedding et al., 2005; Kemp et al., 2008; Gupta et al., 2014; McKean et al., 2017; Rajan and Chawla, 2017).

6.1.1. What are the Types of Atelectasis?

There are two types of atelectasis: obstructive and nonobstructive. When something physically blocks the airway, it results in the reabsorption of air (oxygen and carbon dioxide) from the alveoli, which causes the lung portion in question to collapse. This condition is known as obstructive atelectasis, also known as resorptive atelectasis. Nonobstructive atelectasis, on the other hand, encompasses all other forms that are not connected to an obstruction. Compressive, contraction, and adhesive atelectasis are examples of nonobstructive atelectasis types. When something presses against and compresses the lungs, it results in compressive atelectasis. The cause of contraction atelectasis is fibrosis, or scar tissue that prevents alveoli from expanding and contracting. Lastly, a loss of surfactant on the alveoli results in adhesive atelectasis.

6.1.2. Signs and Symptoms

May have no signs and symptoms or they may include:

- cough, but not prominent,
- chest pain (not common),
- breathing difficulty (fast and shallow),
- low oxygen saturation,
- pleural effusion (transudate type),
- cyanosis (late sign),
- increased heart rate.

There is a widespread misperception and pure conjecture that atelectasis results in fever. According to a study of 100 post-operative patients, fever incidence declined as atelectasis incidence increased. The patients were monitored with serial chest X-rays and temperature readings. The relationship between post-operative fever and atelectasis was found to be unsupported by clinical data.

6.1.3. Causes

The most common cause is post-surgical atelectasis, characterized by splinting, i.e., restricted breathing after abdominal surgery. Atelectasis is a common complication in people undergoing general anesthesia for surgery, occurring in 75–90% of cases. It can also be caused by pulmonary tuberculosis, smoking, and old age. Atelectasis typically involves a blockage in a bronchiole or bronchus, either from something inside the airway (like a foreign object or mucus), a tumor on the airway wall, or pressure from outside (such as a tumor or lymph node). Poor spreading of surfactant during breathing can also lead to collapsed alveoli. Suctioning can exacerbate atelectasis by removing air along with mucus from the lungs. There are different types of atelectasis depending on the cause or pattern of alveolar collapse, such as resorption, compression, microatelectasis, and contraction atelectasis. Relaxation atelectasis occurs when a pleural effusion or pneumothorax interrupts the contact between the parietal and visceral pleurae.

A higher chance of developing atelectasis is linked to certain risk factors, such as the type of surgery (cardiopulmonary or thoracic), the use of muscle relaxation techniques, obesity, high oxygen levels, and lower lung segments. The following variables are also linked to the development of atelectasis: age, anesthesia type, and the existence of asthma or chronic obstructive pulmonary disease.

6.1.4. Diagnosis

On a chest X-ray, clinically significant atelectasis is typically visible; findings may include lung opacification and/or lung volume loss. A biopsy-induced atelectasis will have a bibasal pattern. If the cause of atelectasis is not clinically evident, a bronchoscopy or chest CT scan may be required. The displacement of interlobar fissures and mobile structures within the thorax, overinflation of the unaffected ipsilateral lobe or contralateral lung, and opacification of the collapsed lobe are direct indicators of atelectasis. Apart from the clinically noteworthy results on chest X-rays, patients might also exhibit indirect indications and symptoms like diaphragmatic elevation, tracheal, heart, and mediastinum shifting, hilus displacement, and shifting granulomas shifting.

6.1.4.1. Classification

It is possible for atelectasis to be either acute or chronic. The lung has recently collapsed in acute atelectasis, and its main characteristic is airlessness. The afflicted region in chronic atelectasis is frequently characterized by a complex combination of destruction, bronchiectasis (widening of the bronchi), infection, and scarring (fibrosis).

6.1.4.1.1. Absorption (Resorption) Atelectasis

The primary constituents of the Earth's atmosphere are 78 vol. nitrogen percentage and 21 vol. % oxygen plus one volume. % argon with minor amounts of additional gases). Nitrogen plays a significant role in the alveoli's inflationary state because oxygen is exchanged at the alveoli-capillary membrane. The replacement of a significant amount of nitrogen in the lungs with oxygen may cause the oxygen to be absorbed into the blood, which will decrease the volume of the alveoli and cause absorption atelectasis, a type of alveolar collapse.

6.1.4.1.2. Compression (relaxation) Atelectasis

It is typically linked to a buildup of air, blood, or fluid in the pleural cavity, which causes the lung to mechanically collapse. This is a common occurrence when congestive heart failure (CHF) causes pleural effusion. Compression atelectasis is another consequence of pneumothorax, or the leakage of air into the pleural cavity.

6.1.4.1.3. Cicatrization (Contraction) Atelectasis

It occurs when either local or generalized fibrotic changes in the lung or pleura hamper expansion and increase elastic recoil during expiration. Causes include granulomatous disease, necrotizing pneumonia and radiation fibrosis.

6.1.4.1.4. Chronic Atelectasis

Chronic atelectasis may take one of two forms—middle lobe syndrome or rounded atelectasis.

1. **Right Middle Lobe Syndrome:** The middle lobe of the right lung contracts in right middle lobe syndrome, usually as a result of pressure from enlarged lymph glands or, on occasion, a tumor pressing on the bronchus. The blocked, contracted lung may experience pneumonia, which can cause chronic inflammation, scarring, and bronchiectasis if it does not fully resolve.
2. **Patchy Atelectasis:** It is due to the lack of surfactant, as occurs in hyaline membrane disease of newborns or acute (adult) respiratory distress syndrome (ARDS).
3. **Rounded Atelectasis:** The pleura, or membrane layers covering the lungs, shrinks, and scars in rounded atelectasis (also known as folded lung or Blesovsky syndrome), causing an outer part of the lung to slowly collapse. This condition manifests as visceral pleural thickening and lung tissue entrapment. This causes an X-ray to appear rounded, which medical professionals might confuse for a tumor. Although it can also arise from other forms of chronic scarring and thickening of the pleura, rounded atelectasis is typically a consequence of asbestos-induced disease of the pleura.

6.1.5. Treatment

The goal of treatment is to address the underlying cause. Mucolytic medications like acetylcysteine (NAC) are used in cases of pneumonia and cystic fibrosis patients exhibiting atelectasis symptoms due to mucus plugging the airways. Through the breaking of disulfide bonds in the mucoproteins within the mucus complex, this nebulized treatment helps to facilitate the clearance of mucus by reducing mucous viscosity and elasticity. Physiotherapy is used to treat post-surgical atelectasis; it emphasizes deep breathing and coughing encouragement. One common tool used in the breathing exercises is the incentive spirometer. Another very recommended exercise to enhance lung inflation is walking. Mechanical breathing aids may help people with deformities of the chest or neurological disorders that result in prolonged shallow breathing.

Treating the underlying cause is the main treatment for acute massive atelectasis. A bronchoscopy is often able to remove a blockage that cannot be cleared by coughing or by suctioning the airways. Infections are treated with antibiotics. Since infection is practically a given, antibiotics are frequently used to treat chronic atelectasis. When recurrent or chronic infections become incapacitating or when there is significant bleeding, the affected lung portion may occasionally be surgically removed. Relieving the obstruction caused by a tumor that is obstructing the airway through surgery, radiation therapy, chemotherapy, or laser therapy can stop the development of recurrent obstructive pneumonia and the progression of atelectasis.

6.1.6. Prevention of Atelectasis

Deep breathing exercises designed to maintain lung expansion are usually recommended for the prevention of atelectasis, particularly following surgery. An incentive spirometer, a tool that tracks the quality of breaths taken while a person takes slow, deep breaths, may be used for some of the exercises. Taking pain medication, walking around early, shifting positions frequently, and practicing coughing are some other postoperative preventive techniques. People with chronic illnesses, like cystic fibrosis, may receive chest physical therapy, which clears mucus from the lungs, to avoid atelectasis. Coughing, cupping the hand and tapping on the chest, or sitting in various positions to allow the mucus to move naturally are some methods of chest physical therapy (i.e., percussion) in order to loosen the mucus (Wedding et al., 2005; Kemp et al., 2008; Gupta et al., 2014; McKean et al., 2017; Rajan and Chawla, 2017).

6.2. Respiratory Disorders Associated with Systemic Inflammatory Diseases

Respiratory disorders associated with systemic inflammatory diseases represent a complex interplay between immune dysregulation and pulmonary manifestations. Rheumatoid arthritis (RA), a chronic autoimmune condition, can involve the respiratory system, leading to interstitial lung disease (ILD), pleural disease, and airway complications. ILD in RA often presents as nonspecific interstitial pneumonia (NSIP) or usual interstitial pneumonia (UIP), contributing to progressive dyspnea and impaired lung function. Systemic sclerosis (SSc), another autoimmune disorder, frequently manifests with pulmonary involvement, including ILD (often with a pattern resembling UIP), pulmonary arterial hypertension (PAH), and airway disease. SSc-associated ILD can significantly impact prognosis and requires close monitoring and aggressive management. Systemic lupus erythematosus (SLE) can also affect the respiratory system, with manifestations ranging from pleuritis and pleural effusions to lupus pneumonitis and pulmonary hypertension. Additionally, inflammatory bowel diseases (IBD) such as Crohn's disease and ulcerative colitis can be associated with various pulmonary complications, including airway disease, ILD, and pulmonary vasculitis. Psoriasis, a chronic inflammatory skin disorder, has been linked to an increased risk of respiratory comorbidities such as chronic obstructive pulmonary disease (COPD) and asthma. Understanding the relationship between systemic inflammatory diseases and respiratory disorders is crucial for timely diagnosis and management, often requiring a multidisciplinary approach involving rheumatologists, pulmonologists, and other specialists. Treatment strategies may involve immunosuppressive therapy, anti-inflammatory agents, and targeted therapies tailored to the specific underlying condition and pulmonary manifestations, aiming to alleviate symptoms, preserve lung function, and improve overall outcomes. Early recognition and comprehensive management of respiratory complications in systemic inflammatory diseases are essential to optimize patient care and minimize long-term morbidity and mortality (Wedding et al., 2005; Kemp et al., 2008; Gupta et al., 2014; McKean et al., 2017; Rajan and Chawla, 2017).

6.3. Interstitial Lung Disease

The way that interstitial lung disease (ILD) manifests in adults and children differs significantly. The development and maturation of the pediatric lung is the backdrop against which pediatric ILD occurs. Although little is known about the biology of the development of the postnatal lung, it is probably safe to assume that the normal profiles of cytokine and growth factor expression are very different in childhood compared with adulthood. There are significant differences in the functional behavior of the immune system between adults and children. In fact, a recent study describing an extended kindred with familial ILD found that the disease's adult presentation was consistent with the histology of usual interstitial pneumonitis (UIP), a form of ILD that is essentially unknown in children, while the disease's likely identical childhood manifestation was identified as cellular non-specific interstitial pneumonitis (NSIP). For a more thorough discussion of this phenotype, refer to the section below. Pulmonary interstitial glycogenosis (PIG), another recently identified condition, might potentially be an odd developmental reaction to an unidentified insult. Since pediatric ILD is far less common and less stigmatized than adult ILD, even less is known about treating children with ILD than there is for adults. Lastly, new entities are being found that are either common to adults and children (SP-C deficiency) or unique to infants and occasionally older children (SP-B deficiency, PIG).

Making the diagnosis of pediatric ILD is undoubtedly uncommon. The spectrum can be characterized as including more specific diagnoses that may be linked to immunodeficiencies, for example, as well as inflammatory interstitial diseases of various morphologies without underlying causes. ILD is strictly defined as pathological, meaning that there are more or abnormal inflammatory cells in the interstitium and alveoli. Different cell types may make up the infiltrate. This diagnosis can only be made in a specific case following a lung biopsy, so it is preferable to begin at the clinical end, with presentation.

6.3.1. Classification

The rarity of these conditions and the challenge of comparing across age groups because of variations in immune and pulmonary cell maturity complicate classification. There are numerous practical methods for segmenting the spectrum of pediatric ILD. One classification is summarized in table 6.1.

Those with a known cause make up the first group (Table 6.1).These include the metabolic diseases (e.g., lysinuric acid intolerance and Gaucher's disease), and neurocutaneous syndromes, e.g., tuberose sclerosis. The surfactant protein deficiencies, discussed in more detail below, belong in this category. Drugs (especially chemotherapy for cancerous diseases), radiation, and graft-versus-host disease following bone marrow transplantation are other known specific causes.

Table 6.1. *Distinguishing Features Among Six Common ILD Subgroups*

ILD Subgroup	Medical History Clues	Radiographic Findings	Histologic Patterns	Autoimmune Serology Evaluation	Therapeutic Considerations
Smoking-Related	Prior or current tobacco smoking, biomass combustion exposure	GGO, emphysema with fibrosis, mosaic attenuation	RB, DIP, PLCH, emphysema, fibrosis	Normal or non-reactive	Smoking cessation, removal from exposure, anti-inflammatory therapy in advanced disease
Hypersensitivity Pneumonitis	Exposure to environmental organic antigens (avian proteins, mold, farming-related)	GGO, mosaic attenuation, upper-lobe fibrosis, centrilobular nodules	Poorly-formed granulomas with multinucleated giant cells	Normal or non-reactive; consider serum precipitating antibody panel	Removal from exposure, remediation of environment, anti-inflammatory, and/or immunosuppressive therapy in advanced disease

Connective Tissue Disease-Related	Constitutional symptoms, arthralgia/arthritis, rash, Raynaud's phenomenon	GGO, reticular opacities, consolidation, fibrosis, peripheral sparing	Chronic inflammation, UIP, NSIP, or OP	Autoimmune evaluation recommended	Anti-inflammatory and/or immunosuppressive therapy
Occupation-Related	Current or prior at-risk occupation	GGO, reticular opacities, fibrosis, nodules, pleural plaques (asbestos)	Chronic inflammation, UIP, NSIP, OP, or granulomatous inflammation	Normal or non-reactive; lymphocyte proliferation test if beryllium exposure suspected	Removal from exposure, use of respiratory protective equipment
Medication-Induced	Current or prior use of possible offending medications or therapies	GGO, reticular opacities, consolidation, nodules, fibrosis	Chronic inflammation, UIP, NSIP, OP, or granulomatous inflammation	Usually normal or non-reactive	Medication discontinuation if possible, anti-inflammatory, and/or immunosuppressive therapy in advanced disease
Idiopathic Pulmonary Fibrosis	Male predominance, 7th–8th decade, past history of tobacco smoking or dust exposure	Peripheral and basilar fibrosis with honeycombing (Figure 6.3)	UIP	Normal or non-reactive	Consideration of antifibrotic therapies, lung transplantation evaluation in selected patients

GGO, ground-glass opacities; RB, respiratory bronchiolitis; DIP, desquamative interstitial pneumonia; PLCH, pulmonary Langerhans cell histiocytosis; UIP, usual interstitial pneumonia; NSIP, nonspecific interstitial pneumonia; OP, organizing pneumonia.

Source: Kalchiem-Dekel O, Galvin JR, Burke AP, Atamas SP, Todd NW. Interstitial Lung Disease and Pulmonary Fibrosis: A Practical Approach for General Medicine Physicians with Focus on the Medical History. Journal of Clinical Medicine. 2018; 7(12):476. https://doi.org/10.3390/jcm7120476.

In an effort to reconsider how these conditions are classified, the current author and colleagues have recently reviewed their biopsy experience (Table 6.4). The histological characteristics of desquamative interstitial pneumonitis (DIP), chronic NSIP, and chronic pneumonitis of infancy (CPI), three conditions that have only recently been described (Figure 6.1).

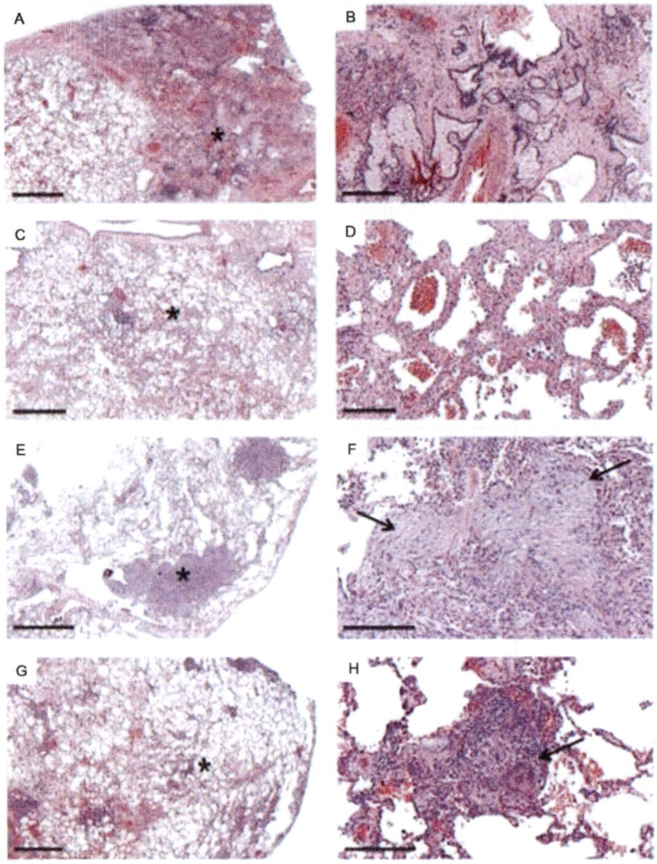

Figure 6.1. *Common histopathologic patterns observed in various forms of ILD. Each pair of horizontal panels represent low (left panel) and high (right panel) magnification images taken from the same tissue section, and the high magnification images are taken from areas identified by an asterisk (*) on low magnification.*

Source: *Kalchiem-Dekel O, Galvin JR, Burke AP, Atamas SP, Todd NW. Interstitial Lung Disease and Pulmonary Fibrosis: A Practical Approach for General Medicine Physicians with Focus on the Medical History. Journal of Clinical Medicine. 2018; 7(12):476. https://doi.org/10.3390/jcm7120476.*

Panels (A, B) demonstrate usual interstitial pneumonia (UIP). Low magnification demonstrates dense fibrotic change and destruction of normal lung architecture on the right side of panel (A), and relatively normal lung on the left side of panel (A). There are widespread areas of honeycomb change observed in the fibrotic areas, as seen on low and high magnification. Panels (C, D) demonstrate non-specific interstitial pneumonia (NSIP). Low magnification demonstrates uniform thickening of the alveolar walls (i.e., the lung interstitium) diffusely throughout the lung, and high magnification demonstrates a combination of cellular inflammation (lymphocytes and macrophages) as well as collagen deposition in these thickened walls. Panels (E, F) demonstrate organizing pneumonia (OP). Low magnification demonstrates preservation of overall lung architecture, but large focal areas of lung abnormality (asterisk in panel (E)) are observed; high magnification demonstrates these focal abnormalities to be areas of organization (arrows in panel (F)). Panels (G, H) demonstrate granulomatous inflammation. Low magnification demonstrates widespread small focal areas of inflammation centered around small airways, and high magnification demonstrates many of these focal areas of inflammation to contain poorly formed granulomas and multinucleated giant cells (arrow in panel H). Horizontal black bars in the lower left of each of the panels (A–H) represent 2 mm (panels A, C, E, G), 300 µm (panel B), and 200 µm (panels D, F, H).

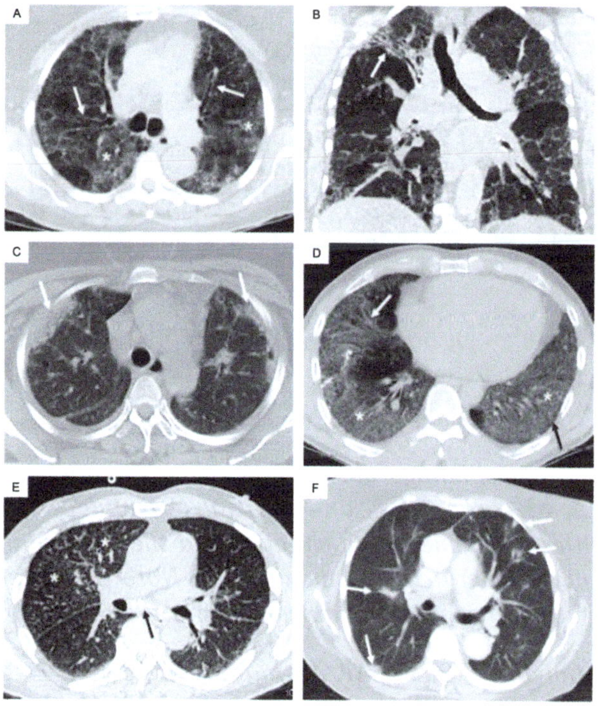

Figure 6.2. *Common radiologic patterns observed on chest CT imaging in various forms of ILD. Panel (A) demonstrates widespread GGO (asterisk) and accompanying traction bronchiectasis (arrows); overall clinical diagnosis was smoking-related ILD. Panel (B) demonstrates findings of fibrosis in the right upper lobe with traction bronchiectasis and volume loss (arrow), and widespread areas of bilateral mosaic attenuation, defined as interspersed areas of hyperattenuated lung (gray) and hypoattenuated lung (black); overall clinical diagnosis was hypersensitivity pneumonitis. Panel (C) demonstrates peripheral areas of consolidation (arrows); overall clinical diagnosis was ILD secondary to systemic lupus erythematosus (SLE). Panel (D) demonstrates widespread areas of GGO (asterisk), mild sparing of the extreme periphery of the lung (black arrow), and mild traction bronchiectasis (white arrow); overall clinical diagnosis was ILD secondary to anti-synthetase syndrome. Panel E demonstrates small nodules, reticular opacities, and prominent interlobular septa in the right upper lobe (asterisk) and to a lesser extent in the left lower lobe, along with calcified mediastinal adenopathy (arrow); overall clinical diagnosis was ILD secondary to chronic beryllium exposure. Panel F* demonstrates multiple ill-defined nodules (arrows) along with surrounding GGO; overall clinical diagnosis was ILD secondary to amiodarone.

Source: Kalchiem-Dekel O, Galvin JR, Burke AP, Atamas SP, Todd NW. Interstitial Lung Disease and Pulmonary Fibrosis: A Practical Approach for General Medicine Physicians with Focus on the Medical History. Journal of Clinical Medicine. 2018; 7(12):476. https://doi.org/10.3390/jcm7120476.

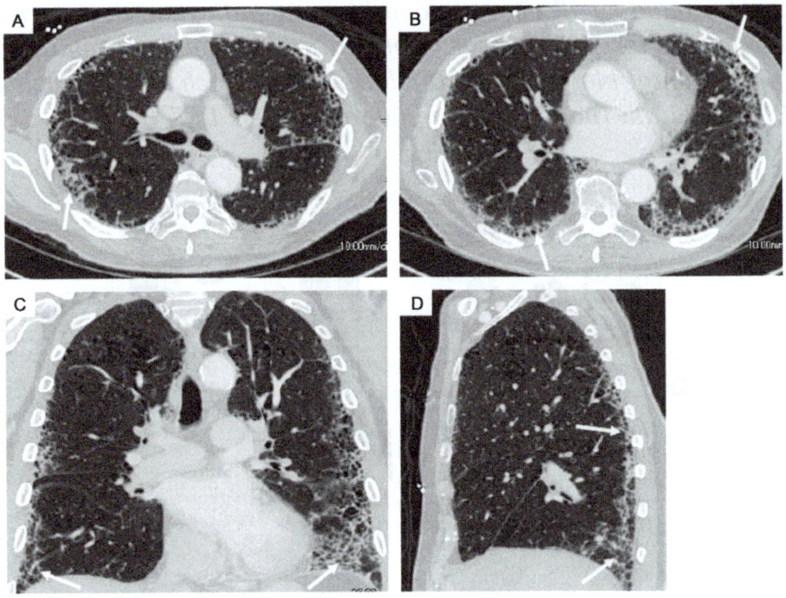

Figure 6.3. *NS Typical radiologic findings observed on chest CT imaging in idiopathic pulmonary fibrosis (IPF), with axial (A, B) coronal (C), and sagittal (D) images. The nature of the opacities (curvilinear reticular opacities and honeycomb change) and their distribution (markedly peripheral and lower lobe-predominant) are very consistent with IPF. Note the absence of subpleural sparing, GGO, consolidation, mosaic attenuation, and nodules which are often observed in other forms of ILD.*

Source: Kalchiem-Dekel O, Galvin JR, Burke AP, Atamas SP, Todd NW. Interstitial Lung Disease and Pulmonary Fibrosis: A Practical Approach for General Medicine Physicians with Focus on the Medical History. Journal of Clinical Medicine. 2018; 7(12):476. https://doi.org/10.3390/jcm7120476.

Age is another useful criterion for sub-typing pediatric ILD; several conditions, some of which have only recently been identified, manifest in early childhood. It is unknown if some of these disorders that appear to be exclusive to infants actually manifest later in life with a different histology. For instance, it is unknown what connection exists between adult idiopathic diffuse hyperplasia of pulmonary neuroendocrine cells and neuroendocrine cell hyperplasia of infancy (NEHI) (Table 6.2).

Table 6.2. *Suggested Serum Serologies in the Evaluation of Patients with ILD*

Serum Markers of Systemic Inflammation
• erythrocyte sedimentation rate (ESR)
• c-reactive protein (CRP)
Autoantibodies
Anti-neutrophil cytoplasmic antibodies (ANCAs)
• c-ANCA, p-ANCA, atypical p-ANCA
• anti-MPO
• anti-PR3
Rheumatoid arthritis

• anti-CCP			
• rheumatoid factor (RF)			
SLE and related autoimmune diseases (MCTD, Sjögren's syndrome)			
• ANA			
• anti-dsDNA			
• anti-SS-A (Ro)			
• anti-SS-B (La)			
• anti-Smith			
• anti-RNP			
Systemic sclerosis			
• anti-Scl-70			
• anti-Centromere			
Myositis-specific and myositis-associated antibodies			
• anti-Jo1	• anti-PL7	• anti-PL12	• anti-EJ
• anti-OJ	• anti-SRP	• anti-Mi-2α	• anti-Mi-2β
• anti-MDA5	• anti-TIF-1γ	• anti-NXP-2	• anti-KS
• anti-Zo	• anti-Ku		
Muscle Enzymes			
• CPK			
• aldolase			

Abbreviations: c, cytoplasmic; p, perinuclear; MPO, myeloperoxidase; PR3, proteinase 3; CCP, cyclic citrullinated peptide; SLE, systemic lupus erythematosus; ANA, anti-nuclear antibody; dsDNA, double stranded DNA; SS-A, Sjögren's syndrome-related antigen A; SS-B, Sjögren's syndrome-related antigen B; RNP, ribonucleoprotein; MDA, melanoma differentiation-associated gene; SRP, signal recognition particle; TIF, transcriptional intermediary factor; NXP, nuclear matrix protein; CPK, creatine phosphokinase.

Source: Kalchiem-Dekel O, Galvin JR, Burke AP, Atamas SP, Todd NW. Interstitial Lung Disease and Pulmonary Fibrosis: A Practical Approach for General Medicine Physicians with Focus on the Medical History. Journal of Clinical Medicine. 2018; 7(12):476. https://doi.org/10.3390/jcm7120476.

6.3.2. How to Identify Children with ILD

6.3.2.1. Clinical Features

ILD in children can manifest at any age. The newborn period is when presentations peak. Their presentation is very nonspecific, usually presenting with cough, tachypnea, and respiratory distress lasting for at least one month. The presence of ILD in other family members, any relationship to feeding or swallowing, potential environmental inhalant triggers, or characteristics suggestive of a multisystem disease—particularly affecting the skin, joints, eyes, or kidneys—are among the specific features that should be looked for. There could be a failure to prosper. Cyanosis is a sign of a more advanced illness. These symptoms have many more common causes, and other diagnoses, like asthma, have typically been ruled out.

Physical examination may show signs of respiratory distress, such as recession and tachypnea; crackles on auscultation occasionally; and digital clubbing, which is often missed and will not be identified unless specifically sought. It is necessary to do a thorough assessment of other systems and to test the urine for protein and blood (Table 6.3).

Table 6.3. *Compilation of Classifications of Interstitial Lung Diseases (ILDs) or Diffuse Parenchymal Lung Diseases (DPLDs)*

Category (This Paper)	ATS/ERS Internatl. Multi-disciplinary Consensus Classification 2002	ATS/ERS Respiratory Society Statement: Update (Travis et al., 2013)	ERS/ATS Research Statement (Fischer et al., 2015)	ERS Task Force on Chronic Interstitial Lung Disease (Clement 2004)	Diffuse Lung Disease in Children (Deutsch 2007)	Incidence and Classification of Pediatric Diffuse Parenchymal Lung Diseases (Griese et al., 2009)	A National Internet-Linked Database for Pediatric Interstitial Lung Diseases (Nathan et al., 2012)	Diffuse Lung Disease in Infancy and Childhood: Expanding the chILD Classification (Rice et al., 2013)	Interstitial Lung Disease in Childhood: Clinical and Genetic Aspects (Kitazawa and Kure 2015)
	adult	adult	adult	pediatric	pediatric	pediatric	pediatric	pediatric	pediatric
Lung only (or native parenchymal) disorders				Congenital disorders	Diffuse developmental disorders	Diffuse developmental disorders (A1)	ILD specific to infancy	Diffuse developmental disorders	Diffuse developmental disorders and growth abnormalities
					Growth abnormalities reflecting deficient alveolarisation	Growth abnormalities deficient alveolarisation (A2)		Growth abnormalities	
					Specific conditions of undefined etiology	Infant conditions of undefined etiology (A3)		Specific conditions of undefined etiology	Conditions specific to infancy
	Idiopathic interstitial pneumonias:			Idiopathic interstitial pneumonias	Surfactant dysfunction disorders	DPLD-related to alveolar surfactant region (A4)	Alveolar disorder related ILD	Histological patterns associated with surfactant disorders	Genetic surfactant dysfunctions

Category (This Paper)	ATS/ERS Internatl. Multi-disciplinary Consensus Classification 2002	ATS/ERS Respiratory Society Statement: Update (Travis et al., 2013)	ERS/ATS Research Statement (Fischer et al., 2015)	ERS Task Force on Chronic Interstitial Lung Disease (Clement 2004)	Diffuse Lung Disease in Children (Deutsch 2007)	Incidence and Classification of Pediatric Diffuse Parenchymal Lung Diseases (Griese et al., 2009)	A National Internet-Linked Database for Pediatric Interstitial Lung Diseases (Nathan et al., 2012)	Diffuse Lung Disease in Infancy and Childhood: Expanding the chILD Classification (Rice et al., 2013)	Interstitial Lung Disease in Childhood: Clinical and Genetic Aspects (Kitazawa and Kure 2015)
	Idiopathic pulmonary fibrosis (IPF), nonspecific interstitial pneumonia (NSIP), cryptogenic organi-zing pneumonia (COP), acute interstitial pneumo-nia (AIP), desquamative interstitial pneumonia (DIP), idiopathic pleuroparenchymal fibroelastosis			Other forms of interstitial pneumonia		Unclear RDS in the mature/ almost mature neonate (Ax/ Ay)		Interstitial pneumonia unrelated to surfactant protein disorder	
	Respiratory bronchiolitis-interstitial lung disease (RB-ILD)							Small airways disease	
		Unclassifiable idiopathic interstitial pneumonias				Unclear RDS in the NON-neonate (Bx)	ILD with no diagnosis		
Systemic disease related disorders	DPLD of known cause (e.g., associated with collagen vascular disease)		Interstitial pneumonia with auto-immune features	DPLD of known association (e.g., connective tissue disorders)	Disorders related to systemic disease processes	DPLD—related to systemic disease processes (B1)	Systemic disease associated ILD	Disorders related to systemic disease	Interstitial lung disease related to a primary systemic disease
	Granulomatous DPLD e.g., sarcoidosis						Granulo-matous diseases		
	Other forms of DPLD (e.g., LAM, HX)						Metabolic disorders		
					Disorders of the immunoco-mpromised host	DPLD—In the immunocompro-mised host or transplanted (B3)	Infectious ILD	Host disorders (presumed immuno-compromised)	

Category (This Paper)	ATS/ERS Internatl. Multi-disciplinary Consensus Classification 2002	ATS/ERS Respiratory Society Statement: Update (Travis et al., 2013)	ERS/ATS Research Statement (Fischer et al., 2015)	ERS Task Force on Chronic Interstitial Lung Disease (Clement 2004)	Diffuse Lung Disease in Children (Deutsch 2007)	Incidence and Classification of Pediatric Diffuse Parenchymal Lung Diseases (Griese et al., 2009)	A National Internet-Linked Database for Pediatric Interstitial Lung Diseases (Nathan et al., 2012)	Diffuse Lung Disease in Infancy and Childhood: Expanding the chILD Classification (Rice et al., 2013)	Interstitial Lung Disease in Childhood: Clinical and Genetic Aspects (Kitazawa and Kure 2015)
	Lymphoid interstitial pneumonia (LIP)	Idiopathic lymphoid interstitial pneumonia				DPLD—Related to reactive lymphoid lesions (B5)		Lymphoproliferative disease	
Exposure-related disorders	DPLD of known cause e.g., drugs			DPLD of known association (e.g., drug, aspiration, infection, enviro-nment)	Disorders of the normal host presumed immune intact	DPLD—In the presumed immune intact host, related to exposures (infect/non-infect) (B2)	Exposure related ILD Hypers-ensitivity pneum-onitis	Host disorders (presumed immune intact)	Exposure-related Interstitial lung disease
Vascular disorders					Disorders masquerading as interstitial disease	DPLD—Related to lung vessels structural processes (B4)	Alveolar vascular disorder related ILD	Disorders masquerading as interstitial disease	

Source: Griese M. Etiologic Classification of Diffuse Parenchymal (Interstitial) Lung Diseases. Journal of Clinical Medicine. 2022; 11(6):1747. https://doi.org/10.3390/jcm11061747.

6.3.2.2. Pulmonary Function Tests

Restrictive physiology, or a reduction in both forced expired volume in one second (FEV1) and forced vital capacity (FVC), with a normal or elevated FEV1/FVC ratio, is typical in children old enough to undergo lung function tests. If there has recently been a pulmonary hemorrhage because of IPH or another pulmonary bleeding disorder, carbon monoxide transfer is typically decreased but may be elevated. In general, exercise testing is probably better for assessing severity, tracking disease progression, or tracking response to treatment than for diagnosing ILD. However, it may reveal desaturation, pointing to the disease. On the other hand, a large number of pediatric ILD cases are in an age group where lung function testing is challenging outside of a research setting. Little research has been done on lung function testing in infants and preschoolers with pediatric ILD, and it would be incorrect to assume that the results would be the same for older children given the wide range of pathologies present in this age group. In fact, there is evidence that suggests the physiology of infantile ILD may be obstructive rather than restrictive. Further investigation is required in this field.

6.3.2.3. Imaging

The chest radiograph typically yields very little information and is not diagnostic. There could be coarse nodular or reticular nodular shadowing, or ground glass shadowing with noticeable air bronchograms; in more severe cases, honeycombing is visible. Nonetheless, chest radiography may not be abnormal in certain ILD children. Generally speaking, the chest radiograph has low sensitivity and specificity and shows little correlation with histology, symptoms, or treatment response. Usually, the high-resolution computed tomographic (HRCT) scan will provide the conclusive evidence that the tachypneic child has an ILD. Occasionally, a primary airway disease, such as bronchiectasis or reflux and aspiration, may be observed, leading to entirely new avenues of inquiry. As an alternative, a child's chest radiograph that appears normal may actually reveal significant ground-glass shadowing or other abnormalities that point to ILD.

Table 6.4. *Classification of Interstitial Lung Diseases (ILDs) Used in the chILD-EU Register (full list available* ***www.childeu.net****, accessed on 29 December 2021)*

Category	Specifier	Subcategories (Major Examples)	Specific Conditions
Lung only (native parenchymal) disorders	Developmental	Diffuse (A1) - Alveolar capillary dysplasia, misalign pulmonary veins (ACDMPV) - Congenital alveolar dysplasia (CAD)	Alveolarization (A2) - Pulmonary hypoplasia - Pulmonary hypoplasia associated with diaphragmatic hernia - Chronic lung disease of prematurity (BPD-cLD)

Category	Specifier	Subcategories (Major Examples)	Specific Conditions
		Infant tachypnea (A3) - Chronic tachypnea of infancy (CTI) (usual, aberrant) - Neuroendocrine cell hyperplasia of infancy (NEHI) - Pulmonary interstitial glycogenosis (PIG)	Surfactant region (A4) - Chronic pneumonitis of infancy (CPI) - Surfactant protein B deficiency - Other surfactant dysfunction disorders - Undefined ILD in mature neonate - Undefined ILD in almost (gest. age 30–36 weeks) mature neonate
	All ages	- ABCA3 deficiency - Surfactant protein C deficiency - Lipoid pneumonitis, cholesterol pneumonia - Nonspecific interstitial pneumonia (NSIP) - Idiopathic pulmonary fibrosis (IPF)/Usual interstitial pneumonitis (UIP) - Cryptogenic organizing pneumonia (COP)	- Acute interstitial pneumonia (AIP) - Desquamative interstitial pneumonia (DIP) - Idiopathic pleuro-parenchymal fibroelastosis - Eosinophilic pneumonitis - Undefined ILD in NON-neonate - Unclassifiable idiopathic interstitial pneumonias
Systemic disease related disorders	Immuno competent	- Collagen vascular/ connective tissue related disorders (CTD-ILD) - Eosinophilic granulomatosis with polyangiitis (EGPA, Churg Strauss) - Granulomatosis with polyangiitis (GPA, Wegener) - Metabolic disorders - Disorders related to chromosomal abnormalities - Aminoacyl-tRNA synthetase (-ARS) deficiency - Birt-Hogg-Dube syndrome - Granulomatous diseases	- Diffuse alveolar hemorrhage due to vasculitic disorders - ITGA3 (Integrin α3) mutations with kidney, lung, skin disease - Niemann-Pick disease - Nkx2.1 gene defect (brain-thyroid-lung syndrome) - Lysinuric proteinuria - PAP secondary to associated diseases - Sarcoidosis - TBX4 mutation (small patella syndrome) - Hoyeral Hreidasson Syndrome (congenital dyskeratosis) - Telomere-related-diseases
	Immuno deficient	- Phagocyte-PAP.CSF2RA or CSF2RB (PAP due to GMCSF receptor deficiency)	- Phagocyte-GATA2 def (MonoMac syndrome).GATA2

Category	Specifier	Subcategories (Major Examples)	Specific Conditions
	Transplanted	- Chronic allograft dysfunction, idiopathic pneumonia syndrome	
	Immune-dysregulated	- Autoimmune pulmonary alveolar proteinosis (PAP) - Antisynthetase syndrome - Celiac disease/pulmonary hemorrhage (Lane-Hamilton) - Anti-basement membrane antibody disease (Goodpasture) - Granulomatous lymphocytic interstitial lung disease (GLILD)	- Follicular bronchitis/ bronchiolitis - Lymphocytic interstitial pneumonia (LIP) - Interstitial pneumonia with auto-immune features (IPAF) - ZNFX1 deficiency - Immune-dysregulated Hermansky Pudlak syndrome
	Auto-inflammatory	- COPA defect - STING-associated vasculopathy, infantile-onset.TMEM173	- OAS1 deficiency - Other interferonopathies
Exposure related disorders	Non-infectious	Exogen allergic alveolitis/ hypersensitivity pneumonitis - Drug induced ILD - Pneumoconiosis	- Radiation lung injury - Respiratory bronchiolitis-interstitial lung disease (RB-ILD) - Occupational lung diseases
	Infectious	- Infectious/post-infectious bronchiolitis obliterans (PIBO) - Diffuse panbronchiolitis	- Mac-Leod-Swyer-James-Syndrome
Vascular disorders		- Diffuse pulmonary (alveolar) hemorrhage (DPH) - Idiopathic pulmonary hemorrhage (hemosiderosis) (IPH) with or without associated features - Pulmonary capillaritis	- Pulmonary capillary hemangiomatosis (PCH) - Pulmonary vena-occlusive disease - Lymphangiomatosis

Source: *Griese M. Etiologic Classification of Diffuse Parenchymal (Interstitial) Lung Diseases.* Journal of Clinical Medicine. *2022; 11(6):1747. https://doi.org/10.3390/jcm11061747.*

In this case, there are three more justifications for executing HRCT. Firstly, HRCT may be diagnostic in very few cases. Although this is far less common than adult ILD, certain patterns, such as pulmonary microlithiasis, pulmonary alveolar proteinosis (PAP), Langerhans cell histiocytosis (LCH), or IPH, may be recognized, avoiding the need for additional testing. The second reason is to identify the location for a lung biopsy, which is most likely going to be necessary. Lastly, it is important to correlate HRCT appearances with the final diagnosis in the hopes that a more accurate interpretation of HRCT will one day eliminate the need for lung biopsies.

6.3.3. The Differential Diagnosis

The majority of pediatric pulmonology is included in the differential diagnosis of ILD. A few sets of conditions are particularly significant in practice. *Pneumocystis carinii* pneumonia, in particular, along with any secondary opportunistic infection, including HIV and hypogammaglobulinemia, can manifest as immune lowering disease (ILD). As part of the diagnostic testing for ILD, an immune work-up may be required. This may involve testing for lymphocyte subsets, immunoglobulins, and subclasses, response to vaccine antibodies, and lymphocyte function. It is required to refer a patient for a more thorough assessment to a pediatric immunologist if the level of suspicion is high. Aspiration, which is typically brought on by gastroesophageal reflux, uncoordinated swallowing, H-type fistula, or laryngeal cleft, is another category of conditions that should be taken into account. This group includes chemical pneumonitis brought on by inhaling oil from nose drops or other medications. Respiratory distress and non-specific chest radiograph shadowing may be caused by any cause of bronchiectasis or chronic bronchial sepsis; however, HRCT should confirm this diagnosis. A further diagnosis that enters the differential is pulmonary edema. The cause is typically cardiac, such as ventricular septal defect or left-to-right shunting brought on by an arterial duct. Non-cardiogenic pulmonary edema typically manifests acutely and is infrequently taken into account for diagnosis in cases of chronic ILD.

Lastly, pulmonary vascular conditions can resemble ILD. These include schistosomal ovuli, intravenous drug abuse, pulmonary embolism (which can be thrombo-embolic or non-thrombotic owing to tumors), etc. pulmonary capillary hemonagiomatosis, pulmonary veno-occlusive disease, and others. The last diagnosis is extremely uncommon. An early examination ought to include an echocardiography. It could make an unanticipated cardiac lesion that caused pulmonary edema visible, or it could allow for a non-invasive assessment of pulmonary artery pressure, which is helpful because pulmonary hypertension can exacerbate pediatric ILD. Regardless of the chest radiography appearances, additional investigations are required if ILD is a plausible diagnosis. The next line of inquiry is HRCT, which ought to come before running a comprehensive panel of blood tests.

6.3.4. Non-Invasive Diagnosis

Once the diagnosis of ILD has been established through history, physical examination, and HRCT, a methodical investigative process ought to be initiated. Serology is the least invasive method. Instead of running a large battery of tests on every case, it is preferable to conduct a few focused investigations and postpone making a final diagnosis while awaiting the results. An opportunistic infection or an unsuspected immunodeficiency may be revealed by a comprehensive immunological work-up. The best methods for diagnosing these conditions are bronchoscopy and bronchoalveolar lavage (BAL). HIV testing is required if opportunistic infection is suspected. The diagnosis of Wegener's granulomatosis or another connective tissue disease may be made using an auto-antibody profile, which should include anti-neutrophil cytoplasmic antibody. This could eliminate the need for a lung biopsy. Renal impairment would indicate Wegener's, Goodpasture's, or another vasculitis, which could be verified by serological testing. Sarcoidosis would be suspected if the angiotensin converting enzyme test came back positive. If there is a compatible history and positive precipitins to, say, pigeon antigen, they would indicate allergic alveolitis and allow treatment to begin without the need for additional testing. After outlining these possibilities, it was discovered that a positive serological diagnosis in pediatric ILD is uncommon (Wedding et al., 2005; Kemp et al., 2008; Gupta et al., 2014; McKean et al., 2017; Rajan and Chawla, 2017).

6.3.4. Role of Bronchoscopy

Fiberoptic bronchoscopy (FOB) enables transbronchial biopsy (TBB), BAL, and airway inspection and biopsy (which are nearly always uninformative in ILD). Nonetheless, a general anesthetic is necessary for the procedure, or a very strong sedative that almost feels like general anesthesia. It should only be carried out if there is a genuine chance that a conclusive diagnosis will be made. When diagnosing opportunistic infections in an immunocompromised host, BAL is a highly valuable tool (Figure 6.4), especially if the child has not previously received antibiotic therapy.

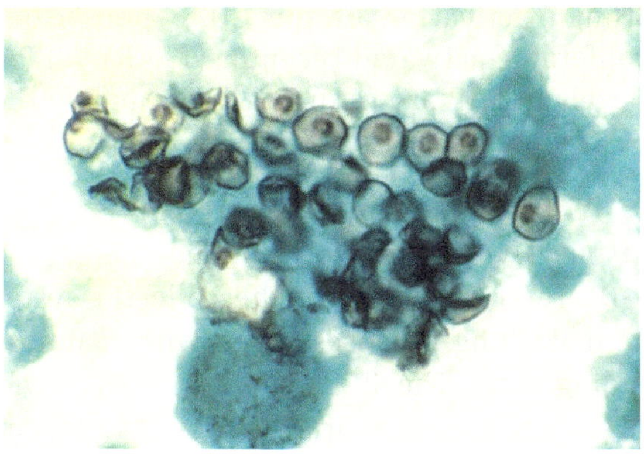

Figure 6.4. *BAL from a child thought to have ILD. Silver stain shows Pneumocystis carinii in a child who ultimately proved to have an immunodeficiency.*

Source: https://upload.wikimedia.org/wikipedia/commons/8/8b/Pneumocystis_carinii_in_smear_from_BAL_01ee046_lores.jpg.

The most recent recommendations regarding bronchoscopy and BAL should be closely followed. The diagnostic yield is low when ILD is present in an otherwise healthy host. BAL can be used to diagnose a few specific conditions, such as lipoid pneumonia caused by aspirating oily medications, IPH, LCH, and PAP. However, in general, BAL is not helpful in other ILDs due to the dearth of normal ranges and the paucity of pediatric BAL experience in ILD.

When it comes to potential lung rejection following a transplant, TBB is invaluable because the small airways—rather than the alveoli—are the main target. It is only beneficial in cases of extremely specific histological features (e.g., microlithiasis of the alveoli). Most pediatric ILDs cannot be diagnosed due to the small sample sizes. In addition, there are safety concerns: pneumothoraxes, which frequently necessitate a chest drain, can occasionally be difficult to control bleeding. Moreover, TBB can only be performed on very young children using a rigid bronchoscope or a modified 2.2-mm bronchoscope. Using this technique, the feeding tube is inserted into a segmental orifice under direct vision, and the bronchoscope is threaded through it. After removing the endoscope and leaving the tube in place, a TBB is performed by passing biopsy forceps down the tube. Furthermore, in the majority of pediatric ILD cases, such samples are probably too tiny to be useful for diagnosis.

6.3.5. Invasive Diagnosis

As can be seen from the above, most pediatric ILD cases will need a biopsy to be diagnosed (figure 6.8), and this should not be put off unless there is a reasonable chance that less invasive procedures will be able to avoid the need for this invasive procedure. Specifically, subjecting the child to multiple anesthetics is not appropriate, e.g., for FOB, followed by HRCT, before proceeding with a biopsy. The tissue's final destination should be considered when performing a biopsy; some tissue should be kept in storage at −70°C for later use. It is always recommended to perform standard histology, immunohistochemistry, electron microscopy, and culture of the biopsy for the presence of fungi and mycobacteria in particular. The limitations of TBB in ILD have already been covered; alternative options include video-assisted thoracic surgery (VATS), open lung biopsy (OLB) via a mini-thoracotomy incision, and percutaneous CT-guided biopsy.

Although percutaneous biopsy has been used in some centers, it is not the best method because it requires a full general anesthesia for the child, takes tissue samples without direct vision even though they are obtained under CT control, and has an unacceptable risk of bleeding and pneumothorax due to its uncontrolled and blind nature. The gold standard for lung biopsies is direct vision because it is a safe and well-tolerated procedure. The surgeon's experience level and the child's size will determine whether a mini-thoracotomy or a VATS procedure is used.

The current author recently discussed his personal experience having a mini-thoracotomy for OLB. In the operating room, the chest drain is typically removed, leaving the child with a small lateral scar. The procedure is well tolerated, and there are very few complications. Large samples can typically be obtained, and a diagnosis can be made. Oral steroids can be empirically trialed as an alternative to biopsy. This isn't ideal, though, as there are known cases of ILDs not responding, and there are risks associated with this therapy. Corticosteroids may actually exacerbate certain conditions that can manifest as ILD, such as an undetected opportunistic infection in a host that was previously believed to be immunocompetent. Furthermore, the healing of the wound may be hampered if OLB is started after a steroid trial fails.

6.3.5.1. Surfactant Protein Abnormalities/PAP Spectrum

The histological appearance of PAP, which shows preserved lung architecture and alveoli filled with granular, eosinophilic material that stains with periodic-acid Schiff, can be caused by three different clinical conditions: congenital, which includes mutations in the genes encoding SP-B or C, or the βC chain of the granulocyte-macrophage colony stimulating factor (GM-CSF) receptor (see below); secondary, in conditions linked to macrophage functional impairment (such as infections, hematological cancers); and later-onset, likely an autoimmune disease, with auto-antibodies targeting GM-CSF. When it was discovered that the GM-CSF knockout mouse had a PAP-like illness with normal surfactant synthesis and recovered after GM-CSF replacement, the significance of GM-CSF in surfactant biology was brought to light. Later, auto-antibodies directed against GM-CSF were discovered in PAP with a late onset. GM-CSF appears to control surfactant homeostasis through activation of the CD36 peroxisome proliferator-activated receptor (PPAR) γ. PPAR γ-levels in PAP are returned to normal by GM-CSF treatment.

Physiology of surfactant proteins is outside the purview of this work. In short, SP-A, and SP-D are components of the collectin system of innate lung defenses along with mannose-binding lectin. The SP-B and SP-C genes provide the surface tension characteristics of surfactant, and mutations in these genes are linked to PAP and other types of ILD.

6.3.5.2. SP-B Deficiency

The congenital form of PAP has been linked to defects in the gene encoding SP-B. The SP-B gene has 11 exons and 9.5 kb. It is found on chromosome 2. The gene product is a prepro-SP-B, about 40 kDa, which is processed to yield mature SP-B (8 kDa), at both the amino and carboxyterminal ends. Numerous mutations have been reported; the most prevalent is a frameshift mutation in exon 4 (1549C-GAA, 121ins2), along with other mutations like 122delC and 457delC. In the population, there is most likely one mutation for every 3000 individuals. A description of the underlying metabolic defect has been obtained. Normal transcription of the mutated gene results in the production of an unstable mRNA. In a term baby, it usually manifests as a respiratory failure that worsens over time, with radiographs displaying established fibrosis or ground-glass shadowing.

The absence of SP-B staining in lung biopsies or tracheal aspirates establishes the diagnosis. A baby with a mutation in one copy of the SP-B gene but a normal copy of the second gene was reported to have a transient absence of SP-B from the tracheal aspirate, but not from a lung biopsy. This suggests that relying solely on the aspirate may be misleading. Misprocessing of SP-C may also lead to diagnostic confusion, but this is a secondary phenomenon.

6.3.5.3. SP-C Deficiency

It has been discovered that both adult and pediatric ILD are linked to defects in SP-C. In the initial instance, a 1-year-old girl was diagnosed with DIP and received corticosteroid treatment until she was 15 years old. Her child had NSIP as well. A lifelong respiratory ailment that went undiagnosed claimed the grandfather of the mother. Other ILD families have reported experiencing the same anomaly. It's possible that inherited surfactant protein issues occur more frequently than anticipated. Infants with SP-C mutations were discovered to have a mutation in 11 of the 34 patients who were examined. The mutations most likely have an autosomal dominant inheritance pattern or be sporadic in nature. An increasing number of cases of ILD with unknown cause should include mutation analysis of the SP-B and -C genes, especially if the condition runs in the family.

6.3.5.4. Other Surfactant Problems

Considering the intricate post-translational processing involved in these molecules, it is probable that additional inherited surfactant protein issues will be reported. It was discovered that two newborns with respiratory failure had significantly lower SP-B but normal SP-C. Normal lamellar bodies were absent. On the other hand, sequencing of the SP-B and -C genes revealed that they were normal. Although the exact cause of the aberrant surfactant accumulations in pneumocytes is unknown, potential explanations include primary secretory defects, abnormal interactions between surfactant proteins and phospholipids, or defects in surfactant phospholipids. In a recent study, 16 infants with normal SP-B and -C gene sequences and severe neonatal surfactant deficiency of unknown cause had mutations in the ATP-binding cassette transporter A3 (ABCA3). Lamellar bodies were noticeably abnormal in the lung ultrastructure. Because ABCA3 is localized to lamellar bodies, it may play a significant part in the metabolism of surfactants. Mutations in numerous other genes that code for proteins crucial to surfactant metabolism are probably going to be connected to ILD as well.

6.3.5.5. PIG

Seven infants with tachypnea, hypoxemia, and diffuse infiltrates with hyperinflation were the first to be described with this condition. A lung biopsy revealed interstitial expansion by spindle cells that contained material consistent with glycogen that was periodic-acid Schiffpositive and diastase labile. Six of the seven patients who received treatment—five with pulse corticosteroids and one with additional hydroxychloroquine—performed well. Given that pulmonary interstitial cells typically do not contain large amounts of glycogen, Canakis hypothesized that this was an aberration in lung cytodifferentiation involving interstitial mesenchymal cells.

6.3.5.6. NEHI

NEHI is another ILD that has only been identified in infants thus far. In addition to hyperinflation and ground-glass opacities on HRCT, infants exhibit respiratory distress. Unless they are stained for bombesin, which shows hyperplasia of the neuroendocrine cells and bodies, lung biopsies appear essentially normal. Given the correlation between NEHI and pediatric ILD cases in infancy with normal histology, bombesin staining ought to be included in the assessment of clinical ILD with an apparently normal lung biopsy (Table 6.5).

Table 6.5. *Advantages of an Etiology-Based Classification of Interstitial Lung Diseases*

Etiology is the driving force for most progress towards treatment of conditions
Etiology, as the one major criterion, is primarily used for all classification-decisions in the system
Hierarchically simple and universal system, which can be easily memorized on a major level
Flat, two-level structure (four major, primary levels and not branched second level, which can accommodate any large number of different entities)
Minimizes contradictions often experienced in hierarchical classifications
Open to further subclassification by convenient specifiers and descriptors
Avoids neglect of unclassifiable conditions by also including conditions with currently not exactly known etiology or even for cases in which the absence of information includes classes as "undefined" or "probable"
Ability to annotate relationships between etiologies at all levels of granularity
The system does not ignore tradition of old classification schemes
Open to all ages, accommodating easily age-specific disease manifestations
Supports closer collaboration of pediatric and adult pneumologists, and, for the patients, an improved transition of grown-ups into adult medical services
Computational methods may overcome the relatively large number of conditions resulting, which is seen by some as a disadvantage
Computations over phenotype, multi-omics, environmental, or psychosocial data easily possible
Proven applicability in electronic databases of a large ILD register
Usage of standardized collections of terms (ontologies) for merging with other machine-based systems (big data analysis)

Source: Griese M. Etiologic Classification of Diffuse Parenchymal (Interstitial) Lung Diseases. Journal of Clinical Medicine. 2022; 11(6):1747. https://doi.org/10.3390/jcm11061747.

6.3.5.7. Conventional Treatment

Naturally, treatment for an underlying cause should begin as soon as one is found, such as extrinsic allergic alveolitis. The first thing to determine is whether treatment is even necessary if there is no underlying cause that can be addressed. Some children with ILD experience months or even years of spontaneous remission, even after they have transitioned to oxygen. In one instance, a young girl was diagnosed with Hamman Rich syndrome (acute rapidly progressive pulmonary fibrosis) not long after birth, despite having two first cousins who had passed away from the same condition, as confirmed by autopsy. After being oxygen dependent for seven years, she naturally recovered, and now, at 30, she is doing well without medication and has normal lung function. Treatment will most likely be taken into consideration. Reducing fibrosis and inflammation are the theoretical goals of treatment. The fact that there are only so many therapeutic options available limits these admirable objectives. The primary treatment for inflammation is prednisolone, sometimes paired with cyclophosphamide for certain types of vasculitides. There are few antifibrotic medications available, with hydroxychloroquine possibly having some effect. Colchicine could be another option in theory, but there is limited experience using it for pediatric ILD. There is a lack of large, randomized, controlled trials to provide treatment guidelines.

Some anecdotal evidence exists that suggests that prednisolone and hydroxychloroquine are the treatments of choice for "chronic pneumonitis" of unknown cause. If they fail, any further therapy is anecdotal, and azathioprine, cyclophosphamide (low-dose or pulsed) and cyclosporin are among the therapies that have been used. There is no consensus as to how much and for how long steroids are to be given to patients. In an ill child, the author would use pulsed methyl prednisolone 500 mg per m^2 daily for 5–7 days, followed by prednisolone 2 mg per kg per day, combined with hydroxychloroquine 6–10 mg per kg per day. The dilemma is always to determine when the child has ceased to be steroid responsive, and time is needed for improvement. One method is to repeat the pulses of steroids for 3 days each month, desisting if there is no further improvement.

Other therapies for specific ILDs that have not been adequately studied include hydroxychloroquine, which is believed to be most effective for IPH. Treatment may involve a combination of hydroxychloroquine and oral corticosteroids, with current recommendations suggesting continuing treatment for 2–3 years after the last relapse and confirming remission with a repeat BAL. While chloroquine is known to cause retinal toxicity, ocular complications from hydroxychloroquine are extremely rare and UK guidelines do not require a formal ophthalmological review. However, most pediatricians may still opt to involve ophthalmic services to monitor for and treat potential ocular complications of ILDs, such as anterior uveitis in sarcoidosis. Large-volume lavage can be used to treat PAP, but the results are typically not as good as they would be for adult PAP. In the future, GM-CSF therapy might be promising for some disease types. Treatments for multisystem LCH with pulmonary involvement include steroids, cotrimoxazole, or cytotoxics like etoposide. Isolated pulmonary LCH, which is uncommon in teenagers, may regress spontaneously if tobacco smoke exposure is stopped. Last but not least, occasionally an unexpected infection—like an undetected case of Pneumocystis carinii pneumonia—may be discovered to have mimicked ILD. It goes without saying that these infections need to be treated with the right chemotherapy. These various treatment options for diseases that are admittedly rare but can manifest as ILD provide a strong argument against prednisolone being used in a blind trial without biopsy in every situation. Therapy monitoring is a contentious topic. All tests are not routinely invasive, with the exception of BAL to see if IPH has resolved. Similarly, this investigation is not appealing due to the radiation associated with serial HRCT scans. Typically, general characteristics are used, such as growth pattern, resting respiratory rate, and oxygen requirement, and when a person is old enough to conduct these tests, lung function and exercise testing are added. Lung transplantation is the only option for children who are rapidly approaching respiratory failure. This has been effectively used in cases of SP-B deficiency, so it may be a possibility even for small infants. The problem with other conditions is that the child frequently takes high dosages of oral steroids, which must be tapered off before the child is approved for transplantation. There is a chance that the underlying lung condition will get worse as a result.

6.3.5.8. Treatment of Sarcoidosis with Infliximab

A chimeric immunoglobulin G monoclonal antibody called infliximab targets tumor necrosis factor (TNF)-α and has shown remarkable efficacy in treating rheumatoid arthritis, including pediatric variants, and Crohn's disease. There is a rationale for this treatment because alveolar macrophages from sarcoidosis patients with active sarcoid secrete high levels of TNF-α. It is frequently used in conjunction with 10 mg/m^2 methotrexate once a week to minimize the formation of antibodies against infliximab. Its application to sarcoidosis is limited to case reports, and a randomized trial is being anticipated. Nonetheless, it would seem sensible to take this into account as a possibility for children with refractory sarcoidosis.

6.4. Bronchopulmonary Dysplasia

Premature babies who have bronchopulmonary dysplasia, a chronic lung disease, are affected. Infants born prematurely (preterm) who need continuous oxygen therapy or supplemental oxygen are more vulnerable. The existing alveoli typically lack the maturity necessary for proper function. Additionally, it is more prevalent in low birth weight (LBW) babies and those who are treated for respiratory distress syndrome with prolonged mechanical ventilation. Significant morbidity and mortality are the outcomes. The population has changed, with more survivors at earlier gestational ages and improved neonatal management including surfactant, antenatal glucocorticoid therapy, and less aggressive mechanical ventilation, leading to a continual evolution in the definition of bronchopulmonary dysplasia. At the moment, bronchopulmonary dysplasia is described with three severity levels: mild, moderate, and severe. This is correlated with the infant's overall illness severity, growth, and maturity. A more accurate description of the underlying pulmonary disease and its severity is provided by the new system.

6.4.1. Bronchopulmonary Dysplasia Affects Your Body

BPD damages the alveoli in the lungs, both the developing and the existing ones. Furthermore, there may be an impact on the small blood vessels that encircle the alveoli, which would complicate blood flow through the lungs. The longer a baby is kept on a ventilator, the more likely it is that their lungs will continue to deteriorate. This is because fewer alveoli are functioning. Pulmonary hypertension may eventually result from elevated pressure inside lung blood vessels and between the heart and lungs. Heart failure can happen in extreme circumstances. BPD-affected newborns may also have difficulties eating, which can delay their development.

6.4.2. Causes of Bronchopulmonary Dysplasia

A newborn's underdeveloped lungs at birth may result in BPD, a respiratory condition that necessitates the use of an oxygen therapy or ventilator. Due to the heightened sensitivity of a newborn's lungs, excessive pressure and oxygen intake can cause the alveoli to overstretch, leading to inflammation and harm to the alveoli, surrounding blood vessels, and the lining of the airways. These effects are especially harmful to the premature lung, and BPD is mostly thought to be a prematurity-related complication. Premature labor can result from various conditions that impact the fetus's growth during pregnancy. Prenatal infections or complications related to the mother, such as drug or smoke use, preeclampsia, inflammation of the fetal membranes, or chorioamnionitis, may be the cause of birth defects. Respiratory distress syndrome (RDS) is associated with a higher risk of borderline personality disorder

(BPD) after birth, though not all RDS infants go on to develop BPD. If a child with patent ductus arteriosus—a heart defect in which the blood vessel that connects the left and right sides of the heart fails to close and stays open—is placed on a ventilator, it may result in brain damage and behavioral problems.

6.4.3. Symptoms of Bronchopulmonary Dysplasia

The symptoms of BPD vary depending on its severity. The most common symptoms of bronchopulmonary dysplasia are:

- Rapid breathing.
- Labored breathing (drawing in of the lower chest while breathing in).
- Wheezing (a soft whistling sound as the baby breathes out).
- The need for continued oxygen therapy after the gestational age of 36 weeks.
- Difficulty feeding.
- Repeated lung infections that may require hospitalization.

6.4.4. Diagnosis of Bronchopulmonary Dysplasia

The diagnosis of BPD is based on the clinical evaluation, the degree of prematurity, and the need for oxygen after a certain age.

As infants with BPD usually have oxygen and mechanical ventilation, they are often in the hospital when diagnosed. Regardless, you should contact your pediatrician if:

- Your infant/child is breathing much faster than usual.
- The breathing is labored (pulling in of the skin between the ribs, below the chest or at the bottom of the neck just above the chest).
- There is bluish discoloration around the mouth or lips.
- There are frequent alarms of the apnea monitor and/or pulse oximeter.

6.4.5. Preventing Bronchopulmonary Dysplasia

The best defense against bronchopulmonary dysplasia is to ensure that your child is born after the lungs have fully developed. Pregnancy-friendly behaviors could make this more likely. The basic precautions that any mother should take are to abstain from drugs, alcohol, and smoking, eat healthfully, avoid getting sick, and visit the doctor frequently. In order to accelerate the development of the baby's lung capacity to produce surfactant, your doctor might inject you with a corticosteroid medication if there is a chance that you will give birth before your due date. This will reduce your baby's chance of respiratory distress syndrome, which has been linked to borderline personality disorder.

6.4.6. Treating and Managing Bronchopulmonary Dysplasia

Although there isn't a known cure for BPD, treatment for the condition aims to prevent additional lung damage and support the developing lungs of the child. BPS-affected newborns are typically treated in a hospital environment where they can receive round-the-clock care. Types of drug therapies that may be used are:

- ***Diuretics***: This class of drugs helps to decrease the amount of fluid in and around the alveoli. They are usually given by mouth one to four times per day.
- ***Bronchodilators***: These medications help relax the muscles around the air passages, which makes breathing easier by widening the airway openings. They are usually given as an aerosol by a mask over the

infant's face and using a nebulizer or an inhaler with a spacer.

- ***Corticosteroids***: These drugs reduce and/or prevent inflammation within the lungs. They help reduce swelling in the windpipe and decrease the amount of mucus that is produced. Like bronchodilators, they are also usually given as an aerosol with a mask, either with the use of a nebulizer or an inhaler with a spacer.
- ***Viral immunization***: Children with BPD are at increased risk for respiratory tract infections especially respiratory syncytial virus (RSV). Infants with moderate or severe BPD receive monthly injections with a medication that helps prevent the infection during the RSV season.
- ***Cardiac medications***: A few infants with BPD may require special medications that help relax the muscles around the blood vessels in the lung, allowing the blood to pass more freely and reduce the strain on the heart.

More seriously ill patients might require oxygen for several months. They might also require assistance in the form of a mask or a machine that applies pressure to the nose using unique prongs. These devices offer bilevel positive airway pressure (BiPAP) or nasal continuous positive airway pressure (NCPAP). A tracheostomy—a breathing tube placed through the neck into the lung—will be necessary for the few patients whose condition is so severe that they must remain on a ventilator for an extended period of time.

6.4.6.1. Managing Bronchopulmonary Dysplasia

Bronchopulmonary dysplasia (BPD) typically presents challenges during infancy and early childhood, with symptoms typically diminishing by 2 or 3 years old and treatment concluding by age 5 at the latest. Nevertheless, abnormal lung development may persist, leading to potential lung issues in the future. It is strongly advised that infants with BPD undergo routine check-ups, timely vaccinations, and consultations with a pediatric lung specialist, especially in the initial years of life. Even mild BPD puts premature babies at risk for additional developmental issues. Breathing pauses (apnea), feeding issues that can be severe enough to require a feeding tube, GERD, pulmonary hypertension, neurological issues, vision or hearing issues, and a variety of learning disabilities are common in newborns diagnosed with BPD. In people with mild to moderate BPD, the majority of these complications are uncommon. Even after being released from the hospital, growth might be impeded. It's possible that your child will have lung issues well into adulthood. Many individuals diagnosed with BPD in infancy may go on to suffer from asthma or reactive airway disease, as well as exercise intolerance for the remainder of their lives. Additionally, they might be more prone to illnesses like the flu or the common cold. These viruses may cause more severe symptoms, and recovery times may be longer. Hospitalizations on a regular basis are not uncommon, particularly in patients with moderate to severe BPD (Wedding et al., 2005; Kemp et al., 2008; Gupta et al., 2014; McKean et al., 2017; Rajan and Chawla, 2017).

6.5. Pleural Effusions (Noninfectious)

An accumulation of too much fluid in the pleural space—the potential area surrounding each lung—is called a pleural effusion. A functional vacuum between the parietal and visceral pleurae is maintained in part by the pleural fluid that is secreted by the parietal pleural capillaries at a rate of 0.6 milliliters per kilogram weight per hour under normal circumstances. The fluid is then cleared by lymphatic absorption, leaving behind only 5 to 15 milliliters of fluid. A fully or partially collapsed lung can be the result of excess fluid in the pleural space disrupting the functional vacuum and hydrostatically increasing the resistance against lung expansion.

- **Epidemiology:** Two% to 12% of children with community-acquired pneumonia and up to 28% of children hospitalized for the illness have parapneumonic effusions. The incidence of pediatric bacterial pneumonia has generally decreased, but the rate of complicated cases—such as those involving parapneumonic effusion or empyema—has increased. Hospitalizations for pneumonia complicated by empyema in children under two years old increased from 3.5 cases per 100,000 admissions in 1996–1998 to 7 cases per 100,000 admissions in 2005–2007. In kids between the ages of two and four, the percentage nearly tripled. Despite the low death rate, parapneumonic effusion and empyema place a significant financial strain on the family, the child, and the healthcare system. Less frequently occurring are other causes of pleural effusion, such as cancer, systemic disease-related effusions, traumatic effusions (blood accumulation in the pleural space), postoperative or congenital chylous effusions (lymph fluid accumulation in the pleural space), and chylous effusions from surgery.
- **Pathogenesis:** Pleural fluid is hypotonic in the normal physiological state, with a pH of 7.6, glucose concentrations akin to serum levels, and protein concentrations of roughly 1.5 g/dL (15 g/L). At the parietal pleural level, pleural fluid is filtered, and parietal pleural lymphatics handle reabsorption. The Starling principle describes movement between the pleural and vascular spaces. In response to increased pleural fluid filtration, the flow rate in the pleural lymphatics increases to prevent excessive accumulation of pleural fluid. The visceral and parietal pleural membranes are subject to opposing hydrostatic and oncotic pressures, which block the flow of pleural fluid from the parietal capillaries. When this equilibrium is upset and fluid builds up in the pleural space as a result of an underlying pathologic process, a pleural effusion develops. Pleural effusions can result from a number of conditions, including increased hydrostatic pressure (CHF), decreased lymphatic drainage, increased capillary permeability (pneumonia), increased intrapleural negative pressure (atelectasis), and decreased colloid osmotic pressure (hypoalbuminemia). Blood can result in a trauma-related pleural effusion (hemothorax), and disruption or blockage of the thoracic duct can result in chyle accumulation in the pleural space (chylothorax). Furthermore, immune cell inflow

brought on by disease processes that induce pleural inflammation triggers the coagulation cascade and results in fibrin deposition. This furthers the accumulation of pleural fluid and increases the permeability of nearby capillaries.

- Pleural effusions have been linked to a variety of medical conditions, the most prevalent of which is pneumonia. Cancer, kidney illness, trauma, congestive heart failure, and systemic diseases are still significant causes that need to be taken into account, though they are far less frequent in pediatric than in adult medicine. Parapneumonic effusions can lead to a number of complications, such as bronchopleural fistula, empyema (which affects about 3% of children hospitalized with pneumonia), and infrequently, pericarditis, and rib osteomyelitis. Three stages comprise the pathogenesis of parapneumonic effusion/ empyema formation: fibrinopurulent, organizational, and exudative. The inflammatory process, which lasts for 24 to 72 hours, causes fluid to leak into the pleural space during the exudative stage. The fibrinopurulent stage takes place during the course of the following 7 to 10 days. Deposits of fibrin in the pleural space can cause thickening of the parietal pleura as well as loculated fluid collections. An empyema is caused by a thicker, more purulent fluid that develops as the white blood cell count rises. In the pleural cavity, fibroblasts multiply at the end of the organizational stage. In this stage, the intrapleural fibrin membranes reorganize into a thick pleural peel as the loculations continue to grow and mature into abscesses (Table 6.6).

Table 6.6. *Summary of Current Recommendations of ATS/STS/STR*

PICO [1]	RECOMMENDATIONS
1. In patients with known or suspected MPE should thoracic USG be used to guide pleural interventions?	Yes
2. In patients with known or suspected MPE, who are asymptomatic, should pleural drainage be performed?	No
3. Should the management of symptomatic known or suspected MPE guided by large volume thoracentesis and pleural manometry?	Yes. Manometry if pleurodesis is contemplated to assess for lung re-expansion
4. In patients with known or suspected symptomatic MPE, with expandable lung and no prior definitive treatment, should IPC or chemical pleurodesis be used as first line intervention?	Yes
5. In patients with known or suspected MPE, undergoing talc pleurodesis, should talc slurry or talc poudrage be used?	Yes, there is no difference in the efficacy between the two
6. In patients with symptomatic MPE with non-expandable lung, failed pleurodesis or loculated effusion, should IPC or chemical pleurodesis be used?	IPC is the preferred method of choice over chemical pleurodesis
7. In IPC associated infection, is catheter removal required?	Not unless infection does not improve

[1] PICO-population, intervention, comparator outcomes format.

Source: Kulandaisamy PC, Kulandaisamy S, Kramer D, Mcgrath C. Malignant Pleural Effusions—A Review of Current Guidelines and Practices. Journal of Clinical Medicine. 2021; 10(23):5535. https://doi.org/10.3390/jcm10235535.

- **Clinical Findings:** Children may initially exhibit no symptoms or symptoms that are in line with the underlying cause of the formation of a pleural effusion. Pleural fluid buildup that occurs quickly is usually not well tolerated. The underlying pathology, as well as the child's cardiovascular and pulmonary conditions, determine the extent of impairment. The diaphragm moves downward and the chest wall expands to make room for the pleural fluid and maintain lung volume. When tidal volumes are reduced, tachypnea is initially needed to sustain minute ventilation in children with intact brains due to large effusions. Children may then experience dyspnea and retractions, requiring more effort to breathe. Ultimately, hypoxia, and hypercapnia may arise from the consequently increased dead space and decreased functional residual capacity. A child with low functional residual capacity and impaired thoracic volume at baseline may experience worsening of these symptoms. For instance, a child's pulmonary reserve and tolerance to pleural fluid accumulation are significantly reduced when they have a thoracic deformity that results in restrictive lung disease. Early bacterial pneumonia signs and symptoms can appear in children with parapneumonic effusions. Fever, malaise, decreased appetite, cough, chest pain, and dyspnea are the most typical symptoms. When inspiration occurs, pleuritic chest pain typically gets worse. These patients very seldom exhibit shock and severe respiratory distress. A physical examination may reveal egophony, a pleural friction rub, diminished or absent breath sounds, and dullness to percussion. However, because of their rapid breathing rates and incapacity to actively participate in the physical examination, infants, and children can be challenging to elicit these examination findings (Wedding et al., 2005; Kemp et al., 2008; Gupta et al., 2014; McKean et al., 2017; Rajan and Chawla, 2017).
- **Laboratory Findings:** The clinician can distinguish between exudative and transudative effusions by analyzing pleural fluid. A transudative effusion is typically straw-colored or clear, and it arises from fluid passing through the visceral pleura into the pleural space and through an intact pulmonary capillary barrier as a result of either decreased colloid osmotic pressure or increased pulmonary capillary hydrostatic pressure. An altered capillary barrier in the lung, pleura, or tissues allows fluid or proteins to pass through, resulting in an exudative effusion that can appear straw-colored or hazy. Since 1972, the Light criteria—which are based on data from adults—have been used to distinguish between exudative and transudative effusions. The criteria in Light's study demonstrated extremely high sensitivity and specificity; however, a meta-analysis of eight additional studies showed

that, when compared to Light's criteria, other tests or criteria used to identify exudative effusions do not significantly differ in diagnostic accuracy. The appearance of pleural fluid may aid the physician in identifying the root cause. Blood indicates trauma or cancer, purulent fluid suggests infection, and thin white milky fluid suggests chyle. Pleural biomarkers are less reliable in children, and diagnostic thoracentesis ought to be reserved for special cases. Suspected resistant organisms, ongoing fever in spite of treatment, and use as a therapeutic intervention are a few indications. Pleural fluid analysis is therefore not always necessary or indicated, even though it can be helpful. Emphyema and parapneumonic effusions are exudative. The fluid has a low glucose concentration, a high leukocyte count with a neutrophil predominance, and a purulent or turbid appearance. Although pleural fluid sent for bacterial culture and Gram staining may reveal bacteria, it is typically sterile due to previous antibiotic use. In cases of bacterial empyema, organism detection by polymerase chain reaction increased from 18% by culture to 67% by polymerase chain reaction detection of bacterial genes. *Serum acutephase* reactants (such as C-reactive protein and erythrocyte sedimentation rate) and a complete blood cell count with differential count may offer supportive evidence of bacterial or viral pneumonia; however, these tests should only be used as adjuncts to the history and physical examination. Low levels of acute-phase reactants and a normal white blood cell count do not rule out infectious causes. Only 1 to 11% of hospitalized children with pneumonia have blood cultures that are found to be positive; however, in patients who also have a parapneumonic effusion or empyema, this yield rises to 13 to 30%. It is significant to remember that when an antibiotic is administered prior to specimen collection, the usefulness of blood culture is reduced. Most bacterial parapneumonic effusions are caused by aerobic pathogens. The most common organisms in kids differ depending on the area, vaccination history, type of lab work, and antibiotic pretreatment. Before the discovery of antibiotics, the most common cause of parapneumonic effusion in infants under six months of age was Staphylococcus aureus. The most common causes of infections in children between the ages of 7 and 24 months were *Streptococcus pneumoniae* and *Haemophilus influenzae*. Because children are vaccinated against H influenzae type b, infections from it are now rare. The most frequent pathogen that causes parapneumonic effusion in children is *S pneumoniae.* Complicated parapneumonic effusions caused by *S. pneumoniae* continue to be common even with pneumococcal conjugate vaccination. In actuality, the frequency of empyemas is rising. Parapneumonic effusions are caused by a variety of other bacterial pathogens, such as group A Streptococcus, Actinomyces, coagulase-negative Staphylococcus, anaerobes (Bacteroides, Fusobacterium), and *Streptococcus viridans*. There are fewer reports of parapneumonic effusions associated with Mycoplasma pneumoniae. In general, the majority of complex parapneumonic effusions in children are caused by *S. pneumoniae* and *S. aureus* (Figure 6.5).

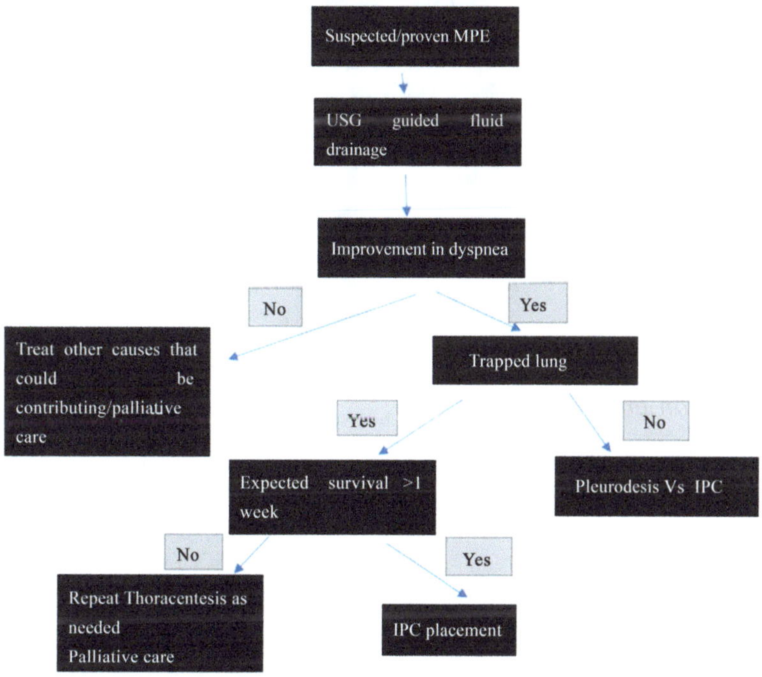

Figure 6.5. *Algorithm suggested for the management of suspected/proven recurrent malignant pleural effusion.*

Source: Kulandaisamy PC, Kulandaisamy S, Kramer D, Mcgrath C. Malignant Pleural Effusions—A Review of Current Guidelines and Practices. Journal of Clinical Medicine. 2021; *10(23):5535. https://doi.org/10.3390/jcm10235535.*

- **Radiologic Findings:** Pleural effusions are diagnosed with the use of radiographs, specifically posteroanterior and lateral or posteroposterior. Chest radiographs taken with the lateral decubitus technique can reveal whether an effusion layers dependently. As seen in Figure 6.6, blunting of the costophrenic angle is the first radiographic sign of pleural effusion (in adults, this finding requires the presence of about 200 mL of fluid). It is not always possible to distinguish between a large effusion and atelectasis, consolidation, or tumor when the lung is completely opacified. Ultrasonography can be used to assess the extent of an effusion and distinguish between straightforward and complex effusions. Effusions with floating pinpoint echoes may look echoic or anechoic. Septations, pleural thickening, or fibrinous strands adhered to the pleural surface can all be signs of fibrin deposition. When the fluid is not moving freely, locution may be detected. This can be observed more clearly by scanning the patient while they are seated and then in the supine position. Chest tube insertion or thoracentesis can be guided by ultrasound. The use of ultrasonography has several advantages over computed tomography (CT) scans in terms of early loculation detection, radiation-free radiation exposure, patient tolerance, and increased availability, especially at the bedside.

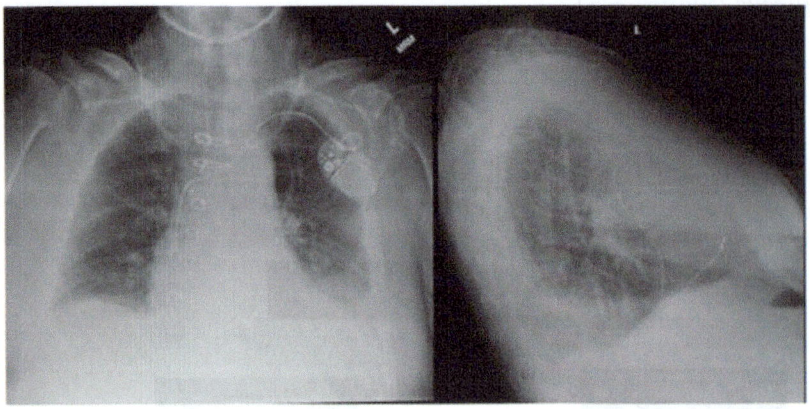

Figure 6.6. *Pleural effusion on chest radiograph.*

Source: Nicholson MJ, Manley C, Ahmad D. Thoracentesis for the Diagnosis and Management of Pleural Effusions: The Current State of a Centuries-Old Procedure. Journal of Respiration. 2023; 3(4):208-222. https://doi.org/10.3390/jor3040020.

Although a chest CT scan can be used to assess pleural fluid, it shouldn't be done frequently because of the expense and radiation risk. Furthermore, research indicates that CT scanning does not routinely influence management decisions or help characterize pleural fluid any more than ultrasonography does. The pleura can be identified with the use of intravenous contrast material. On a CT scan, pleural thickening and enhancement, internally convex pleural collections, and elevated extra pleural subcostal fat density are all indicative of empyema. Most of the time, the risks associated with a CT scan may exceed the advantages of the investigation. On the other hand, results from CT scans could help physicians make decisions about how to treat complex cases and could even be helpful prior to surgery.

- **Treatment:** Initial management of pleural effusion should focus on supporting the patient and addressing the underlying cause. If there is suspicion of an infectious cause, antibiotics should be chosen based on factors such as the suspected pathogen, local resistance patterns, patient age, and medical history. It is important to choose antibiotics that cover common organisms like S pneumoniae and group A Streptococcus. Vancomycin should be added to the treatment regimen in severe cases of pneumonia caused by S pneumoniae in critically ill children. Antimicrobial therapy should be adjusted based on susceptibility test results and unnecessary antibiotics should be stopped. Macrolides are preferred when an atypical organism is suspected in school-age children with pneumonia. Most cases of parapneumonic effusion can be managed with antibiotic therapy alone, without the need for drainage.

  Decisions about draining a pleural effusion should be based on the child's clinical condition, rather than solely on radiographic size classifications. Pediatric specialists such as surgeons, intensivists, or radiologists typically place thoracostomy tubes when needed, as routine thoracentesis is not recommended in children. Consultation with a pulmonologist may be helpful in diagnosing the cause of the effusion, but therapeutic procedures like thoracentesis are usually not performed by pediatric pulmonologists. In the past, complicated parapneumonic effusions were routinely drained based on fluid analysis results, but current evidence does not strongly support this approach. Drainage should be considered in cases of large effusions, worsening symptoms, sepsis, or lack of improvement with antibiotics (Wedding et al., 2005; Kemp et al., 2008; Gupta et al., 2014; McKean et al., 2017; Rajan and Chawla, 2017).

6.5.1. Noninfectious Causes of Pleural Effusions

6.5.1.1. Chylous Effusions

Chylous effusions are brought on by the thoracic duct and lymphatic collaterals being damaged or obstructed, which allows chyle (lymphatic fluid) to leak into the pleural space. One of the most frequent causes of pleural effusion in newborns is congenital chylothorax. Most chylous effusions in children are caused by subclavian vein thrombosis, thoracic duct damage from surgery, obstruction of the superior vena cava, Fontan surgery, cancer, and abnormalities of the pulmonary or thoracic lymphatic systems.

- **Pathogenesis:** The thoracic duct allows chyle, which is mainly made up of long-chain triglycerides, proteins, and lymphocytes, to enter the bloodstream. At the fifth thoracic vertebral body, the thoracic duct crosses over to the left hemithorax and empties into the venous circulation near the left jugular and subclavian veins. The thoracic duct ascends to the right of the vertebral column. Chyle may leak into the pleural space if the thoracic duct is disrupted at any point by trauma (including surgery), extrinsic compression (from a tumor), or spontaneous causes (cough, vomiting, hyperextension). Furthermore, aberrant lymphatic vessels and reduced venous return may result in collateral lymphatic rupture and chyle leakage.
- **Clinical Findings:** Children exhibit the signs and symptoms of pleural effusion. A physical examination may reveal decreased breath sounds, tachypnea, and cough. Patients who have had surgery may have a continuous or milky-looking chest tube drainage. A chest radiograph usually reveals bilateral opacifications as well as various degrees of unilateral opacification.
- **Laboratory Findings:** Chyle is usually milky-appearing, with a high concentration of triglycerides as chylomicrons. Pleural fluid is typically exudative but may appear serous in neonates, malnourished or fasting children, and children on a low-fat diet. The pleural fluid of a chylothorax classically has a triglyceride concentration greater than 110 mg/dL (1.24 mmol/L) with a white blood cell count of more than 1000/mL (1.109/L) and greater than 80% lymphocytes. Chyle has

a high protein concentration and immunoglobulin content.

- **Treatment:** The management of childhood chylothorax is based on small case series. Until spontaneous healing takes place, the objective is to drain fluid from the pleural space and reduce lymphatic flow via the thoracic duct. It is typically recommended to drain the chyle by thoracentesis in order to diagnose and relieve symptoms. As the main source of dietary fat, medium-chain triglycerides are used in dietary treatment to reduce lymphatic flow and promote enteric rest while long-chain fatty acids are avoided. Patients requiring enteric rest may need to have their lost nutrients and electrolytes replaced; parenteral nutrition can help with this. Treatment for chylous effusions in children has included the use of somatostatin and a synthetic analog called octreotide. Although the exact mechanism is unknown, these medications cause the splanchnic circulation to vasoconstrict and most likely reduce the production of lymphatic fluid. No randomized, controlled trials have been carried out to ascertain the safety and effectiveness of this treatment, although case series have documented successful treatment with these agents using various dosage and timing of initiation. The use of octreotide in neonates was the subject of a Cochrane review, which found insufficient evidence to support a recommendation. If chylothorax does not improve with drainage and dietary changes, surgical procedures (pleurodesis or ligation of the thoracic duct via thoracotomy or VATS) should be considered. Although there are no set guidelines for when to have surgery, most doctors decide to do so when medical therapy has failed for two to four weeks.

6.5.2. Cardiovascular Causes of Pleural Effusion

Compared to adults, children are much less likely to have CHF. Myocardial dysfunction (cardiomyopathies and myocarditis), arrhythmias, myocardial ischemia, congenital heart disease, and systemic illnesses like sepsis can all lead to congestive heart failure (CHF). Restrictive pericarditis, obstruction of the superior vena cava, and cardiac surgery are other cardiovascular causes of pleural effusions in children.

- **Pathogenesis**: The main cause of the buildup of pleural fluid is either elevated pulmonary capillary wedge pressure from left heart failure or left atrial hypertension. Fluid seeps into the pleural space as a result of elevated capillary hydrostatic pressure. In contrast to adults, pleural effusion in children is rarely caused by pulmonary arterial hypertension or right heart failure.
- **Clinical Findings**: In addition to the symptoms of pleural effusion, children also exhibit signs and symptoms of heart failure. A child with low cardiac reserve may suffer hemodynamic collapse if they are unable to tolerate a large pleural effusion. The radiographic results reveal opacification that is consistent with a bilateral, most

common type of pleural effusion.

- **Laboratory Findings**: Bilateral and transudative pleural fluid is the norm. Typically, there is not much protein present. Adult CHF patients' pleural fluid has been found to contain higher levels of N-terminal pro-brain natriuretic peptide, according to studies. When diuresis is performed and there is a pleural effusion, this test might be useful because the pleural fluid analysis could be unclear and seem exudative.
- **Treatment**: Pleural effusions due to CHF usually resolve with treatment of the underlying condition causing CHF and improvement in cardiac function. If patients have substantial clinical signs (dyspnea, large effusion, hemodynamic compromise), thoracentesis may improve symptoms but is not routinely recommended.

6.5.3. Malignancy-Related Pleural Effusions

The most common cause of malignancy-related effusions in children is lymphoma. Pleural effusion in children is not commonly associated with leukemia or carcinoma.

- **Pathogenesis**: Effusion may result from pleural invasion by the tumor, obstruction of lymphatic flow, pneumonia, or atelectasis from extrinsic compression of the tumor or lymphadenopathy.
- **Clinical Findings**. Children with malignancy-related effusions show many of the symptoms previously described for children with pleural effusions. In addition, they may have systemic signs of lymphoma, including lymphadenopathy, cough, shortness of breath, fever, unexplained weight loss, and fatigue. Effusions may be unilateral or bilateral on imaging. The clinical signs and symptoms differ based on the type of cancer and the size of the effusion.
- **Laboratory Findings**. Pleural fluid is exudative and may be bloody or chylous. Cytopathologic studies documenting the presence of malignant cells help in diagnosis.
- **Treatment**: Drainage of large effusions in patients with moderate-to-severe respiratory symptoms is indicated. However, children with lymphoma may present with mediastinal masses. Therefore, the risks and benefits of surgical intervention and administration of anesthetics should be carefully considered before proceeding with intervention. Treatment of the underlying malignancy often results in improvement of the effusion.

6.5.4. Pneumothoraces

Epidemiology: An air buildup in the pleural space, known as a pneumothorax, can occur spontaneously and have no known underlying cause or it can be associated with a number of different medical conditions. 3.41 out of every 100,000 children under the age of 18 experience spontaneous pneumothoraces. Male incidence is higher than female incidence, with 7.4 to 18 cases per 100,000 versus only 1.2 to 6 cases per 100,000 females. One to two% of term neonates have been reported to experience spontaneous pneumothorax. There is insufficient information available regarding the prevalence of secondary pneumothorax in children.

- **Pathogenesis:** A pneumothorax is a condition in which air enters the intrapleural space through the parietal pleura and causes partial or complete lung collapse. Because of the pressure gradient that favors gas absorption into the circulation between the pleural space and the total gas pressure in the venous system, the pleural space is typically air-free. Anatomic anomalies like blebs, bullae, and pneumatoceles are linked to both primary and secondary causes of spontaneous pneumothoraces, which happen in the absence of trauma. According to theory, blebs, and bullae are caused by alterations in the lung's connective tissue that occur gradually over time and put the patient at risk for a spontaneous rupture. Males experience spontaneous pneumothoraces more frequently than females, but pediatric patients experience them far less frequently than adult patients. Children with asthma, cystic fibrosis (Figure 6.7), and connective tissue disorders (a1-antitrypsin deficiency, Marfan syndrome, and Ehlers-Danlos syndrome) are more likely to experience secondary pneumothoraces. It is thought that localized lung tissue alterations or systemic inflammation linked to these illnesses are the direct causes of secondary causes. Children with underlying connective tissue disorders, such as Marfan syndrome, have been found to exhibit a variety of pulmonary histologic changes, including bronchiectatic changes that raise the risk of pneumothoraces, pulmonary bullous dysplasia, patchy cystic changes, and emphysematous changes. Bleb rupture and pneumothorax are likely caused by the coexistence of inflammation, bronchospasm, and hyperinflation in children with asthma.

  When the lungs, esophagus, chest wall, or tracheobronchial tree are injured, air can enter the pleural space and cause a traumatic pneumothorax. One-third of pediatric thoracic trauma cases result in pneumothoraces, which also happen at a similar rate in cases of blunt and penetrating trauma. Compared to blunt trauma, where hemothorax is infrequent, penetrating trauma is more likely to result in pneumothorax associated with hemothorax. In conclusion, medical procedures such as central venous cannulation, thoracentesis, thoracic surgery, or mechanical ventilation are the causes of iatrogenic pneumothoraces. Specifically, neonates on mechanical ventilation may develop pulmonary interstitial emphysema or a pulmonary air leak as a result of pneumothoraces. Because of the uneven distribution of alveolar inflation, preterm neonates and pediatric patients with heterogeneous lung disease who require mechanical ventilation are even more vulnerable to pneumothorax.

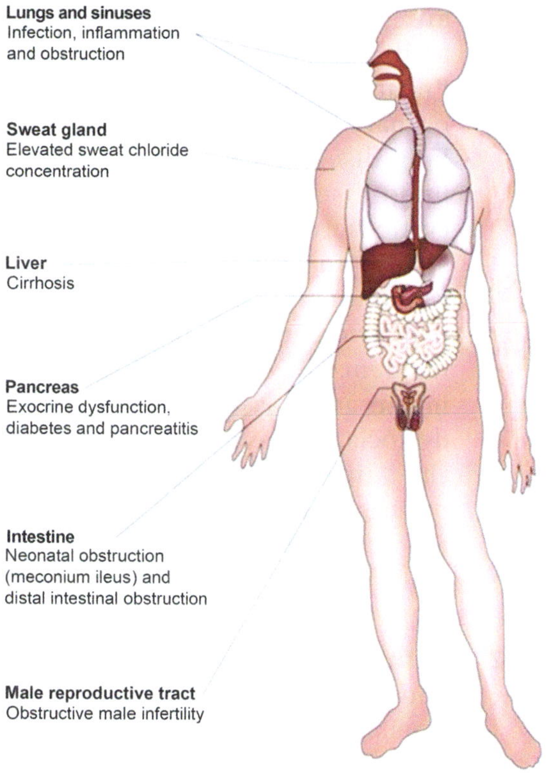

Figure 6.7. *Cystic fibrosis.*

Source: Meoli A, Fainardi V, Deolmi M, Chiopris G, Marinelli F, Caminiti C, Esposito S, Pisi G. State of the Art on Approved Cystic Fibrosis Transmembrane Conductance Regulator (CFTR) Modulators and Triple-Combination Therapy. Pharmaceuticals. 2021; 14(9):928. https://doi.org/10.3390/ph14090928.

3. **Clinical Findings:** In children, a minor pneumothorax might not cause any symptoms. However, signs of respiratory distress appear as a result of growing air accumulation and the compression of the lung parenchyma that follows. Cough, chest pain, hypoxia, tachypnea, and the use of accessory muscles could all be presenting signs or symptoms. Upon physical examination, the patient might exhibit reduced breath sounds, hyperresonance, and decreased chest excursion. Tension physiology could emerge if the pleural space's air volume keeps rising. If left untreated, tension pneumothorax can lead to hypotension, bradycardia, and cardiac arrest in addition to vascular compromise, decreased cardiac return, and tachycardia. Additional physical examination findings related to tension pneumothorax include shifting of the apical impulse (toward the contralateral side), tracheal deviation, and diminished heart sounds. Tension pneumothorax is more common in the context of trauma than it is in spontaneous Pneumothoraces.
4. **Radiologic Findings:** Pneumothorace detection with a chest CT scan has long been thought to be the gold standard. This investigative modality has the additional disadvantage of increased radiation exposure, and it may not be feasible or practical. Radiography of the upright chest reveals pleural line displacement. When performed by a skilled clinician, ultrasonography is more sensitive than chest radiography and can be used on a seated or supine patient. The absence of lung sliding in the B mode of ultrasonography, along with the presence of a linear, laminar pattern in the tissue superficial to the pleural line and a similar linear pattern in the M mode (barcode sign) deep to the pleural line, all point to the absence of lung sliding and the possible presence of pneumothorax at this interspace. Lastly, research on newborns supports the diagnosis of pneumothorax using transillumination.
5. **Treatment:** The cause and contributing factors, as well as the child's size and respiratory status, all play a role in the management of pneumothorax in neonates and children. Children who are hypoxic and experiencing

respiratory distress should receive additional oxygen. Angio catheter or large-bore needle decompression is necessary for the prompt treatment of tension physiology. According to adult guidelines, stable patients with small spontaneous pneumothoraces should be observed on chest radiographs, and stable patients with large spontaneous pneumothoraces should be admitted to the hospital and have a chest tube placed. There is a lack of guidelines tailored specifically for the initial management of pneumothoraces in children. Pigtail catheters and small-bore catheters are safe and effective for use in children, and large-bore thoracostomy tubes are rarely required. The goals of treatment are to treat chronic air leaks, permit lung reexpansion, and prevent pneumothorax from recurring. It has been noted that children experiencing primary spontaneous pneumothorax have a recurrence rate of between 40 and 61%. However, this strategy is debatable due to the higher expense and morbidity linked to primary VATS with blebectomy and pleurodesis in pediatric patients. Surgical treatment, which includes pleurodesis and VATS, is often saved for patients who have recurrent pneumothoraces or persistent air leaks (Orenstein, 2004).

6.5.5. Pneumomediastinum/ Pneumopericardium

1. **Epidemiology**: Air or gas in the pericardium (pneumopericardium) and mediastinum (pneumomediastinum) can occur spontaneously or as a result of trauma, surgery, esophageal disturbance, infection, or other conditions. It typically occurs in conjunction with other air leaks like pneumothoraces and pneumomediastinum. Pneumomediastinum is classified as primary (no risk factors or underlying lung disease) or secondary (known lung disease such as asthma or cystic fibrosis). This classification is similar to that of pneumothoraces. Pneumomediastinum is rare in pediatric patients. In newborns, the incidence is 1.7 to 2.5 per 1000 infants and is associated with shoulder dystocia. In the pediatric population, the incidence of spontaneous pneumomediastinum has been reported to be 1 in 8000 to 1 in 15,000 children consulting the emergency department.
2. **Pathogenesis:** Pneumomediastinum and pneumopericardium resulting from traumatic events include blunt or penetrating injuries to the chest, injuries to the tracheobronchial tree, and iatrogenic injuries sustained during procedures or surgery. When there is an abrupt rise in intrathoracic pressure, the intra-alveolar pressure also rises, leading to alveolar rupture and air leakage into the interstitium, bronchoalveolar tissue, and mediastinum. This condition is known as spontaneous pneumomediastinum. Pneumomediastinum may be caused by air from the gastrointestinal tract, intrathoracic airways, and upper respiratory tract. Vascular sheaths allow air to pass through subcutaneous tissues in the neck and thorax, into the mediastinum, and even into the pericardium. Pneumopericardium rarely develops on its own. Asthma, Valsalva maneuvers (related to strenuous activities like weightlifting, coughing, and drug-induced exertion), vomiting, respiratory infections,

ingestion of foreign bodies, scuba diving, and inhalation of helium or inhalation drugs are risk factors for pneumomediastinum and pneumopericardium. Infectious pericarditis with gas-producing organisms, entrainment of air with pericardial drain placement, and pericardiocentesis are additional causes of pneumopericardium. Additionally, preterm birth, severe respiratory distress syndrome, and mechanical ventilation have been linked to pneumopericardium.

3. **Clinical Findings:** Children that develop spontaneous pneumomediastinum may complain of breathing difficulties, coughing, and chest pain that travels to the back or neck. This pain usually gets worse when one is inspired. Reports have also been made of dysphagia. In addition to having subcutaneous emphysema, many affected children may also exhibit clinical symptoms associated with the course of the disease if pneumomediastinum is the result of an underlying lung condition like asthma. Furthermore, reports of hoarseness, coughing, wheezing on auscultation, facial or neck swelling, and cervical emphysema have been made. It has also been described how to auscultate the precordium and hear the Hamman crunch, which is a crunching or rasping sound that matches the heartbeat. In secondary pneumomediastinum, tachypnea, and tachycardia are frequently observed. Patients who have a large pneumomediastinum or pneumopericardium may experience poor venous return, tension pneumomediastinum, muffled heart sounds, and tamponade physiology. While some children may appear healthy, others may exhibit nonspecific symptoms and normal vital signs.

4. **Radiologic Findings:** A chest radiograph in pneumomediastinum outlines the mediastinal structures with radiolucent gas. Infants may exhibit the spinnaker sign, which is an upward and outward displacement of the thymic lobes. The continuous diaphragm sign is the outline of mediastinal gas that divides the diaphragm from the heart. Furthermore, gas can be observed extending laterally between the medial left hemidiaphragm and the parietal pleura, as well as defining the lateral border of the descending aorta. When there is pneumopericardium, the parietal pleura may protrude as a thin, radiopaque line that delineates the air surrounding the heart on a chest radiograph. Due to the anatomic boundaries of the pericardium, unlike in pneumomediastinum, the air in pneumopericardium does not extend to the aorta or great vessels. Both pneumomediastinum and pneumopericardium may have associated subcutaneous emphysema, pneumothorax, and pneumoretroperitoneum. Pneumomediastinum can rarely be diagnosed without a CT scan, but when a lung disease needs to be evaluated, one should use one. An echogenic interface that blocks the view of the cardiac structures in the pneumomediastinum can be found via ultrasonography. During diastole, pneumopericardium can be seen as bright echogenic foci that are moving along the pericardial layer.

5. **Treatment:** Supportive care is provided, and isolated spontaneous pneumomediastinum typically resolves with little chance of recurrence. The

goal of secondary pneumomediastinum and pneumopericardium therapy is to address any underlying lung pathologies, traumatic injuries, or additional reasons why air is introduced. It is important to make an effort to reduce airway pressures in children on mechanical ventilation. Large air collections very rarely require pericardial or mediastinal drainage. Activities involving strong inspiration or elevated positive end-expiratory pressure should generally be avoided during the recovery phase; however, no published guidelines have been made to help with the timing of these recommendations (Wedding et al., 2005; Kemp et al., 2008; Gupta et al., 2014; McKean et al., 2017; Rajan and Chawla, 2017).

A Closer Look

Inflammatory Bowel Disease (IBD)

Either Crohn's disease ulcerative colitis or indeterminate colitis is the diagnosis of inflammatory bowel disease for your child. These illnesses affect your child's stomach as well as the small and large intestines, causing pain and discomfort. Even though the illnesses are typically identified in adults, research indicates that up to 30% of adult cases may have their origins in childhood.

While the two diseases are classified as inflammatory bowel disorders, Crohn's disease can affect any region of the digestive system, while ulcerative colitis is confined to the large intestine (colon). In both diseases, immune cells are dysfunctional and damage the lining of the digestive system. While it is sometimes difficult to distinguish between the two if the inflammation is confined to the large intestines, if other regions are involved, it is clearly Crohn's disease.

Children often have more severe symptoms or flare-ups when they are under stress or when exposed to certain environmental conditions.

- Stomach cramping and pain.
- Diarrhea and persistent feeling of need to eliminate stool.
- Bloody, watery stool.
- Delayed growth and onset of puberty.
- Decreased appetite.
- Feeling of constant tiredness, joint pain and eye problems.
- Fever with infection.
- Anemia due to blood loss.
- Vomiting.

When inflammatory bowel disease is suspected in children, our pediatric gastroenterologist will order tests that may include:

- Complete Blood Count (CBC) and other blood tests that can confirm inflammation in the body and antibodies (proteins) found with IBD.
- Stool tests to look for blood, bacteria, and inflammation.
- Upper endoscopy that looks at the esophagus, stomach, and the upper portion of the small intestine.
- Colonoscopy that visualizes the lower small intestine, colon, and anus.
- X-rays, ultrasound, CT scan, MRI or capsule endoscopy (depending if previous test results are inconclusive).

Considering that IBD is a chronic illness, many parents and kids find the diagnosis upsetting. It is imperative to bear in mind that these ailments can be managed in conjunction with your pediatric gastroenterologist, who will prescribe the most appropriate courses of action following the gravity and progression of the illness. Education, maintaining a healthy diet, and taking medication to control symptoms and prevent distress are all crucial because these conditions worsen during flare-ups. Kids can lose weight and stop growing taller at times. These kids frequently have an increased risk of developing early bone thinning. Under these circumstances, the gastroenterologist treating your child might suggest strict dietary regimens, extra calcium and vitamin D supplements, and in the worst situations, IV therapy.

Summary

- Atelectasis is the partial collapse or closure of a lung resulting in reduced or absent gas exchange. It is usually unilateral, affecting part or all of one lung.
- Respiratory disorders associated with systemic inflammatory diseases represent a complex interplay between immune dysregulation and pulmonary manifestations.
- Fibreoptic bronchoscopy (FOB) allows inspection and biopsy of the airways (almost invariably not informative in ILD), BAL, and transbronchial biopsy (TBB). However, the procedure requires a general anesthetic or such heavy sedation as it almost amounts to general anesthesia.
- Bronchopulmonary dysplasia is a chronic lung disease that affects premature infants. Premature (preterm) infants who require treatment with supplemental oxygen or require long-term oxygen are at a higher risk.
- BPD is a respiratory disease that can occur when a newborn's lungs are undeveloped at birth, requiring the use of a ventilator or oxygen therapy for support.
- Parapneumonic effusions are found in 2% to 12% of children with community-acquired pneumonia and in up to 28% of children hospitalized for community-acquired pneumonia.
- Common symptoms include progressive dyspnea (shortness of breath), dry cough, fatigue, and reduced exercise tolerance. These symptoms result from impaired gas exchange and decreased lung function.
- Diagnosis typically involves a combination of medical history, physical examination, imaging studies (such as high-resolution CT scans), pulmonary function tests, and sometimes lung biopsy. Management often includes addressing underlying causes (such as autoimmune disorders or environmental exposures), medications to reduce inflammation and fibrosis, oxygen therapy, pulmonary rehabilitation, and in severe cases, lung transplantation.

References

1. Aguayo, S. M., Miller, Y. E., Waldron, J. A., et al. (1992). Brief report: Idiopathic diffuse hyperplasia of pulmonary neuroendocrine cells and airways disease. *New England Journal of Medicine, 327*(18), 1285–1288.
2. Barbato, A., Panizzolo, C., Cracco, A., et al. (2000). Interstitial lung disease in children: A multicentre survey on diagnostic approach. *European Respiratory Journal, 16*(3), 509–513.
3. Bush, A., & duBois, R. (1996). Congenital and pediatric interstitial disease. *Current Opinion in Pulmonary Medicine, 2*(4), 347–356.
4. Canakis, A. M., Cutz, E., Manson, D., & O'Brodovich, H. (2002). Pulmonary interstitial glycogenosis: A new variant of neonatal interstitial lung disease. *American Journal of Respiratory and Critical Care Medicine, 165*(11), 1557–1665.
5. Clement, A., Allen, J., Corrin, B., et al. (2004). Task force on chronic interstitial lung disease in immunocompetent children. *European Respiratory Journal, 24*(4), 686–697.
6. Fan, L. L., & Langston, C. (1993). Chronic interstitial lung disease in children. *Pediatric Pulmonology, 16*(3), 184–196.

7. Fan, L. L., Mullen, A. L., Brugman, S. M., Inscore, S. C., Parks, D. P., & White, C. W. (1992). Clinical spectrum of chronic interstitial lung disease in children. *Journal of Pediatrics, 124*(6), 867–872.

8. Feldman, D., Nava, A., Myers, D., & Mayer, R. (2019). Emergencies in the rehabilitation unit. In R. Mitra (Ed.), *Principles of Rehabilitation Medicine*. McGraw-Hill.

9. Gupta, N., Matta, E., & Oldham, S. (2014). Cardiothoracic imaging. In K. Elsayes & S. Oldham (Eds.), *Introduction to Diagnostic Radiology*. McGraw-Hill.

10. Katzenstein, A. L., Gordon, L. P., Oliphant, M., & Swender, P. T. (1995). Chronic pneumonitis of infancy. *American Journal of Surgical Pathology, 19*(4), 439–447.

11. Kemp, W., Burns, D., & Brown, T. (2008). *Pathology: The Big Picture*. McGraw-Hill.

12. Madappa, T. (2017). Atelectasis. *Medscape*. Retrieved from: https://www.medscape.com (accessed on 22 October 2024).

13. McKean, S., Ross, J., Dressler, D., & Scheurer, D. (2017). *Principles and Practice of Hospital Medicine* (2nd ed.). McGraw-Hill.

14. Midulla, F., Strappini, P. M., Ascoli, V., et al. (1998). Bronchoalveolar lavage cell analysis in a child with chronic lipid pneumonia. *European Respiratory Journal, 11*(2), 239–242.

15. Moore, J., & Mancuso, N. (2017). Respiratory distress. In C. Stone & R. Humphries (Eds.), *Current Diagnosis & Treatment: Emergency Medicine* (8th ed.). McGraw-Hill.

16. Nicholson, A. G., Kim, H., Corrin, B., et al. (1998). The value of classifying interstitial pneumonitis in childhood according to defined histological patterns. *Histopathology, 33*(3), 203–211.

17. Orenstein, D. M. (2004). *Cystic Fibrosis: A Guide for Patient and Family*. Lippincott Williams & Wilkins.

18. Parto, K., Svedstrom, E., Majurin, M. L., Harkonnen, R., & Simell, O. (1993). Pulmonary manifestations in lysinuric protein intolerance. *Chest, 104*(4), 1176–1182.

19. Payne, C. R., Jaques, P., & Kerr, I. H. (1980). Lung folding simulating peripheral pulmonary neoplasm (Blesovsky's syndrome). *Thorax, 35*(12), 936–940.

20. Qadir, N., & Mathew, R. (2017). Imaging of the critically ill patient: Radiology. In J. Oropello, S. Pastores, & V. Kvetan (Eds.), *Critical Care*. McGraw-Hill.

21. Rajan, P., & Chawla, S. (2017). Bronchoscopy. In J. Oropello, S. Pastores, & V. Kvetan (Eds.), *Critical Care*. McGraw-Hill.

22. Restrepo, R., & Braverman, J. (2015). Current challenges in the recognition, prevention, and treatment of perioperative pulmonary atelectasis. *Expert Review of Respiratory Medicine, 9*(1), 97–107.

23. Thomas, A. Q., Lane, K., Phillips, J. III, et al. (2002). Heterozygosity for surfactant protein C gene mutation associated with usual interstitial pneumonitis and cellular nonspecific interstitial pneumonitis in one kindred. *American Journal of Respiratory and Critical Care Medicine, 165*(9), 1322–1328.

24. Wedding, M. E., & Gylys, B. A. (2005). *Medical Terminology Systems: A Body Systems Approach*. Philadelphia, PA: F. A. Davis Company.

25. Woodring, J. H., & Reed, J. C. (1996). Types and mechanisms of pulmonary atelectasis. *Journal of Thoracic Imaging, 11*(2), 92–108.

Chapter 7

PEDIATRIC SLEEP MEDICINE

Contents

Introduction

The process of sleep has a significant impact on one's functioning and overall health. Children need healthy sleep that is uninterrupted, of sufficient length and timing, and free from disruptions. In children, sleep issues are thought to affect at least 25% of the population. If left untreated, these sleep issues cause serious impairment that affects kids' physical and mental health.

Sleep is most abundant during infancy, childhood, and adolescence, making up a significant percentage of daily life during these stages. This is when various sleep disorders and disturbances in circadian rhythms can first appear, leading to important behavioral and biological changes. It is crucial to understand the normal development of sleep and wake patterns during childhood to accurately diagnose these disorders. Early detection and appropriate treatment can greatly impact the progression of the disease and improve a child's future. Since adult sleep patterns are often established in the first two decades of life, early intervention is key. Neurologists who understand the developmental aspects of sleep and circadian rhythms are in a unique position to address complex cases that may be challenging for other medical professionals (Allen et al., 2000; Allen et al., 2001; Allen et al., 2003; Blunden et al., 2005).

Orientation and Directional Terms

Term	Definition	Illustration
Polysomnography	Polysomnography refers to a systematic process used to collect physiologic parameters during sleep. A polysomnogram (PSG) is a procedure that utilizes electroencephalogram, electro-oculogram, electromyogram, electrocardiogram, and pulse oximetry, as well as airflow and respiratory effort, to evaluate for underlying causes of sleep disturbances.	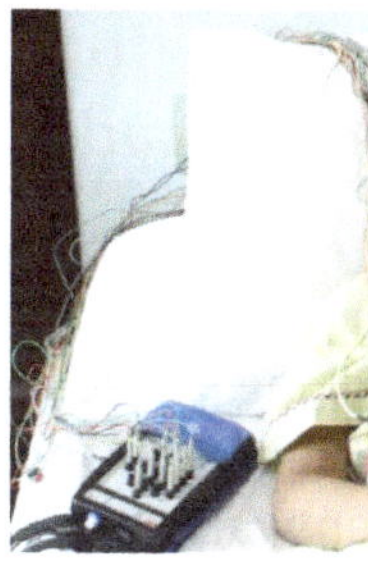
Insomnia	Insomnia is a common sleep disorder that can make it hard to fall asleep or stay asleep. It also can cause you to wake up too early and not be able to get back to sleep. You may still feel tired when you wake up.	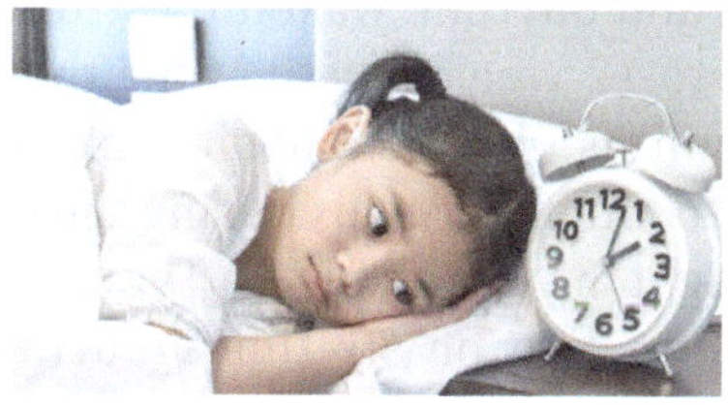
Parahippocampal gyrus	The parahippocampal gyrus (or hippocampal gyrus) is a grey matter cortical region of the brain that surrounds the hippocampus and is part of the limbic system. The region plays an important role in memory encoding and retrieval. It has been involved in some cases of hippocampal sclerosis.	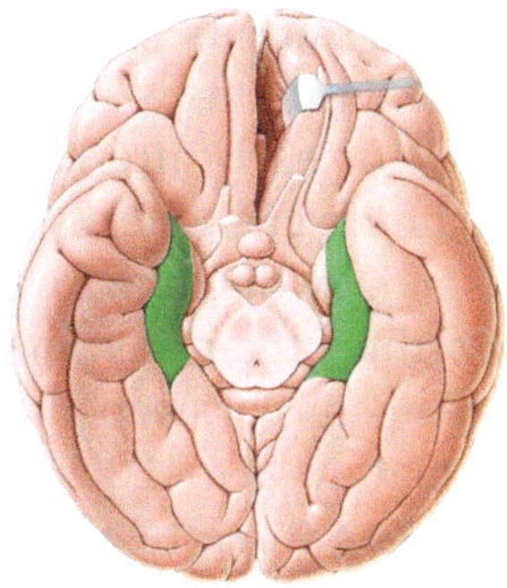
Somnambulism	Somnambulism is a phenomenon of combined sleep and wakefulness. It is classified as a sleep disorder belonging to the parasomnia family. It occurs during slow wave stage of sleep, in a state of low consciousness, with the performance of activities that are usually performed during a state of full consciousness.	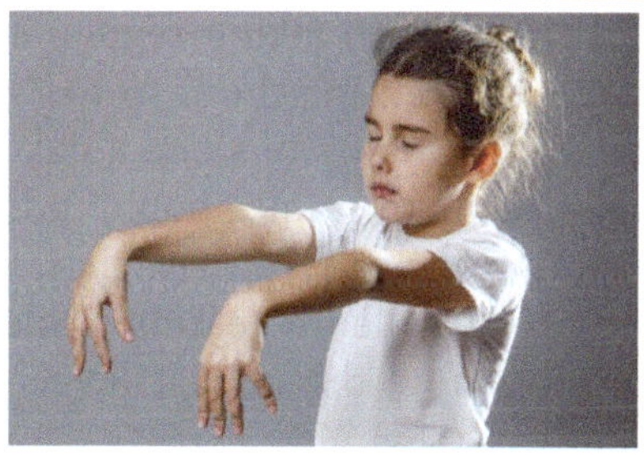
Sleep apnea	Sleep apnea is a serious sleep disorder that happens when your breathing stops and starts while you're asleep. If it goes untreated, it can cause loud snoring, daytime tiredness, or more serious problems like heart trouble or high blood pressure.	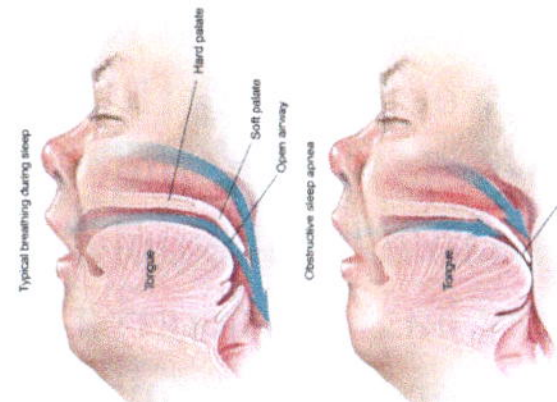

7.1. Sleep in the Context of Development

7.1.1. Sleep and Wakefulness, Sleep Stages, and Circadian Rhythms

At birth, a person's sleep and wake cycles consist of one to three-hour waking periods interspersed with two to five-hour sleep episodes over a 24-hour period. Short sleep-wake intervals combine into longer, recognizable periods of nocturnal sleep and daytime wakefulness during the first eight to 12 weeks. By the time they are four or six months old, most babies take two or three two- to four-hour naps during the day and sleep for eight hours at night. Typically, newborns wake up five or six times during the night, which does not necessitate but frequently draws attention from parents. Most infants have cut down their daytime naps to one or two in the late morning or early afternoon, lasting up to one or two hours at a time, by the time they are 12 months old. By the time a child is 18 months old, most reduce their daytime naps to once a day, and the nocturnal sleep phase has stabilized at approximately 8 to 10 hours. Children in preschool (ages three to five) sleep 11 to 12 hours a day on average, and during this time most of them stop taking regular naps during the day. Children in school (6 to 12 years old) need 10 to 11 hours of sleep a day on average, so naps during this time should indicate a weak arousal system or sleep restriction. Based on objective somnolence testing, children in this age group show the lowest levels of daytime sleepiness.

During early infancy, sleep is divided equally between active (REM-like) sleep and quiet (non-REM) sleep. Indeterminate sleep is a term used to describe polysomnogram (PSG) activity that has characteristics of both active and quiet sleep. By 6 months old, active/REM sleep decreases to 35% to 40% of total sleep time, and four distinct non-REM sleep stages begin to appear with regular 40- to 50-minute REM sleep cycles. Infants at this stage start to enter sleep through non-REM stages instead of the active/REM stage. In early childhood, REM sleep occurs around 40 to 50 minutes after falling asleep and eventually matures to adult-like timing (90 to 120 minutes) in late childhood (ages 10 to 12). In adolescence, REM sleep makes up 20% to 30% of total sleep time, reaching adult levels.

Non-REM sleep increases as a percentage of total sleep time throughout childhood, reaching its peak in preschool and young school-aged children at 30% to 40% of total sleep. Slow-wave sleep is mostly found in the first half of the sleep period. Sleep efficiency peaks during the school-age years, with daytime sleepiness at its lowest. Slow-wave sleep decreases by 40% in adolescence, making up 15% to 20% of total sleep time in early adulthood.

Adolescents typically need between 5 and 8 hours to 10 hours of sleep per night. The timing of the main sleep epoch, rather than the amount of sleep, is the main change in this age group. The majority of teenagers tend to inherently postpone going to sleep and waking hours due to variations in their circadian cycles. This shift is reflected in biological sleep and wake markers, which corroborate the notion that adolescents need later sleep and wake times.

At first, babies sleep for brief periods of time and wake up again, which is frequently related to biological cravings for food. Up until day-night differentiation happens between two and three months, the amount of sleep during the day usually equals the amount of sleep during the night at this point. Certain people have a preference for either an earlier or later start time for sleep or wakefulness (advanced and delayed sleep phases, respectively), which can be attributed to biological variation in the circadian regulatory mechanisms for sleep and wake in the suprachiasmatic nucleus of the anterior hypothalamus. Regarding sleeping patterns, the majority of school-age children report going to bed earlier (between 8:00 and 9:00 PM), and on the Sleep Habit Questionnaire, a validated test of sleep-phase preference, they exhibit significantly more "morningness" than "eveningness" types (corresponding to advanced and delayed sleep-phase types). The transition from morningness to eveningness chronotypes is significantly correlated with school grade level, as evidenced by the study's finding that there is a dramatic increase in eveningness between the fourth and eighth grades. Adolescents who exhibit behavioral changes during the sleep phase also show a measurable delay in the onset of sleep, as indicated by temperature nadirs and melatonin secretion. The homeostatic sleep drive and the response to sleep restriction appear to be blunted during adolescence, along with the delay in the circadian phase for both sleep and wake. Sleep tendency in prepubescent versus postpubescent adolescents shows that younger adolescents have a much stronger sleep drive than older adolescents, even when controlling for the circadian phase (using dim light melatonin onset measures). This implies that there is a reduction in sleep drive in addition to the maturational delay in the circadian phase for wake and sleep, which may exacerbate insufficient sleep regulation during adolescence.

7.1.2. CNS: Behavior

Even though the exact function of sleep is still unknown, the brain primarily produces it, most likely for its own advantage. It is clear at any age, but especially in childhood, how poor sleep affects brain functions such as behavior, cognition, and emotional regulation. In contrast to adults with sleep disorders, who frequently experience easily characterized or observed daytime sleepiness, children with sleep disorders are less likely to present with this symptom. A thorough history can frequently elicit subjective sleepiness, and in certain cases, objective evidence of sleepiness as well. However, school-aged children are more likely to exhibit attention deficit, hyperactivity, aggression, an inability to control their emotions, or other externalizing behaviors during the day as symptoms of sleep problems. Correlated cognitive impairments have also been reported. A possible phenomenologic explanation for sleepy children could be that they still have a strong desire to stay awake during a developmental stage where learning is essential. These kids exhibit high levels of physical activity and stimulus-seeking behavior in an attempt to stay awake. Neurobiologically speaking, the prefrontal cortex—which mediates executive functioning and is involved in numerous behaviors impacted by sleep deprivation—is the region that produces slow-wave sleep the strongest. There may be a specific vulnerability of the prefrontal cortex to sleep deprivation.

7.1.3. Respiratory Tract: Tonsils and Adenoids

Compared to adults, children's upper airways are substantially smaller. Children's etiologies of sleep-disordered breathing (SDB) differ significantly from those of adults, as evidenced by the higher upper airway muscle tone in children. Most children's tonsils and adenoids' lymphoid tissue hypertrophies between the ages of 2 and 6. A lot of pediatricians, ear, nose, and throat surgeons, and sleep specialists use visual grading scales to help assess the size of these tissues and any associations with symptoms of SDB, even though the absolute size of tonsils may not correlate to increased upper airway resistance in all people. Furthermore, children's normal anatomical and physiological changes in their upper airways may also put them at risk for SDB and higher upper airway resistance. These include retrognathia, a short neck, edema, and erythema of the posterior oropharynx and nasopharynx brought on by recurrent infections of the nose, throat, and ears, and lateral narrowing of the hard and soft palates.

7.1.4. Cardiovascular System: Heart Rate and Blood Pressure

Even when they sleep, an infant's heart rate is significantly higher and typically ranges from 100 to 140 beats per minute. During development, there seems to be a dynamic shift in the cardiovascular response to nocturnal arousal through the developing sympathetic nervous system, with the heart rate decreasing and blood pressure rising. One well-known consequence of adult untreated obstructive sleep apnea (OSA) is hypertension. In fact, up to 85% of adults with treatment-resistant hypertension have underlying OSA, which may be the cause or a contributing factor in this issue. It is also known that children with OSA can develop hypertension. In children, SDB is linked to left ventricular hypertrophy, pulmonary hypertension, and hyperactivity of the sympathetic nervous system. It's unclear if a predisposition to these disorders, the severity or chronicity of SDB, or both contribute to cardiovascular complications. There is very little research on the cardiovascular problems that arise from SDB therapy in adults, and even less in children.

7.1.5. Growth and Metabolism

Height, Weight, and Obesity: Growth hormone is primarily secreted in the early hours of deep, non-REM sleep. Reduced growth hormone secretion may be linked to sleep disturbance or deprivation. For instance, growth is restricted by OSA, and following treatment for this sleep disorder, a rebound growth spurt is seen.

Exciting correlations have been found in studies on how sleep disorders affect metabolism. A prospective study that evaluated various obesity risk factors in 150 children aged 0 to 9 1/2 years found that getting less sleep raises the risk of childhood obesity. Although there isn't yet an established biological correlate for this result, theories about metabolic rates, sympathetic tone, and underlying sleep disorders point the way for further investigation. Adults with untreated OSA have a higher risk of developing type II diabetes. There may be a connection between the current "epidemic" of childhood obesity and the rise in type II diabetes cases in young people. Notably, there is a higher likelihood of adult-onset SDB in obese children. It is yet unknown if the rise in type II diabetes and obesity is directly linked to an increase in SDB in children. However, following treatment for SDB in children, weight loss and a drop in type II diabetes markers are observed (Allen et al., 2000; Allen et al., 2001; Allen et al., 2003; Blunden et al., 2005).

7.2. Evaluation of Childhood Sleep Complaints

7.2.1. History and Physical

The majority of children who have sleep issues can be diagnosed primarily based on their medical history. It is easy to overlook sleep-related questions in a busy clinical setting. BEARS, a straightforward screening algorithm consisting of five questions, can be utilized to evaluate various aspects of sleep-related issues and yield more insightful data than a single sleep-related question.

Certain sleep-related disorders, like many parasomnias, tend to manifest more frequently or even exclusively in childhood. When a child or adolescent is being interviewed regarding strange behaviors or arousals that occur during sleep, it is helpful to find out which part of the night is typically problematic. While sleep disorders that happen during REM sleep, like nightmares, usually happen later at night or early in the morning, those that happen during non-REM sleep, like sleep terrors, are more common in the early hours of sleep.

Specific elements of the standard pediatric interview are helpful when figuring out the causes of sleep and wakefulness disorders. A possible explanation for behavioral or respiratory complaints during sleep could be found in the mother's pregnancy history, with special attention to placental abnormalities, premature birth, or birth complications related to fetal distress or hypoxia. These slight respiratory disturbances around birth result in behavioral patterns of hyperactivity and inattention later in life, as intermittent hypoxia experiments in neonatal rat pups show. This remarkable behavioral shift in these animals is thought to be the result of a modification in the dopaminergic innervation of the cortex.

Given the possibility of diagnosing and treating many sleep disorders with genetic components in childhood, family history plays a significant role in the pediatric sleep history. Even in the absence of comorbid obesity, SDB has been observed to run in families. In such families, one may expect genes that confer a reduction in upper airway muscle tone or one of several anatomic risk factors linked to SDB (e.g., midline facial or maxillary and mandibular hypoplasia). Additionally, the genetic pattern of inheritance for restless legs syndrome (RLS) is compatible with either an autosomal dominant or pseudo dominant mode of inheritance. There is evidence to suggest that children with a family history of the idiopathic form of this disorder are more likely to have genetic components that lead to dysfunctional dopaminergic innervation of sensory.

The timing of sleep and wakefulness as well as the sleep-related behaviors are other important aspects of the pediatric and adolescent sleep history. Parents generally set bedtimes and wake hours for their children, in one way or another. The circadian cycle for sleep and wake naturally lengthens as children grow and approach adolescence, and the homeostatic drive for sleep and wake diminishes, delaying the timing of sleep and wake patterns. As a child grows older, their sleep length decreases and they consolidate their sleep into a single, long nocturnal epoch rather than sleeping in short bursts during the day and night. There is a tiny reduction in sleep duration from childhood to adolescence, but it is much less than the drop from infancy to childhood. Teenagers therefore still need long major sleep epochs—nine hours on average—but ironically, sleep length is frequently shortened by waking up earlier for activities like work, sports, or school.

Having an informed adult or parent to help with reporting bedtime routines, nocturnal, and daytime symptoms and behaviors is crucial during the pediatric sleep interview. Children with insomnias seldom exhibit conscious awareness of their condition, and even parents may be blind to snoring, restlessness, and other nocturnal behaviors. In certain situations, home videos of behaviors and nocturnal movements can help with diagnosis. Sleeping in class, missing school, or behavioral issues related to sleep deprivation can all be signs of declining grades or social problems. Critical information about daytime hyperactivity, inattention, and sleepiness may be added by teachers. Furthermore, a history of depression or attention deficit hyperactivity disorder (ADHD) in a psychiatric or behavioral context may also point to a sleep-related issue like delayed sleep-phase syndrome, behavioral insomnia, RLS, or SDB.

Physical causes of the primary sleep and wake complaint should be the main focus of the examination. For breathing issues, this might involve a thorough examination of the face, mouth, nose, ears, and lungs. It might also entail keeping a close eye out for symptoms of atopy, allergic shiners, and Dennie lines. SDB may be more common in kids with hypotelorism, midline hypoplasia, or just a hypoplastic nasal bridge. Standard procedure involves routine examination of the central and peripheral nervous systems in cases of suspected SDB, RLS, headaches, seizures, nocturnal movement disorders, and parasomnias. Examining the skin, tongue, and mucosa for pale coloring or uneven surfaces suggestive of anemia or vitamin deficiencies is necessary in cases of excessive somnolence during the day. Frequent weeping episodes in infants may indicate the need for additional testing for gastroesophageal reflux, but they may also show signs of acidic damage to the oropharynx, such as reddened soft tissues. When evaluating developmental milestones, it can help direct further testing in infants and children who have delays in their language, motor skills, or other developmental domains.

Additional elements of the physical examination that support the diagnosis include body mass index (BMI), weight, and height measurements. Regular growth tracking along percentiles during development could be useful in illustrating how a sleep disorder affects a person. A three-year-old child with large tonsils and adenoids may have the effects of SDB if their height and weight do not progress. A child's growth frequently accelerates to the prior height and weight percentile following successful therapy. Early-life BMI (kg/m^2) readings in the 95th percentile raise the risk of childhood obesity, which in turn raises the chance of late-life and adolescent SDB.

7.2.2. Sleep Questionnaires and Diaries

To screen for signs of childhood sleep disorders, any of a number of validated questionnaires can be helpful in clinical and especially research settings. A number of categories of pediatric sleep issues are screened for using the Sleep Disturbance Scale for Children. There are subscales on the Pediatric Sleep Questionnaire for OSA and restless legs/periodic limb movements. The Children's Sleep Habits Questionnaire is a screening tool used to determine whether a child's sleep issues are behavioral or medical in nature. It is intended for use with school-aged children. A modified Epworth Sleepiness Scale, the Pediatric Daytime Sleepiness Scale, or a component of the Pediatric Sleep Questionnaire can all be used to measure subjective sleepiness.

To diagnose and treat nocturnal events such as parasomnias, restlessness, enuresis, or even headaches, it can be useful to use sleep diaries to track how frequently these events occur. Sleep diaries are notebooks that track the times each day that you go asleep, wake up from sleep, and finally, wake up. Diaries ought to be used for a set amount of time (a few weeks to a few days), and they ought to be easy enough for older kids and teenagers to use on their own. Clear instructions for parents should be provided, along with details about previous daytime activities, medications, and other regular sleep-related information. Sleep diaries can help confirm poor sleep hygiene and sleep and wake patterns consistent with specific circadian rhythm diagnoses in children and especially adolescents complaining of insomnia or symptoms associated with the circadian rhythm.

7.2.3. Actigraphy

Actigraphy, also known as actometry, is the recording of movement from an apparatus that resembles a large wristwatch. This method can be used to objectively document patterns of sleep and wake activity on a daily and weekly basis, in addition to sleep diaries. Actigraphy recorded from a leg can be used to confirm periodic leg movements in periodic limb movement disorder, which may be linked to sleep fragmentation. Actigraphy continuously records arm and leg movements for a predefined number of hours or days using a triaxial accelerometer. The gadget can be set up to collect data at intervals of up to several minutes or as little as one microsecond. Children of all ages tolerate these commercially available devices quite well.

7.2.4. Polysomnogram

To diagnose sleep breathing disorders, numerous parasomnias, seizures, certain movement disorders (like periodic limb movements), and therapeutic continuous positive airway pressure (CPAP) titrations, the polysomnogram (PSG) is the gold standard for testing sleep disorders. The PSG technique for children is comparable to that for adults in that it involves transduction of the respiratory movements of the chest and abdomen in addition to recording EMG, EEG, electrooculography, and EKG. Sensors that are sensitive to temperature are used to monitor nasal and oral airflow, while cannulae attached to transducers are used to measure nasal pressure. In contrast to adult PSG, children's end-tidal carbon dioxide is frequently measured, and esophageal pH monitoring can be used to connect respiratory or arousal events to reflux disease (Figure 7.1).

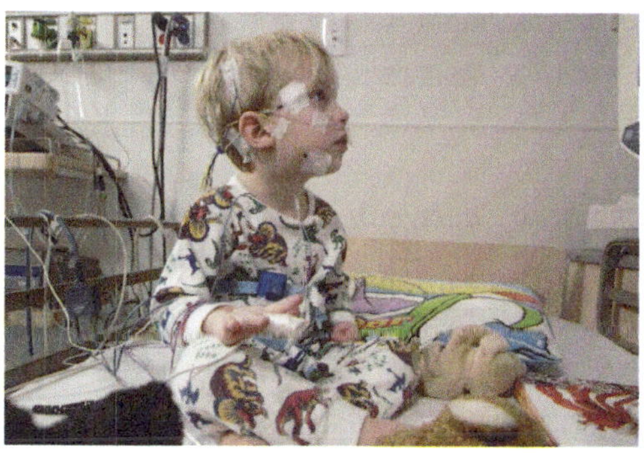

Figure 7.1. *Polysomnography sleep test.*

Source: By Robert Lawton – Own work, CC BY-SA 2.5, https://commons.wikimedia.org/w/index.php?curid=741662.

Infant sleep-stage scoring is different from adult and child sleep-stage scoring; many pediatric PSG textbooks provide details on this. It may not be optimal to score respiratory, movement, and arousal events using adult criteria. Children breathe more quickly than adults do, so apneas or hypopneas that last less than two respiratory cycles, regardless of how many seconds have passed, should definitely be recorded. Unlike in adults, when it lasts for 10 seconds, central apneas in infants typically lasts for at least 20 seconds. Recent research indicates that an apnea/hypopnea index as low as 1.5 may work best to distinguish significant SDB. In children, an obstructive apnea index (number of apneas per hour of sleep) greater than 1 is frequently used as a threshold for clinically significant OSA. To determine the best cutoffs, more outcomes-based research will be needed. In any case, to deliver the best care, the cutoffs must be interpreted in conjunction with clinical histories.

7.2.5. Multiple Sleep Latency Test

The multiple sleep latency test (MSLT) is the most widely used objective test for excessive daytime sleepiness. It is suggested that someone lie in a quiet, dark room and attempt to fall asleep. Daytime sleepiness is reflected in the sleep latency, which is averaged over four or five of these nap attempts spaced out throughout the day. In clinical settings, children as young as 8 years old are treated with the MSLT. However, recent studies have indicated that the tool can be useful for kids as young as 3 or 5 years old. Results should be interpreted with consideration for the fact that children's mean sleep latencies are significantly longer than those of adults. Another useful tool for supporting a narcolepsy diagnosis is the recording of two or more sleep-onset REM periods during the MSLT's quick naps (Allen et al., 2000; Allen et al., 2001; Allen et al., 2003; Blunden et al., 2005).

7.3. Insomnia

A sleep disorder called insomnia makes it

difficult to go asleep, stay asleep, and wake up too early. Short-term insomnia can last a few days or weeks and be caused by medication, anxiety following a stressful event, or a medical condition. It may also be a chronic illness that affects the child for the rest of their life.

7.3.1. Behavioral Insomnia of Childhood

7.3.1.1. Sleep-Onset Association Type

Clinicians frequently ignore actions that either cause or exacerbate childhood sleep disorders, such as those that occur before bedtime and following nocturnal awakenings. Environmental cues like temperature, noise level, and lighting help babies and kids fall asleep by setting the right mood. Adults often participate during this time by singing, rocking, feeding, rubbing, or even lying down with their children as they fall asleep. Unfortunately, the association many infants and children make is that sleep onset occurs with the parent in the room actively soothing them to sleep. When they wake during the night—and most children do this four or more times per night—they invariably cry or fuss until the adult restores the exact condition (e.g., rocking, feeding) that was present at sleep onset. We refer to this prevalent form of behavioral insomnia as sleep-onset association disorder (Figure 7.2).

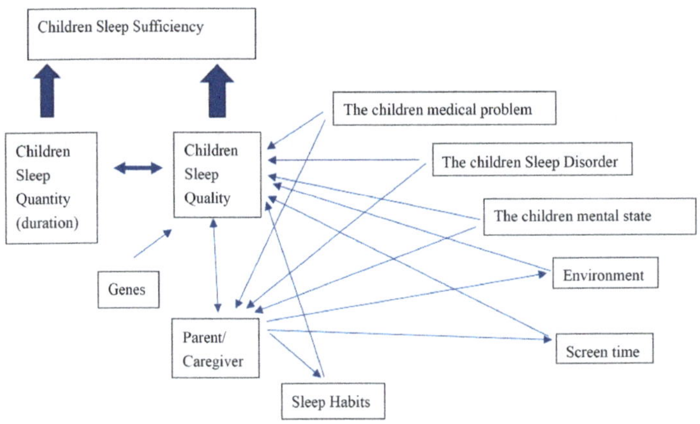

Figure 7.2. *Factors that affect sleep quality and the interactions between factors.*

Source: Fadzil A. Factors Affecting the Quality of Sleep in Children. *Children. 2021; 8(2):122. https://doi.org/10.3390/children8020122.*

Sleep-onset association disorder in infants is characterized by excessive sleep fragmentation brought on by soothing behaviors from parents. Extrinsic calming techniques like feeding, rocking, singing, or engaging in other stimulating activities have been shown to cause nocturnal awakenings in young children and may exacerbate chronic sleep issues in both the child and the adult. Parents' actions and presence need to be disengaged from the process of falling asleep to treat this conditioned response in infants and children. Therapy aims to assist a child in developing the ability to "self-soother." This can happen almost instantly with "extinction," where the child is let to "cry it out," or it can happen more gradually, as suggested by some, or very quickly with "graduated extinction," as demonstrated by the so-called Ferber method.

7.3.1.2. Limit-Setting Type

Children in preschool and school are also susceptible to behavioral insomnia. Research indicates significant variations in sleep duration between weekday and weekend sleep periods, which can be attributed to recuperating from sleep deprivation during the week. However, these variations are also linked to sleep environments that are unmonitored or uncontrolled during the week. The term "limit-setting sleep disorder" refers to the absence of a clear structure imposed by parents regarding behaviors at the onset of sleep and following awakenings.

Youngsters with this issue frequently "push the envelope" and don't have enough boundaries in place to stop demanding food, beverages, attention, or playtime activities right before or right after bedtime. Restoration of parental authority is the goal of treatment. Time and behavioral restrictions during the 20 to 30 minutes before bedtime can be helpful, as can a regular schedule that the child can grow accustomed to. Furthermore, older kids might gain from receiving praise for appropriate bedtime behaviors.

7.3.2. Sleep Deprivation and Inadequate Sleep Hygiene

Many kids exhibit a hyperactive state with inattention and poor impulse control after experiencing sleep deprivation. Because of this, daytime sleepiness may not be as evident as it is in adults, but it is frequently discernible through a thorough interview. Preschoolers and early school-age children who experience sleep disturbances have much higher injury rates than children who do not.

The phrase "sleep hygiene" refers to both positive and negative actions that people take either before bed or during their actual sleep period. There is usually a relaxing phase involved in the regular process of falling asleep. This period of relaxation is disrupted by poor sleep habits or behaviors, which can result in "insomnia" symptoms that have the potential to spread on their own. Children who don't have a calming, regular routine as bedtime draws near frequently have poor sleep hygiene. Excessive roughhousing, late-night eating, prolonged homework assignments, and prolonged use of phones, computers, televisions, and electronic games are all factors that contribute to arousal and hinder the transition to sleep. It's critical to recognize poor sleep hygiene since it can worsen behavioral insomnia, behavioral issues during the day, and family dissatisfaction.

Childhood insomnia is also linked to several neurologic and psychiatric disorders, such as Asperger syndrome, depression, ADHD, autism, and post-traumatic stress disorder. It has also been observed that precocious kids experience insomnia related to sleep onset and maintenance, which isn't always connected to behavioral insomnia or poor sleep hygiene. According to survey studies, patients with special needs are more likely than the general pediatric population to take medication for treating childhood insomnia. In a double-blind, placebo-controlled trial, the use of melatonin in conjunction with sleep hygiene therapy has been shown to be an effective treatment for children with ADHD and insomnia. In the general pediatric clinical setting, benzodiazepines, alpha-2 agonists, and antihistamines are frequently utilized as additional therapies. Sadly, children's safety and efficacy of many drugs used to treat adult insomnia have not been thoroughly investigated. It is obvious that research on the pharmacologic treatment of pediatric insomnia with prescription and over-the-counter medications is required (Allen et al., 2000; Allen et al., 2001; Allen et al., 2003; Blunden et al., 2005).

7.4. Parasomnias: Disorders of Arousal

A group of sleep-related behaviors that can happen during REM or non-REM sleep are called parasomnias. The classic nightmare, which usually happens in the later half of the night when REM is most prominent, is a common REM parasomnia in childhood. Periods of maximal nonREM sleep occur in the first half of the major sleep epoch, coinciding with nonREM parasomnias, also known as arousal disorders. While some parasomnias, like enuresis, can happen during non-REM or REM sleep, slow-wave non-REM sleep is usually linked to them.

7.4.1. Enuresis

Most authorities view enuresis, or sleep-related bedwetting, as developmentally inappropriate after the age of six or seven years old. Before the age of 11, boys are impacted twice as frequently as girls, and during adolescence, this gender disparity appears to vanish. The presentation of symptoms distinguishes between primary and secondary forms of enuresis.

	Patients with nocturnal enuresis	Normal controls
Total sleep time	Decreased	No difference
REM sleep	Higher variability	Not increased
Depth of sleep	Light sleep but difficult to wake up during enuresis. Deeper depth in children with NMNE	Normal sleep circle
Wake %	Frequent in PNE	Rarely
Sleep efficiency	Lower sleep efficiency especially with comorbidity	No difference between primary monosymptomatic NE with normal controls
Abnormal EEG detected	Show changes similar to sleep–wake transition before enuresis; increased delta power	Not detected
Cortical arousal index (CAI)	A decreased CAI in NREM An increased CAI in refractory patients	Fewer sleep fragmentation
Cyclic alternating pattern (CAP)	Increase in CAP rate during N3 (slow wave activity)	No significant disruption

Figure 7.3. *Comparing children with enuresis vs. controls.*

Source: Zhu B, Zou K, He J, Huang X, Zhu W, Ahmad Harb AK, Wang J and Luo A (2021) Sleep Monitoring of Children With Nocturnal Enuresis: A Narrative Review. Front. Pediatr. 9:701251. doi: 10.3389/fped.2021.701251.

Primary enuresis, which is more prevalent and affects 60–70% of children with enuresis, is defined as sleep-related urine incontinence that has not had a remission interval since birth. It is implied by secondary enuresis that interfering periods of continence have lasted for at least three months. Organic or psychological factors such as recurrent UTIs, seizures, SDB, genetic, and anatomic abnormalities, abdominal masses, constipation, sleep restriction, anxiety, and situational stress are often linked to the secondary form of enuresis. Both types of enuresis can recur in a single night, but they usually only happen once. Although REM sleep-related enuresis is also documented, the majority of studies indicate that enuresis arises from slow-wave non-REM sleep

(Figure 7.3). Children diagnosed with ADHD or SDB have a higher likelihood of experiencing enuresis compared to their peers. While the exact connection between these conditions is unclear, it provides an opportunity for additional research and potential treatment options. Studies have also found that children with enuresis may experience delays in motor and language development milestones. The root cause of primary enuresis remains unknown, with theories pointing to factors such as immature neurologic control of the urinary tract, inadequate arousal response during slow-wave sleep, and a genetic predisposition based on family and twin studies.

As mentioned above, evaluating for secondary causes is a necessary part of diagnosing and treating enuresis. In certain situations, urologic testing could be helpful, and full remission is frequently the result of treating underlying psychological or medical issues. Children who have other sleep disorders, like SDB, should be evaluated. Numerous accounts point to a marked decrease in enuresis following SDB treatment.

There are several options for treating primary enuresis once secondary causes have been ruled out. Reducing liquid intake before bedtime, emptying the bladder before bed, and using waking techniques to prevent bedwetting are examples of non-medical therapeutic approaches. Due to a lower relapse rate (less than 50%) following therapy cessation, a Cochrane Database review of the literature indicates that bell and pad techniques involving liquid-sensitive alarms are more effective than medical treatments. A watch-and-wait strategy is frequently used because children with primary enuresis exhibit a 15% annual spontaneous remission rate between the ages of 5 and 16. Studies indicate that the majority of young children with mild symptoms (less than three nights per week) will go away on their own before reaching adolescence. Compared to their less affected peers, severe (nightly) primary enuretics are more likely to experience this issue well into adolescence. For over 30 years, desmopressin has been used to treat pediatric enuresis. A significant positive effect was seen in all treated individuals in a recent double-blind, placebo-controlled trial involving 84 children with primary enuresis and low-dose, fast-melting oral desmopressin. Similar to desmopressin, tricyclic antidepressants (TCAs) can also be an effective treatment for enuresis; however, most children relapse after stopping the medication. Furthermore, the effectiveness of TCAs as enuresis treatments for kids is frequently limited by the side effects associated with tricyclic drugs.

7.4.2. Nightmare Disorder

Childhood nightmares are frequent and frequently linked to the emergence of adaptive fear reactions to external threats. 24% of children aged 2 to 6 years, 41% of children aged 6 to 10 years, and 22% of teenagers report having nightmares. Because there is more REM sleep during the second half of the sleep cycle, nightmares tend to happen during this time.

Studies on human functional imaging during sleep show that, in comparison to other stages of sleep, REM sleep is when limbic memory structures like the amygdala, parahippocampal gyrus, and anterior cingulate gyrus are most active. This could be connected to the main characteristic of nightmares, which is the capacity to recollect a highly charged emotional event or memory. Even though nightmares are common in childhood, a diagnosis of nightmare disorder is based on persistent problems that cause insomnia in the second half of the night. The diagnosis entails ruling out any secondary causes, which may include drug interactions, seizures, non-REM parasomnias, SDB, other sleep disorders, and mental health issues like PTSD. An expanded EEG montage can be beneficial when the differential diagnosis suggests seizures and video PSG is useful in complex cases.

Treating secondary causes of nightmare disorder, such as SDB and seizures, is part of therapy. Although the effects of medications have not been thoroughly investigated, a small double-blind, placebo-controlled study involving adults with posttraumatic stress disorder suggests that the alpha-1 antagonist prazosin can considerably lessen recurrent nightmares. Additional treatments that have been documented include lucid dreaming, hypnosis, relaxation techniques, psychotherapy, and REM suppression using TCAs and selective serotonin reuptake inhibitors.

7.4.3. Non-REM Parasomnias

Sleepwalking, sleep terrors, and confusional arousals fall into the category of non-REM parasomnias. Even though they are all classified as distinct parasomnias, they can all be attributed to dominant modes of inheritance, involve behavior arising from deep non-REM sleep, and frequently occur in combination. Research utilizing a sizable Finnish twin cohort comprising more than 11,200 individuals revealed a 50% phenotypic covariance between sleepwalking and sleep talking. For non-REM parasomnias in this cohort, structural equation modeling revealed a strong additive and dominant effect. When children are asked what arouses them, they usually don't remember, and non-REM parasomnias usually appear in the first few hours after sleep onset.

7.4.3.1. Sleepwalking

All age groups of children experience somnambulism. According to prevalence studies, between the ages of three and 10, between nine and 10% of children report sleepwalking at least once. Peak prevalence is reached at age five, and it is believed to decline from 7% in children aged 11 to 3% in teenagers aged 13. Up to 24% of teenagers with a past history still engage in sleepwalking, which is linked to a history of confusional arousals. Guilleminault et al. provided evidence that SDB could potentially trigger sleepwalking. In a prospective one-year study, sleepwalking was completely eliminated after one year of effective therapy for 50 young adult chronic sleepwalkers with different SDB diagnoses (from upper airway resistance syndrome to OSA). It has also been demonstrated that other sleep disorders like periodic limb movement disorder and RLS can cause children to start sleepwalking. Other non-REM parasomnias, psychiatric conditions, and nocturnal frontal lobe epilepsy are also included in the differential diagnosis.

Safety is the main worry when it comes to sleepwalking. Evidence of kids and teenagers running, falling, and walking into potentially fatal situations points to the importance of monitoring and helping vulnerable people. The goal of therapy is to lessen the risk factors that could lead to a somnambulistic event, such as anxiety, sleep deprivation, and situational stress. Bells and other alarming devices can be used to keep an eye on children who have a history of sleepwalking. These devices alert others to the child's arousal from sleep. Redirecting sleepwalking children without fully waking them is advised by parents because it is frequently linked to confusion, tantrums, and difficulty falling back asleep. Clonazepam-based medical therapy may be beneficial in certain circumstances. Typically, episodes of sleepwalking are self-limiting and endure for a few to several minutes.

7.4.3.2. Sleep Terrors

Sleep terrors also referred to as Pavor nocturnus, are characterized by an abrupt awakening from slumber accompanied by a scream or other sudden display of fear. The event is startling to witness and frequently wakes others who are sleeping. Kids seem to be afraid for no apparent reason; they frequently yell, kick, punch, and even flee from imaginary attackers. Parents may be present in the room and try to calm the child, but the child usually responds poorly and the incident ends on its own in a matter of minutes with the child going back to sleep. Children usually don't remember these things and appear perplexed when they wake up later. Children rarely experience multiple sleep terror episodes in a single night. The majority of sleep terror episodes are singular.

Similar to sleepwalking, precipitating factors like periodic limb movement disorder, RLS, and SDB should be ruled out of the differential diagnosis. Furthermore, a history of posturing, enuresis, or rhythmic movements may indicate nocturnal seizures, which can be assessed with an extended EEG video PSG. Safety is the most crucial component of therapy. Children who are more prone to sleep terrors should be watched during stressful times, such as the beginning of a new school year, or when they experience sleep restriction, as they may display aggressive and harmful behaviors. Preventing sleep loss and excessive stress in situations could potentially lower the frequency of sleep terrors. Drugs like clonazepam are given to people who experience sleep terrors frequently.

7.4.3.3. Confusional Arousals

A sleep disorder called confusional arousals makes you act very strangely and confusedly when you wake up or shortly after waking up. You might come across as being unaware of your surroundings or your actions.

Your behavior may include the following:

- Slow speech.
- Confused thinking.
- Poor memory.
- Blunt responses to questions or requests.

The confusional arousal is the mildest type of non-REM parasomnia. Children may sit up and even look around the room during this brief (seconds to minutes) interruption of apparent wakefulness, but they will stay in bed and go back to sleep without further explanation of the arousal. Confusional arousals, like other nonREM parasomnias, are harmless in and of themselves, but they can indicate that an underlying sleep disorder needs to be investigated to determine what is causing the partial arousals. When confusional arousals occur on their own, therapy is typically not necessary; however, it might be if an underlying sleep disorder is found.

When a confusional arousal happens, you might appear to be awake despite having a disoriented mental state. When someone else has to physically wake you up, episodes frequently begin (Figure 7.4).

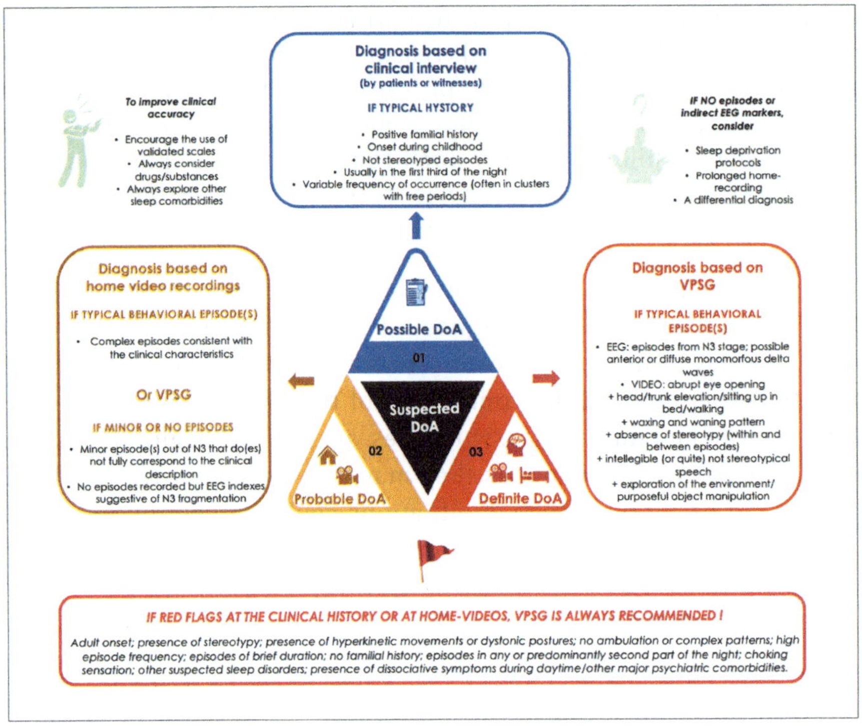

Figure 7.4. *Coping with confusional arousal.*

Source: Mainieri G, Loddo G, Provini F, Nobili L, Manconi M, Castelnovo A. Diagnosis and Management of NREM Sleep Parasomnias in Children and Adults. Diagnostics. 2023; 13(7):1261. https://doi.org/10.3390/diagnostics13071261.

7.4.3.4. Risk Factors for Confusional Arousals

You are more likely to experience confusional arousals if you have a relative with this sleep disorder. Other factors that can increase your risk for arousals include:

- Rotating shift work.
- Night shift work.
- Other sleep disorders (hypersomnia, insomnia, circadian rhythm sleep disorders).
- Not enough sleep.
- Stress.
- Worry.
- Bipolar and depressive disorders.

7.4.3.5. Diagnosis

Parents should monitor their child's sleep and wake schedule as well as the dates, times, and details of their events. This can be useful in determining the kind of incident and in formulating a treatment plan. The child must undergo a sleep evaluation to rule out any additional sleep issues that might be preventing them from getting the recommended amount or quality of sleep. In certain circumstances, polysomnography might be advised.

A sleep specialist will frequently ask you to keep a two-week sleep journal if you're an adult. This will help the physician determine the potential causes of your issues. She may also ask you to complete a brief questionnaire rating how well you sleep. This will demonstrate how your sleep is impacting your day-to-day activities. Your whole medical history will need to be disclosed to the doctor. Make careful to let her know if you currently or previously used drugs or medications. Inform the doctor if you or a family member has ever experienced a sleep disturbance.

A sleep doctor will try to determine if there is something else that is causing your arousals or making the symptoms worse, such as:

- Another sleep disorder.
- A medical condition.
- Medication use.
- A mental health disorder.
- Substance abuse.

A sleep study may be recommended by the sleep specialist to assess your sleep. A sleep study also referred to as polysomnography, records your respiration, heart rate, and brain waves while you sleep. It also records your movements with your arms and legs and captures your behavior on video while you sleep. This will assist in demonstrating whether you move during your sleep study or get out of bed (Allen et al., 2000; Allen et al., 2001; Allen et al., 2003; Blunden et al., 2005).

7.5. Sleep-Disordered Breathing

A healthy childhood depends on getting enough sleep, and sleep-disordered breathing (SDB), which is defined as abnormal breathing and ventilation during sleep, has been linked to many behavioral and physical health problems. Despite mounting evidence linking untreated, long-term obstructive sleep apnea (OSA) to obesity, metabolic disorders, hypertension, neuropsychiatric disorders, and developmental problems, many clinicians still fail to recognize the full impact of SDB on health.

7.5.1. Obstructive Sleep Apnea

The term "severe breathing disorders" (SDB) encompasses a variety of breathing irregularities that occur during sleep. Primary snoring (without gas exchange abnormalities or obvious arousals), upper airway resistance syndrome, OSA, and obstructive hypoventilation during sleep are all considered forms of obstructive sleep disorder breathing (SDB). Among the various forms of central SDB are central sleep apnea and hypoventilation resulting from central nervous system causes (Table 7.1).

The anatomical caliber of the upper airway, the gradient of pressure across the upper airway (inner airway versus surrounding tissue pressure), neuromuscular coordination of contractions that occur with each inspiration, and adequate muscle tone in the pharyngeal walls are all factors that contribute to upper airway patency. The inner airway pressures decrease during breathing, and fast, turbulent airflow may result in the tissue vibrations that cause snoring. Complete or nearly complete upper airway collapse (apnea) can be caused by sufficient reductions in upper airway muscle tone or caliber, as can happen with enlarged tonsils and adenoids. Similar to breathing pauses, central apneas are caused by the cessation of breathing effort, which is typically produced by the central nervous system and peripheral sensorimotor components of the ventilatory control system.

Table 7.1. *Frequency of Sleep Disturbances Compared by Groups of Different Age Ranges 206 Children Between the Ages of 7 and 17 Who Attended A Dental Office*

	Group	n	%	*p*-Value	OR	95% CI	
Initiating and maintaining sleep	A	68	33.0	0.003 *	2.554	1.360	4.797
	B	75	36.4				
Respiratory Sleep disorders	A	30	14.6	0.888	1.045	0.565	1.935
	B	26	12.6				
Arousal disorders	A	53	25.7	0.702	1.113	0.643	1.927
	B	47	22.8				
Sleep–wake transition disorders	A	70	34.0	0.784	0.924	0.526	1.624
	B	57	27.7				
Excessive somnolence disorders	A	38	18.4	0.013 **	2.032	1.158	3.567
	B	48	23.3				
Hyperhidrosis	A	53	25.7	0.402	0.789	0.454	1.372
	B	39	18.9				

SD: standard deviation; A: children aged 7 to 11 years; B: children aged 12 to 17 years; *p*-value: X^2 significance level; *: X^2 significance = 8.757; **: X^2 significance = 6.17; OR: odds ratio; CI: confidence interval.

Source: Diéguez-Pérez M, Burgueño-Torres L, Reichard-Monefeldt G, Tapia-Sierra FE, Ticona-Flores JM. Prevalence and Characteristics of Sleep Disorders in Children Aged 7–17: Insights from Parental Observations at the Dental Office. Children. 2024;11(5):609. https://doi.org/10.3390/children11050609.

The anatomical size of the upper airway, the gradient of pressure across the upper airway (inner airway versus surrounding tissue pressure), neuromuscular coordination of contractions that occur with each inspiration, and adequate muscle tone in the pharyngeal walls are all factors that contribute to upper airway patency.

In children, the most common form of SDB is known as OSA syndrome, which is characterized by a combination of obstructive apneas, hypopneas, and occasionally central apneas. Adenotonsillar hypertrophy and lymphoid hyperplasia cause OSA, which affects 1–3% of preschool-aged children. It peaks between the ages of 2 and 6 years. The risk of OSA can increase during adolescence, most likely in connection with rising obesity rates. Children who identify as African American and boys may be more susceptible to developing OSA. Children with asthma or atopic dermatitis may also be more susceptible.

7.5.1.1. Effects of Snoring and Obstructive Sleep Apnea on Children

It's unclear how snoring affects health in general, and until recently, primary snoring in children was thought to be a benign condition that didn't need medical attention. Research on sleep-related brain disorders in young children and infants now indicates that snoring on its own, whether or not there are detectable apneas or hypopneas, is linked to behavioral, cognitive, and psychosocial morbidity. Increased snoring during sleep is associated with more arousals during sleep and lower scores on standardized mental development assessments in infants without observable apneas or hypopneas on PSG. There is a known correlation between snoring in kids and lower scores on executive function tests, verbal IQ, global IQ, selected, and sustained attention tasks, and multiple memory scales. Such findings may be explained by upper airway resistance syndrome, which some sleep specialists classify as a component of OSA. In this condition, respiratory effort-related arousals occur without frank apneic events. These children's notable increases in attention deficit disorder, hyperactivity, social problems, and depressive and anxious symptoms may be related to their increased sleep fragmentation. A prospective, longitudinal study involving 229 children found that baseline symptoms of snoring and SDB were predictive of the emergence or worsening of hyperactivity four years later.

Increased arousals from sleep and decreased arterial oxygen saturation may be linked to the etiology of the neurocognitive and behavioral abnormalities associated with SDB. The slight (less than 3%) intermittent hypoxic episodes that are associated with SDB are directly linked to a growing deficit in working memory and other cognitive functions. Arterial oxygen saturation nadirs consistent with intermittent hypoxemic events are highly correlated with neurocognitive deficits and subpar academic performance, according to pulse oximetry measurements taken during sleep. However, children with SDB who do not exhibit elements of hypoxia are still found to have behavioral impairment, including hyperactivity, inattention, excessive daytime sleepiness, poor behavior, emotional symptoms, and trouble with peers. Gozal and Kheirandish's more formalized model of this process and its implications aligns with the idea that increased upper airway resistance is a critical pathophysiologic element in SDB. They propose that upper airway resistance rises and SDB deteriorates as a result of a local inflammatory response in the upper airway. As SDB worsens, there is an increased inflammatory response throughout the body, which can lead to end =-organ morbidity (such as hypertension), as seen in both adults and children with SDB.

SDB is also linked to childhood growth deficiencies. The height and weight growth curves of children with SDB may "fall off" for no apparent reason. This is assumed to be caused by SDB's higher metabolic "cost." Another reason for this could be that SDB causes frequent sleep arousals. Arousals that interfere with slow-wave sleep can affect growth hormone secretion. Growth hormone is released in the early hours of the regular sleep cycle during slow-wave sleep. Significant variations in insulin-like growth factor-1 and insulin-like growth factor-binding protein-3 are linked to impaired growth hormone secretion. Growth hormone indices and growth resume following appropriate therapy for sickle cell disease (SDB), and children typically resume their pre-disease developmental patterns.

7.5.1.2. Diagnosis

The method used to diagnose SDB in children is different from that used in adults in several ways. While daytime sleepiness is not typically a complaint of school-aged or preschool-aged children with SDB, it can often be inferred by carefully probing the parents. Children who are past puberty, younger people who are severely affected, and obese children frequently complain of being sleepy in a way that is more akin to that of adults with OSA. Observed apneas or labored breathing during sleep, excessive sweating during the night, daytime sleepiness, hyperactivity, impulsivity, inattentiveness, small stature, mouth breathing, or recurrent sinus, throat, and ear infections are additional symptoms of sleep disturbance in children. Adenotonsillar hypertrophy is the most common risk factor for SDB in children, but other significant risk factors include obesity, neuromuscular weakness, and craniofacial abnormalities. SDB is predisposed to numerous other medical and neurological disorders. To effectively plan therapy for children with SDB, it can be helpful to identify the probable causes of the condition.

It is advised to obtain objective confirmation, typically through PSG, when clinical suspicions of SDB exist. Regarding what cutoffs in results should be used to define SDB, there is still a great deal of uncertainty in borderline cases. The fact that the tools and scoring systems employed in various sleep laboratories frequently vary adds to this uncertainty. On the other hand, current data indicates that apnea/hypopnea index (rate per hour of sleep) greater than 1.5 is a rough cutoff point for significant childhood SDB. In actual practice, PSG results should only be used in conjunction with other clinical data to inform patient care, especially when objective results are close to borderline values. In addition, oxygen desaturations, paradoxical breathing—in which the chest contracts rather than expands—flow limitation detected by a sensitive nasal pressure cannula, increased effort to breathe as indicated by intrathoracic pressure monitoring via an esophageal catheter, and increased arousals in connection with such respiratory difficulties are other PSG indicators that children with SDB may exhibit.

When tonsillar hypertrophy is not evident but there is suspected adenoid hypertrophy, a lateral neck X-ray or nasopharyngoscopy may be helpful. These studies can also yield important information for comparison in the future, as adenoid tissue can regenerate following incomplete surgical resection.

7.5.1.3. Therapy

A proper diagnosis is necessary for SDB treatment to be effective. In the majority of cases, tonsillectomy, and adenotonsillectomy (T&A) are regarded as the best course of action. Although T&A is frequently used in various contexts, therapy based solely on a direct inspection of the tonsils does not guarantee an accurate diagnosis in children who do not also exhibit other signs and symptoms of SDB. The majority of cases with suspected SDB should use diagnostic PSG, which is currently the gold standard. With reported cure rates of 80%, T&A therapy has generally been deemed to produce excellent results. T&A is still thought to be the best course of action for the majority of children with SDB, despite recent data suggesting that subtle residual SDB may affect many more children.

According to the case series, T&A lowers other PSG indicators of SDB, such as the apnea/hypopnea index. Many of the neurobehavioral issues linked to SDB appear to be resolved by the process as well. A battery of neuropsychological tests and PSG were used to evaluate 105 children (27 unrelated surgical patients and 78 with suspected SDB) before and one year after T&A. Neuropsychological testing also revealed reductions in hyperactivity, inattention, ADHD, and excessive daytime somnolence measures. PSG evidence also showed effective resolution of SDB at one year. Significant before-and-after effects on behavioral and neuropsychological testing in children have also been shown in other studies.

Alternative therapies are available that, depending on the situation, might be better or equal to T&A. For instance, mandibular or maxillary advancement may be advantageous for kids with craniofacial abnormalities, even mild nonsyndromic abnormalities. In studies on pediatric OSA, two modalities that have been used with some success are oral appliance therapy and rapid palatal expansion. For infants and young children with SDB, CPAP is a fantastic therapeutic option. It has been shown that CPAP is a safe and effective treatment for infants and children with SDB who have failed T&A therapy, obesity, neuromuscular disease, and craniofacial abnormalities. Although up to 80% of children find CPAP therapy to be effective and well-tolerated, compliance is the main factor that limits its effectiveness. Losing weight is a useful tactic for obese kids as well, though it's typically combined with other, faster therapies.

It has been observed that children with recurrent throat infections and OSA have higher levels of glucocorticoid receptor (GCR) expression in their tonsillar and adenoid tissues. The GCR isoform GCR-alpha exhibits notably higher levels of GCR expression in the tissue of OSA patients. These results imply a biological basis for the potential treatment of adenotonsillar hypertrophy in children with OSA through topical steroid therapy.

Based on reports of children with habitual snoring who showed mild or no elevations of PSG parameters, such as oxygen desaturations and the apnea-hypopnea index, regular use of budesonide can reduce both PSG evidence of SDB and clinical symptoms, despite the paucity of studies in this area. Nasal inhaled steroids could be a good treatment option for mild SDB or elevated arousals associated with snoring.

7.5.2. Central Sleep Apnea

The solitary tract of the medulla, which in turn drives respiration, integrates several afferent signals from the pons, peripheral chemoreceptors, and mechanoreceptors at the ventral and dorsal respiratory groups. This intricate physiology underlies respiratory control. There may be some underlying maladaptation in children with central sleep apnea (CSA) to the change from waking control of breathing to sleep control. A dysregulated central respiratory drive causes a cessation or reduction in airflow, which is known as central sleep apnea. A common reason for a sleep consultation in the NICU is apnea of prematurity, which is linked to immaturity or dysmaturity of the brain's respiratory control in newborns and infants. Uncertainty surrounds the connection between sudden infant death syndrome (SIDS) and BRUEs (brief, resolved, unexplained events, formerly known as "ALTE"). Congenital central hypoventilation syndrome (CCHS) and brainstem abnormalities like Chiari malformation are rare causes of CSA that need to be ruled out in addition to the relatively common idiopathic and transient causes that affect very young children.

7.5.2.1. History and Physical Examination

Parents of young infants frequently present with concerns regarding a history of breathing pauses during sleep. The first few months of life are when irregular breathing patterns are more common than not. In particular, periodic breathing is a common neonatal respiratory pattern that consists of 5- to 10-second breathing pauses followed by 10- to 15-second compensatory tachypnea. Infants experience periodic breathing during the rapid eye movement phase of sleep and can continue to do so for up to two months after term gestational age. However, it may be challenging to differentiate between true CSA and periodic breathing based only on the history when the parental report of the infant's unusual breathing is complex or otherwise not comfortingly typical for an infant.

When a parent notices a prolonged episode of apnea, or when the history is linked to a sudden change in color or other symptoms of respiratory distress, a PSG should be conducted. Apneas lasting longer than 20 seconds are usually a sign of preterm CSA. Patients with CSA may exhibit symptoms or be able to report a morning headache, just like those with OSA. When older patients awaken from sleep, they may report feeling as though they are "drowning" in CSA arousals. CSA is linked to several syndromes, most notably Rett syndrome. Despite hypoxemia and hypercapnia during cyanotic episodes, patients with congenital central hypoventilation syndrome often present in infancy and may not exhibit respiratory distress.

Tone assessment should be part of the physical examination for infants suspected of having CSA. When examining a patient with suspected CSA in an older child, the goal is to rule out any brainstem or intracranial abnormalities that could be physically affecting the medulla or pons, which are the centers of respiratory control. A basic fundal examination for papilledema, although potentially challenging in the pediatric patient, can be informative.

7.5.2.2. Diagnosis

7.5.2.2.1. PSG Findings

Formally speaking, CSA in children is defined as follows: a decrease in airflow of 90% or more for a minimum of 20 seconds; if linked to an arousal, for two breath cycles; a decrease in arterial oxygen saturation of three% or more; a decrease in heart rate to less than 50 beats per minute for a minimum of five seconds; or, in the case of infants, a heart rate less than 60 beats per minute for 15 seconds.

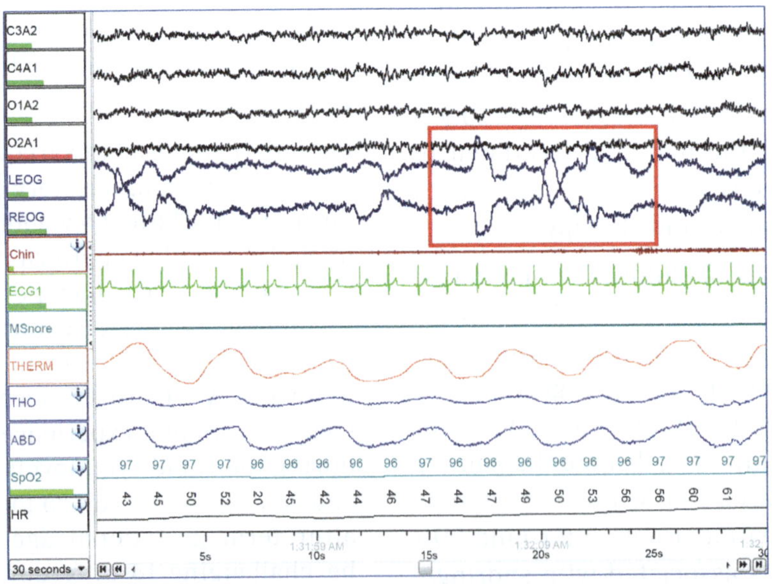

Figure 7.5. *Example of central sleep apnea as seen on polysomnography.*

Source: By NascarEd – Own work, CC BY-SA 3.0, https://commons.wikimedia.org/w/index.php?curid=24506939.

The absence of respiratory effort during these episodes is a defining characteristic of CSA. A CO_2 stimulation challenge is not routinely performed, but it could help distinguish intractable chemosensory dysfunction associated with CCHS from abnormal periodic breathing or other forms of idiopathic central apneas in young infants.

7.5.2.2.2. Laboratory Tests and Imaging

There may be no need for additional assessment in newborns in the first few months of life who exhibit brief bouts of irregular breathing or classical periodic breathing without aberrant neurologic examination findings. A blood gas test may be useful in determining the serum partial pressure of carbon dioxide in premature infants exhibiting symptoms of particularly persistent or frequent episodes of apnea of prematurity. Genetic testing for PHOX2B mutation should be used to rule out CCHA, a syndrome of dysregulated physiologic response to hypoxemia and hypercarbia resulting in hypoventilation during sleep, in patients with severe and refractory CSA in the neonatal period. Magnetic resonance imaging of the head and neck is a crucial imaging modality for ruling out Chiari malformation and other brainstem problems in older children with CSA of unknown cause.

7.5.2.2.3. Management

Oral caffeine is a reassuring intervention for preterm apnea, as studies have shown that treated infants may benefit modestly from neuroprotective effects. In cases of idiopathic CSA of infancy that last longer than the corrected gestational age of 37 weeks, caffeine therapy is typically not recommended. Acetazolamide, a carbonic anhydrase inhibitor that increases respiratory drive by altering the partial pressure of the CO_2 threshold, may be helpful for patients with idiopathic CSA. Supplemental oxygen helps some patients even when there is no overt nocturnal hypoxemia by stabilizing or decreasing the responsiveness of the peripheral chemoreceptors; however, patients treated with oxygen alone frequently experience significant sleep fragmentation. Nocturnal positive airway pressure (PAP), usually bi-level with a backup respiratory rate or an assist-control ventilator mode, is necessary for the management of patients with refractory CSA or CCHS. Individuals who exhibit symptoms of a Chiari I malformation—a compression of the brain stem and related center of respiratory control—benefit from an immediate neurosurgical evaluation to discuss the possibility of surgical decompression.

7.6. Disorders of Movement

7.6.1. Restless Legs Syndrome and Periodic Limb Movement Disorder

Consensus criteria developed at the National Institutes of Health for the diagnosis of RLS in children use the four essential adult criteria as follows:

(1) An irresistible urge to move the legs or a sensation that compels movement,

(2) Accentuation of these symptoms at rest,

(3) Amelioration of these symptoms with movement or physical stimulation of the legs, and

(4) Increased symptoms in the evening or night.

Children must also express in language appropriate for their age the sensory or captivating leg experience. In lieu of this requirement, a child may demonstrate one or more other secondary criteria, including:

(1) Sleep disturbance,

(2) Excessive periodic leg movements (PLM) on PSG, or

(3) A family history of RLS.

Owing to the subjective character of this syndrome and the stricter pediatric criteria, supporting data from the more objective secondary criteria is frequently needed for a diagnosis. According to recent epidemiologic studies, RLS affects 10% of the adult US population and is linked to depression and hypertension. Picchietti and Winkelman recently used a combined US and European sample to show a prevalence of 1% to 2% using the National Institutes of Health consensus criteria for RLS in children. Two types of RLS are identified by epidemiologic and genetic linkage studies: primary RLS, which manifests early, and secondary RLS, which manifests late. The early-onset form is more common in females (2:1), usually starts in childhood or young adulthood, develops slowly, is inherited in an autosomal dominant manner, exhibits genetic anticipation, and has been linked to at least two distinct human genetic loci (12q and 14q). In this form, PLMs are assumed to be more prevalent. According to prevalence studies, the prevalence of RLS rises with age, from 3% in adults 30 years of age and 20% in adults 80 years of age.

In contrast to RLS, periodic limb movement disorder (PLMD) only causes an increase in PLMs above five per hour of sleep on PSG testing (in children); it does not exhibit any other RLS symptoms. In the general population, PLMs are more common than RLSs, and they are known to get worse with age. It is arguable how PLMs affect behavior during the day and while sleeping. Although EEG arousals linked to PLMs are observed and may be a factor in sleep disturbance and dysfunction during the day, there is currently insufficient evidence to conclusively support this theory in either adult or pediatric populations. Case studies show that PLMs are linked to SDB and ADHD in kids in addition to a distinct relationship with RLS.

ADHD and iron deficiency are two common medical disorders in children with RLS. According to a cross-sectional questionnaire study conducted on 866 children aged 2 to 14 in a general pediatric clinic, symptoms of PLM and RLS are linked to high scores for hyperactivity and inattention. According to a review of the literature, up to 26% of children with RLS and up to 44% of children with ADHD also experience symptoms related to RLS. Dopamine may be the neurotransmitter that these two child groups have in common. The bilateral A11 cell group of the dorsal posterior hypothalamus is the source of the spinal cord's dopaminergic innervation. The clinical manifestations of primary RLS may be caused by a relative deficiency of A11 dopaminergic activity, according to current models. Research on both humans and animals has linked dopamine hypofunction to the genesis of ADHD. Although hypothalamic dopamine systems are not linked to RLS, frontal lobe dopamine systems are known to influence behaviors in ADHD. Additional research on humans and animals is required to describe the neural systems underlying these two unique disorders.

Even in the absence of concomitant anemia, iron deficiency is linked to a heightened occurrence of RLS symptoms in adults. Adult RLS patients have been shown to have deficiencies in brain iron content or metabolism through postmortem neuropathologic procedures, CSF analysis, and MRI. Serum iron and ferritin levels in a study of 39 kids with periodic limb movements during sleep (PLMS) showed a relative lack of body iron stores. PLMs per hour were higher in children with serum iron concentrations below 50 mg/dL than in those with levels above 50 mg/dL. Following a three-month course of oral iron sulfate treatment, PLMs per hour significantly decreased in 76% (n = 19) of the children whose serum iron concentration was less than 50 mg/dL. It is believed that there is a connection between RLS/ PLMS symptoms and iron deficiency because iron functions as a cofactor in the brain during dopamine transport. The function of dopamine transport is significantly diminished in animal models of iron deficiency. Additionally, tyrosine hydroxylase, which is necessary for the synthesis of dopamine, is activated by iron. Currently, studies on humans are being conducted to find genetic targets in adults and children that could lead to particular RLS phenotypes, like RLS associated with iron deficiency.

7.6.1.1. Diagnosis

These days, the four primary features and the three secondary features listed above are used to diagnose RLS. Specifically, a family history of RLS and the use of one night of PSG or multiple nights of home ambulatory accelerometer measures (actigraphy or actometry) to demonstrate PLMs may be beneficial. When complaints of sleep disturbance or daytime fatigue are present, the diagnosis of PLMD is typically established based on PSG evidence of five or more PLMs per hour of sleep. Accelerometry is another method that is employed, and it has the benefit of providing a more comprehensive description of PLM variability, along with any connections to medications, daytime activities, and sleep deprivation over multiple nights in the home. In the appropriate clinical setting, serum testing for concomitant diseases or causes such as low ferritin, hypothyroidism, B12 deficiency, anemia, uremia, and diabetes is recommended. Children diagnosed with an ADHD subtype may exhibit suggestive symptoms like "growing pains" or insomnia. When considering these diagnoses, it is important to keep in mind that caffeine, sleep deprivation, and certain antidepressants can exacerbate the symptoms of RLS and PLMD.

7.6.1.2. Treatment

The current treatments for PLMD and RLS in children are comparable to those for adults. Dopamine agonists are the most specialized treatment option, even though no clinical trials have been conducted to examine their safety or effectiveness in pediatric patients. Therapy should include maintaining regular sleep and wake times, supplementing for vitamin or iron deficiency, and avoiding substances that worsen RLS symptoms. Other drugs that treat dopaminergic neuropathy include gabapentin, clonazepam, opioids, and other medications.

7.6.2. Sleep-Related Rhythmic Movement Disorder

A portion of children's REM sleep, which often lasts into light non-REM sleep, is characterized by rhythmic movements or rocking of the arms, hands, trunk, or head. The head banging, body rocking, or other behavior can be anything from a harmless self-soothing habit to a dangerous and violent issue (such as jactatio capitis nocturna). Usually starting before the age of three, rhythmic movements seem to diminish as stage 2 sleep takes hold. Movements also occur during REM sleep in a subgroup of children and adolescents with rhythmic movement disorder (RMD), indicating the possibility of an independent neural mechanism. ADHD and less common neurologic conditions like Tourette syndrome, autism, Rett syndrome, and Angelman syndrome are noted to be present in many children with RMD.

The results of the sleep history and the rule out of other conditions like dystonia, nocturnal seizures, behavioral issues, and parasomnias like confusional arousals are used to make the diagnosis of RMD. Other methods to distinguish between these entities include routine EEG testing and overnight video PSG with additional EEG leads. Furthermore, since certain antidepressants, antihistamines, antiemetics, and neuroleptic agents can cause excessive movement before or during sleep, it is important to rule out the possibility of medication side effects. Treatment for RMD includes (1) maintaining a regular sleep and wake schedule to avoid sleep loss, (2) addressing safety concerns if violent movements occur, and (3) considering medication to help reduce the intensity of RMD in some cases. One way to be safe is to place the mattress on the floor, away from any walls or hard objects that could hurt someone. Another way to be safe is to wear a helmet if someone is severely beating their head. There are case reports of several RMD treatments, such as clonazepam, relaxation methods, and consolation. Parents may find RMD strange and unsettling, but children are generally fine with the movement and even enjoy the self-soothing aspects of the activity (Allen et al., 2000; Allen et al., 2001; Allen et al., 2003; Blunden et al., 2005).

7.7. Hypersomnia: Disorders of Arousal

7.7.1. Narcolepsy with Cataplexy

7.7.1.1. Diagnosis

For specific clinical details regarding hypersomnia and narcolepsy, refer to that chapter. It is common for narcolepsy to be identified for the first time in childhood and adolescence; research indicates that the condition has two incidence peaks, at ages 14.7 and 35. A family history of narcolepsy and a younger onset age are linked to more severe symptoms, which include cataplexy and excessive daytime sleepiness. The two main clinical signs of narcolepsy are cataplexy and excessive daytime somnolence. Narcolepsy with and without cataplexy are the two diagnoses for narcolepsy that happens without provocation (which can happen following physical or medical trauma to particular subcortical structures). A small or large group of muscles can suddenly lose their tone or strength in response to emotional situations, a condition known as cataplexy. Cataplexy is a symptom that about 60% of narcoleptics experience, although it is uncommon in children. For children, isolated hypersomnolence is the most common presentation of narcolepsy, with or without cataplexy. A structured interview-based study including 157 narcoleptics and 164 controls showed that daytime sleepiness was the initial symptom in 65.5% of cases and that over 50% of narcoleptics report symptom onset before the age of 20. Large surveys of individuals with narcolepsy actually show an average 10.5-year delay in diagnosis following the onset of symptoms. Making this diagnosis therefore depends on identifying additional clinical symptoms that excessively sleepy narcoleptic children may display.

When cataplexy is not yet evident, other signs of hypothalamic dysfunction in children with narcolepsy have been observed and may aid in the diagnosis. The BMI of narcoleptic children is found to be significantly higher than that of controls in a small case-control series involving children with and without narcolepsy. Medication or any other factor that could have been included in the analysis was not the cause of this increase. Therefore, early-onset narcolepsy and modifications in metabolic regulation mediated by the hypothalamus may indicate a more widespread hypothalamic dysfunction in narcoleptic children.

When compared to controls, narcolepsy patients report significantly more issues with depression, cognitive impairments, and difficulties focusing their attention. Narcolepsy-related behavioral and emotional abnormalities can make children and teenagers with the disease seem to have psychiatric problems. Just 20% of the 51 children with narcolepsy (mean age of 7:09 years) in this small descriptive study displayed cataplexy, but every child showed signs of depression related to their illness. This emphasizes how crucial it is to rule out narcolepsy in children who appear melancholy, drowsy, or "lazy."

7.7.1.2. Testing

Although the clinical diagnosis of narcolepsy in children can be difficult, clinical findings can be supported by PSG testing in conjunction with the MSLT. When put through PSG testing, adults with narcolepsy show a reduction in REM latency from sleep onset (typically less than 60 minutes) as well as fragmentation of sleep structure. REM latencies of 50 to 60 minutes are common in children under the age of eight, and adult latencies of 80 to 120 minutes may not develop until late childhood or early adolescence. In clinical settings, polysomnograms (PSGs) can help rule out other sleep-related conditions like PLMD or apnea even though they rarely provide conclusive evidence of REM sleep dysregulation.

However, MSLT testing might be just as helpful for diagnosing conditions in kids as it is in adults. Traditionally, MSLT examinations have been limited to kids eight years of age and up. A decrease in mean sleep latency over four or five tests and the occurrence of REM sleep during two or more naps are two characteristics of MSLT results that are consistent with narcolepsy. It has been observed that younger narcoleptics have a lower mean sleep latency than older subjects. This result contradicts reports that children who do not have narcolepsy have longer mean sleep latencies than do adolescents and adults. Because of this, a child's modest decrease in mean sleep latency may have far greater implications than it would for an adolescent or adult. The measurement of naps that involve REM sleep is another helpful feature of the MSLT. It is believed that two or more REM naps in an MSLT are indicative of adult narcolepsy. It has been observed that younger narcoleptics experience more REM sleep naps on MSLTs than older narcoleptics. Therefore, REM sleep dysregulation testing with MSLT may be even more useful in diagnosing narcolepsy in children than in adults.

Testing for the human leukocyte antigen (HLA) may occasionally be used to help diagnose childhood narcolepsy. While no single HLA marker has been found to be specifically associated with childhood narcolepsy, 88–98% of subjects with narcolepsy who also have cataplexy show a strong association with HLA DQB1-0602. The clinical usefulness of this test for narcolepsy detection is unfortunately limited because estimates indicate that up to 99% of individuals with this HLA marker do not have narcolepsy. Given the high false-positive rate, it seems possible that this type of testing could help identify people who do not have a genetic propensity for narcolepsy and cataplexy. A negative test can raise doubts about the diagnosis of narcolepsy with cataplexy in the diagnostic workup of children, who frequently do not exhibit it. This is because a negative test would raise the possibility of an increased genetic (HLA-associated) component in this population. Of course, pediatric narcolepsy may also be caused by additional hereditary factors that have not yet been identified with the apparent apoptotic loss of hypocretin neurons in the posterior lateral hypothalamus.

Children with cataplexy and narcolepsy are reported to have very low to undetectable levels of hypocretin-1 in CSF, similar to adult cases. This finding is linked to HLA DR2 in children, and since very few other neurologic disorders show low levels of CSF hypocretin-1, it may help confirm narcolepsy.

7.7.1.3. Therapy

The symptomatic relief sought in adult narcolepsy is comparable to the treatment for childhood narcolepsy. Amphetamine-based drugs and modafinil are examples of stimulants that are first-line treatments for excessive daytime sleepiness. When there is cataplexy or other severe REM dysregulatory behaviors (hypnagogic or hypnopompic hallucinations, sleep paralysis), REM-suppressant drugs like selective serotonin reuptake inhibitors and TCAs are also usual. Research on modafinil in adults with narcolepsy has shown safety and effectiveness for excessive daytime sleepiness; however, small case series have only shown modest efficacy and safety in children.

In children with narcolepsy, REM-suppressant drugs have not been investigated. Children with severe narcolepsy with cataplexy showed a significant reduction in both excessive daytime sleepiness and the frequency and intensity of cataplexy, according to a recent small, uncontrolled, open-label study using sodium oxybate (approved for use in adult narcolepsy with cataplexy). Suicidal ideation, dissociative episodes, tremor, and constipation were among the side effects; however, more research is required to accurately determine safety precautions for children.

Hypocretin replacement therapy and reversing the presumed autoimmune process that is believed to be destroying hypocretin neurons in the hypothalamus are potential future treatments for narcolepsy. An 8-year-old boy with a documented hypocretin deficiency and a quick onset of symptoms (less than two months) did not respond to immune-suppressant therapy, and the disease did not progress as expected. Three adult patients with rapid-onset narcolepsy who also had cataplexy showed a significant and long-lasting (7 months) reduction in the frequency and intensity of cataplexy after receiving IV immunoglobulin therapy. In animal models of narcolepsy, intrathecal hypocretin infusion has been used to treat the underlying hypocretin deficiency with encouraging outcomes. Humans have not yet attempted this.

7.7.2. Idiopathic Hypersomnolence

In both children and adults, excessive diurnal somnolence without indications of REM dysregulation has a wide differential diagnosis. Psychiatric issues, medical conditions, and sleep disturbances can all contribute to excessive somnolence during the day. In certain instances, screening, and testing for these additional disorders may not show any clear cause. Idiopathic hypersomnolence (IH) is the diagnosis made for patients whose excessive daytime somnolence has no apparent cause.

Identification of narcolepsy without cataplexy, delayed sleep-phase syndrome, mild SDB, and depression are important because IH is diagnosed by a process of exclusion and has few characteristic features. Individuals with IH frequently report regular, long-lasting sleep, but they also consistently exhibit excessive somnolence during the day, both subjectively and objectively. PSG readings typically show long-term, very effective sleep without any obvious anomalies. Because a significant percentage of familial cases are reported, reports point to a genetic component of IH. There are no CSF hypocretin-1 deficiencies in IH patients, and the scant research on this uncommon illness has not revealed a particular diagnostic procedure.

Medications used to treat narcolepsy include stimulant medications. It is common to observe a lack of response to therapy, and managing symptoms with medicine can be challenging. There haven't been any non-medical or medical treatment trials carried out on patient populations with IH.

7.7.3. Kleine-Levin Syndrome

Clinically, Kleine-Levin syndrome (KLS) is a rare form of recurrent hypersomnolence characterized by discrete, recurrent episodes of excessive sleep and sleepiness, eating disturbances, and cognitive changes. A recent large-scale systematic review of the literature suggests that the age of onset is between 16 and 17 years old, with a median of 15 years. The mean is 16 points 9 plus or minus 8 points 5 years. In total, 81% of KLS cases began in the second decade; the male to female ratio was 2:1, and there may have been a predisposition among Jews. The average duration of a hypersomnolence episode is approximately 12 plus or minus 9 days, and the average interepisode interval is 6 +/- 10 months. The review found that the average number of episodes was 12 plus or minus 15 and that the majority of KLS patients had their recurrent symptoms stop within 4 years on average. KLS was found to last a median of 8 years from the onset of symptoms using Kaplan-Meier analysis. Additionally, transient symptoms of compulsive behaviors (29%), depression (48%), and hypersexual behaviors (43%) may be present during episodes of hypersomnolence. Although female subjects exhibit more severe and prolonged courses than males, male subjects are more frequently observed to exhibit these symptoms.

In between episodes, neurologic testing, brain imaging, and serum and CSF analysis of immune, endocrine, and metabolic processes show that 96% of KLS patients are completely normal.

During episodes, studies demonstrate variable findings including:

(1) PSG evidence of decreased sleep efficiency, diffuse slowing of EEG activity, and increased cortical delta and theta activity;

(2) increased REM episodes during MSLT testing;

(3) autonomic dysfunction;

(4) cerebral hypoperfusion in diencephalic regions, especially the thalamus; and

(5) diminished hypothalamic responses to thyroid-releasing hormone and reduced hypoglycemic stimulation of cortisol and adrenocorticotropic hormone.

Although 98% of KLS cases are sporadic, a genetic predisposition with a potential autoimmune trigger is suspected because European KLS patients have an association with the HLA subtype DQBI*02, and 43% of cases have an overall incidence of a predisposing infection or fever.

Treatment studies for KLS are limited to open-label trials, which infrequently employ case controls due to the disorder's rarity. Numerous treatments, including insulin coma, electroconvulsive therapy, and symptomatic use of neuroleptics, amphetamines, and antiepileptics, have not shown any discernible advantages. The only treatment that has been shown to produce unquestionable results is the use of the mood stabilizer lithium. Weighing the advantages of ongoing lithium therapy against the risks and need for frequent monitoring that come with this drug is necessary (Allen et al., 2000; Allen et al., 2001; Allen et al., 2003; Blunden et al., 2005).

7.8. Circadian Rhythm Sleep Disorders—Delayed Sleep-Phase Type

Circadian rhythms alter from childhood to adolescence as a result of maturation. As we age, we gradually experience increasingly later wakefulness and sleep onset times. Children entering adolescence have later bedtimes and rise times as a result of this circadian rhythm delay. Children may not feel sleepy until 10:00 PM or 11:00 PM and may not wake up feeling rested until 9:00 AM or 10:00 AM, in contrast to the past when they went to bed at 8:00 PM or 9:00 PM and woke up at 7:00 AM or 8:00 AM. If you have to wake up early for school or other obligations, this could be very troublesome. The term "delayed sleep-phase syndrome" (DSPS) refers to the naturally occurring maturational delay in the sleep phase that is amplified in many teenagers and young adults with a genetic predisposition for eveningness, leading to abnormally late sleep-onset and wake times.

It is estimated that between 5 and 10% of teenagers have DSPS, with puberty being the typical time of onset. Genetic factors that regulate the intrinsic timing of the brain's circadian rhythm generator in the suprachiasmatic nucleus are thought to be the cause of this excessive delay in circadian rhythm, at least in part. The activity of particular intracellular DNA-regulating proteins causes the rhythmic expression of proteins in lengthy feedback loops in the anterior hypothalamus of humans, flies, and many other species. The oscillations produced by these molecular feedback loops are not precisely 24 hours. It takes daily light activation via the retinohypothalamic tract to entrain to a 24-hour period.

By noting that the delay is not brought on by bad sleep hygiene, other sleep disorders (like RLS or primary insomnia), or psychiatric conditions like anxiety and depression, one can distinguish between DSPS and a natural maturational delay. Furthermore, some children's preference for a later wake-up and bedtime is not always indicative of DSPS. Patients with DSPS usually experience normal sleep and no noticeable symptoms during the day when they sleep according to their natural schedule. The distinctive characteristic of DSPS is that sleep and wake timing are changed, but not actual sleep. In addition to complaints of insomnia and excessive daytime sleepiness, a long-standing personal history of delayed sleep phase and additional family history are suggestive of delayed sleep phase syndrome (DSPS). In addition, DSPS is typified by circadian timing delays for numerous biological markers of sleep onset, including temperature nadirs and melatonin production. Up to 50% of people may exhibit a preference for sleep start times between 4:00 AM and midnight and wake up times after 10:00 AM in some families with DSPS. A multifactorial or incomplete penetrant autosomal dominant mode of inheritance can be seen in pedigrees.

Teens with DSPS may have chronic school tardiness, sleep-onset insomnia, daytime sleepiness, depression, and avoidance of school behaviors. They also frequently report feeling best in the evening and at night. According to studies, the average age at which chronic insomnia manifests itself is 11 years old, and 52% of teenagers who experience insomnia symptoms also have comorbid psychiatric disorders. An important preventive measure during adolescence may be to diagnose and treat DSPS as a cause of insomnia and possibly co-occurring mental illnesses. In addition to historical information gleaned from interviews, sleep-wake diaries—with or without actigraphy—may be used to diagnose DSPS to highlight the persistent nature of the issue.

With the goal of phase-advancing the underlying circadian rhythm, behavioral therapy, light therapy, and medication therapy are used to target cues that signal the onset of sleep for individuals with DSPS. DSPS is tenacious, and for the benefits to last over time, a motivated participant must continue therapy. A regular schedule and good sleep hygiene are critical for the effective treatment of DSPS (Allen et al., 2000; Allen et al., 2001; Allen et al., 2003; Blunden et al., 2005).

A Closer Look

Mechanism of Polysomnography

Generally, a polysomnogram will record on at least 12 channels, meaning that the patient will need to have at least 22 wire attachments made. Every lab has different channels, and these can be modified to satisfy the needs of the physician. The EEG has at least three channels; one or two measure airflow; one or two measure chin muscle tone; one or more measure leg movements; two measure eye movements (EOG); one or two measure heart rate and rhythm; one measures oxygen saturation; and one or two measure the movement of the chest and upper abdominal walls through the belts. Usually, respiratory inductance plethysmography or piezoelectric sensors are used to measure the movement of the belts. As the patient inhales and exhales, this movement—which is equivalent to effort—produces a low-frequency sinusoidal waveform.

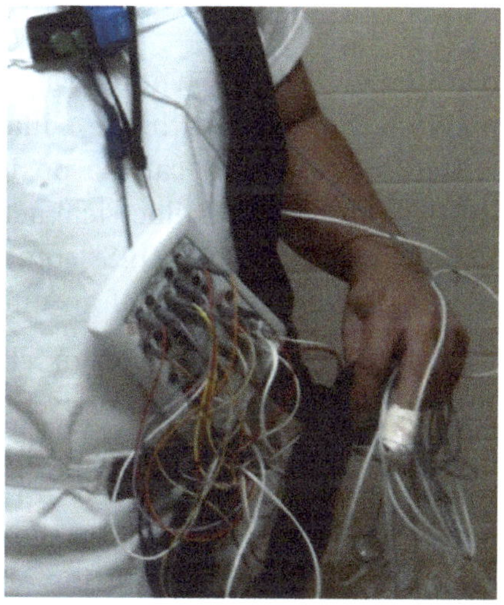

(By Z22 – Own work, CC BY-SA 4.0, https://commons.wikimedia.org/w/index.php?curid=34459662).

Each recorded data channel's wires originate from the patient and come together in a central box. This box is then connected to a computer system that records, stores, and displays the data. The computer monitor can show several channels at once while it is sleeping. Most labs also have a tiny video camera installed so the technician can watch the patient in person from a nearby room.

The electroencephalogram (EEG) will generally use six "exploring" electrodes and two "reference" electrodes unless a seizure disorder is suspected, in which case more electrodes will be applied to document the appearance of seizure activity. The exploring electrodes are usually attached to the scalp near the frontal, central (top) and occipital (back) portions of the brain with a paste that will conduct electrical signals originating from the neurons of the cortex. These electrodes will provide a readout of the brain activity that can be "scored" into different stages of sleep (N_1, N_2, and N_3 - which combined are referred to as NREM sleep - and Stage R, which is rapid eye movement sleep, or REM, and Wakefulness). The EEG electrodes are placed according to the International 10–20 system.

The EOG utilizes two electrodes positioned 1 cm above the outer canthus of the right eye and 1 cm below the outer canthus of the left eye. These electrodes detect eye activity based on the electrical potential difference between the cornea and the retina (where the cornea is positively charged compared to the retina). This information is used to identify the occurrence of REM sleep, characterized by rapid eye movements, and to help determine sleep onset.

Four electrodes are usually used in an electromyogram (EMG) to measure muscle tension in the body and to check for excessive leg movements while sleeping, which could be a sign of periodic limb movement disorder or PLMD. On the chin, one lead is positioned above the jawline and the other below. This aids in determining both the onset and duration of REM sleep, much like the EOG. There is a noticeable reduction in muscle tension during sleep because sleep usually involves relaxation. During REM sleep, skeletal muscle tension further decreases. To act out dreams, a person must become partially paralyzed; however, REM behavior disorder can develop in those without this paralysis. To measure leg movements, two additional leads are finally positioned on each leg's anterior tibialis.

A polysomnogram uses two or three electrodes, whereas an electrocardiogram (ECG or EKG) typically uses 10. They can be positioned one beneath the collarbone and the other six inches above the waist on either side of the body, or they can be positioned under the collarbone on each side of the chest. These electrodes measure the electrical activity of the heart as it contracts and expands, recording such features as the "P" wave, "QRS" complex, and "T" wave. These can be analyzed for any abnormalities that might be indicative of an underlying heart pathology.

Pressure transducers and/or thermocouples placed in or close to the nostrils can be used to measure nasal and oral airflow; the pressure transducer is thought to be the more sensitive. This makes it possible for the doctor or researcher to gauge breathing rate and spot breathing irregularities. Using belts, respiratory effort is also measured in relation to nasal and oral airflow. When breathing is exerted, these belts stretch and contract. On the other hand, false negatives could also result from this respiration technique. When experiencing obstructive apneas, some patients will open and close their mouth. As a result, air is forced into and out of the mouth but stays out of the lungs and airway. Because of this, the respiratory event may be mistakenly diagnosed as a hypopnea—a brief period of reduced airflow—rather than an obstructive apnea by the pressure transducer and thermocouple.

Changes in blood oxygen levels, which frequently accompany sleep apnea and other respiratory issues, can be measured with pulse oximetry. The pulse oximeter is designed to fit over the earlobe or fingertip.

Snoring may be recorded with a sound probe over the neck, though more commonly the sleep technician will just note snoring as "mild," "moderate" or "loud" or give a numerical estimate on a scale of 1 to 10. Also, snoring indicates airflow and can be used during hypopneas to determine whether the hypopnea may be an obstructive apnea.

Summary

- Sleep is an important process that critically impacts health and functioning. Children require good quality sleep that is adequate in duration and timing and free of sleep disturbances.
- Sleep and wake patterns begin at birth as 1- to 3-hour bouts of wake followed by 2- to 5-hour episodes of sleep over a 24-hour period.
- In early infancy, sleep is evenly divided between active (REM-like) sleep and quiet (non-REM) sleep. Indeterminant sleep is a term given to polysomnogram (PSG) activity that appears to have elements of active and quiet sleep. By 6 months, the amount of active/REM sleep declines to 35% to 40% of the total sleep time, and the four definable non-REM sleep stages emerge with regular 40- to 50-minute REM sleep cycles.
- Children have higher upper airway muscle tone compared with adults, which underscores a major difference between the etiologies of sleep-disordered breathing (SDB) in children versus adults.
- During infancy, the heart rate is much higher, even during sleep, and usually falls between 100 and 140 beats per minute.
- When interviewing a child or adolescent about odd behaviors or arousals during sleep, useful information includes the portion of the night most often associated with the problem.
- The PSG is the gold standard for sleep disorders testing and is indicated for diagnosing sleep breathing disorders, many parasomnias, seizures, some movement disorders (such as periodic limb movements), and therapeutic continuous positive airway pressure (CPAP) titrations.
- The most commonly used objective test for excessive daytime sleepiness is the multiple sleep latency test (MSLT). An individual is instructed to lie in a dark, quiet room and try to fall asleep.
- Parasomnias are a collection of sleep-related behaviors that occur during REM and/or non-REM sleep. A common REM parasomnia in childhood is the classic nightmare, which occurs most frequently in the latter half of the night when REM is most prominent.
- Sleep-related bed-wetting, or enuresis, is considered developmentally inappropriate by most authorities after the age of 6 or 7 years.
- Nightmares are common during childhood and are often associated with the development of adaptive fear responses to real-world threats.
- Confusional arousals is a sleep disorder that causes you to act in a very strange and confused way as you wake up or just after waking.
- Current therapies for pediatric RLS and PLMD are similar to those used in adults. While no clinical trials have been completed to investigate safety or efficacy in children, dopamine agonists constitute the most tailored therapeutic alternative.

References

1. Agras, W. S., Hammer, L. D., McNicholas, F., & Kraemer, H. C. (2004). Risk factors for childhood overweight: A prospective study from birth to 9.5 years. *Journal of Pediatrics, 145*(1), 20–25.
2. Alexopoulos, E. I., Kaditis, A. G., Kalampouka, E., et al. (2004). Nasal corticosteroids for children with snoring. *Pediatric Pulmonology, 38*(2), 161–167.
3. Allen, R. P., & Earley, C. J. (2000). Defining the phenotype of the restless legs syndrome (RLS) using age-of-symptom-onset. *Sleep Medicine, 1*(1), 11–19.
4. Allen, R. P., Barker, B. P., Wehrl, F., et al. (2001). MRI measurement of brain iron in patients with restless legs syndrome. *Neurology, 56*(2), 263–265.
5. Allen, R. P., Picchietti, D., Hening, W. A., et al. (2003). Restless legs syndrome: Diagnostic criteria, special considerations, and epidemiology. A report from the restless legs syndrome diagnosis and epidemiology workshop at the National Institutes of Health Sleep Medicine. *Sleep Medicine, 4*(2), 101–119.
6. Ancoli-Israel, S., Schnierow, B., Kelsoe, J., & Fink, R. (2001). A pedigree of one family with delayed sleep phase syndrome. *Chronobiology International, 18*(5), 831–840.
7. Arnulf, I., Zeitzer, J. M., File, J., et al. (2005). Kleine-Levin syndrome: A systematic review of 186 cases in the literature. *Brain, 128*(pt 12), 2763–2776.
8. Baehr, E. K., Revelle, W., Eastman, C. I., et al. (2000). Individual differences in the phase and amplitude of the human circadian temperature rhythm: With an emphasis on morningness-eveningness. *Journal of Sleep Research, 9*(2), 117–127.
9. Baeyens, D., Roeyers, H., D'Haese, L., et al. (2006). The prevalence of ADHD in children with enuresis: Comparison between a tertiary and non-tertiary care sample. *Acta Paediatrica, 95*(3), 347–352.
10. Baeyens, D., Roeyers, H., Demeyer, I., et al. (2005). Attention-deficit/hyperactivity disorder (ADHD) as a risk factor for persistent nocturnal enuresis in children: A two-year follow-up study. *Acta Paediatrica, 94*(11), 1619–1625.
11. Basha, S., Bialowas, C., Ende, K., & Szeremeta, W. (2005). Effectiveness of adenotonsillectomy in the resolution of nocturnal enuresis secondary to obstructive sleep apnea. *Laryngoscope, 115*(6), 1101–1103.
12. Bediwy, A. S., El-Mitwalli, A., Zaher, A. A., Belal, T., & Saleh, A. B. M. (2014). Sleep apnea in children with refractory monosymptomatic nocturnal enuresis. *Nature and Science of Sleep*, 6, 37–42.
13. Beebe, D. W., & Gozal, D. (2002). Obstructive sleep apnea and the prefrontal cortex: Towards a comprehensive model linking nocturnal upper airway obstruction to daytime cognitive and behavioral deficits. *Journal of Sleep Research, 11*(1), 1–16.
14. Berger, K., von Eckardstein, A., Trenkwalder, C., et al. (2002). Iron metabolism and the risk factors of restless legs syndrome in an elderly general population—The MEMO-study. *Journal of Neurology, 249*(9), 1195–1199.
15. Blunden, S., Lushington, K., Lorenzen, B., et al. (2005). Neuropsychological and psychosocial function in children with a history of snoring or behavioral sleep problems. *Journal of Pediatrics, 146*(6), 780–786.

16. Bushby, K., Finkel, R., Birnkrant, D. J., et al. (2010). Diagnosis and management of Duchenne muscular dystrophy, part 2: Implementation of multidisciplinary care. *The Lancet Neurology, 9*(2), 177–189.

17. Chervin, R. D., Archbold, K. H., Dillon, J. E., Pituch, K. J., et al. (2002). Associations between symptoms of inattention, hyperactivity, restless legs, and periodic leg movements. *Sleep, 25*(2), 213–218.

18. Chervin, R. D., Hedger, K., Dillon, J. E., & Pituch, K. J. (2000). Pediatric sleep questionnaire (PSQ): Validity and reliability of scales for sleep-disordered breathing, snoring, sleepiness, and behavioral problems. *Sleep Medicine, 1*(1), 21–32.

19. Chervin, R. D., Ruzicka, D. L., Giordani, B. J., et al. (2006a). Sleep-disordered breathing, behavior, and cognition in children before and after adenotonsillectomy. *Pediatrics, 117*(4), e769–778.

20. Chervin, R. D., Weatherly, R. A., Ruzicka, D. L., et al. (2006b). Subjective sleepiness and polysomnographic correlates in children scheduled for adenotonsillectomy vs other surgical care. *Sleep, 29*(4), 495–503.

21. Connor, J. R., Boyer, P. J., Menzies, S. L., et al. (2003). Neuropathological examination suggests impaired brain iron acquisition in restless legs syndrome. *Neurology, 61*(3), 304–309.

22. Dauvilliers, Y., Carlander, B., Rivier, F., et al. (2004a). Successful management of cataplexy with intravenous immunoglobulins at narcolepsy onset. *Annals of Neurology, 56*(6), 905–908.

23. Decker, M. J., Hue, G. E., Caudle, W. M., et al. (2003). Episodic neonatal hypoxia evokes executive dysfunction and regionally specific alterations in markers of dopamine signaling. *Neuroscience, 117*(2), 417–425.

24. Decker, M. J., Jones, K. A., Solomon, I. G., et al. (2005). Reduced extracellular dopamine and increased responsiveness to novelty: Neurochemical and behavioral sequelae of intermittent hypoxia. *Sleep, 28*(2), 169–176.

25. Spilsbury, J. C., Storfer-Isser, A., Kirchner, H. L., et al. (2006). Neighborhood disadvantage as a risk factor for pediatric obstructive sleep apnea. *The Journal of Pediatrics, 149*(3), 342–347.

Chapter 8

GENETIC DISORDERS

Contents

Introduction

The significance of genomic medicine is growing in all medical fields, including pediatric pulmonology. In the pediatric pulmonary clinic, lung manifestations are often complex in nature and can be linked to certain genetic conditions. Phenotypes such as neonatal respiratory distress, interstitial lung disease, bronchiectasis, pulmonary fibrosis, vascular abnormalities, and pneumothorax have a strong genetic component, necessitating a genetic differential diagnosis in these patients.

Orientation and Directional Terms

Term	Definition	Illustration
Cystic fibrosis	Cystic fibrosis is a genetic disorder. A child who has cystic fibrosis has received a mutated cystic fibrosis transmembrane conductance regulator (CFTR) gene from both parents.	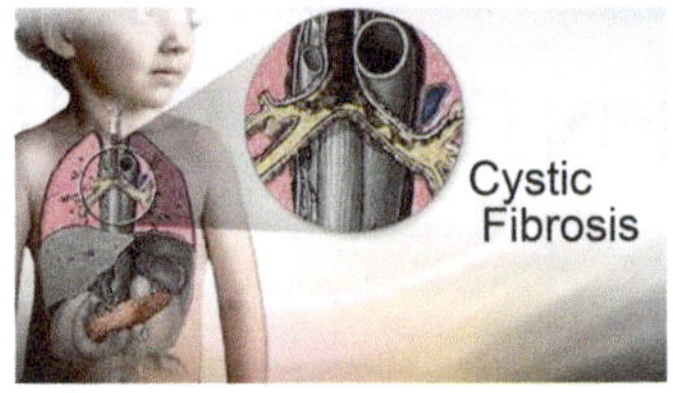
Bronchopulmonary Dysplasia (BPD)	Bronchopulmonary dysplasia (BPD), sometimes called chronic lung disease, is a problem with how a baby's lung tissue develops.	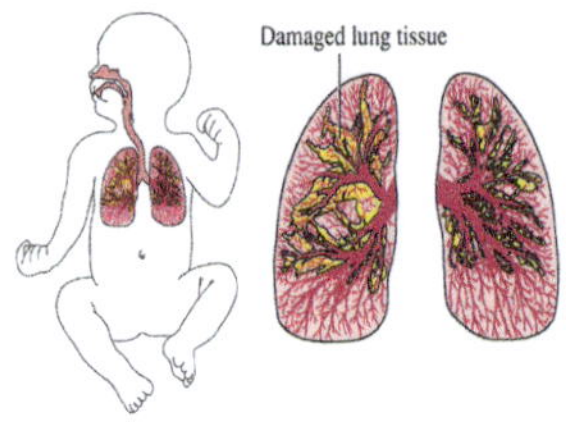
Asthma	Recurrent episodes of coughing, wheezing, chest tightness and trouble breathing, often triggered by infections and allergies in children.	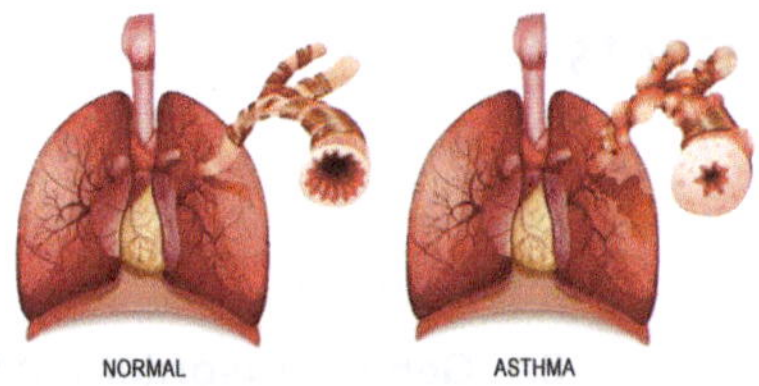
Primary Ciliary Dyskinesia	A rare genetic disorder that affects the function of cilia, the tiny structures that line the airways, ears, sinuses, and other organs, leading to frequent respiratory infections.	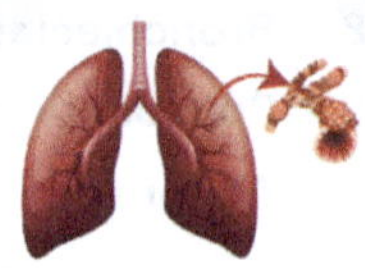

8.1. Genetic Disorders of Neonatal Respiratory Function

In the United States, the most common respiratory cause of death and morbidity for children under one year of age is respiratory distress syndrome in newborns. Additionally, it predicts a child's risk of developing chronic lung diseases. Asthma and bronchopulmonary dysplasia survivors of respiratory distress syndrome spend 20 times more annualized dollars ($19,104 versus $955) and 5.9% of all money spent on children under the age of 18 years. Respiratory distress syndrome has most frequently been linked to the developmental immaturity of pulmonary surfactant production since the initial description of surfactant deficiency. Type II pneumocytes that line the distal airways synthesize, package, and secrete a mixture of proteins and phospholipids known as pulmonary surfactant. At the air-liquid interface, this mixture creates a monolayer that reduces surface tension during respiratory cycle expiration, preventing atelectasis and ventilation-perfusion mismatch. The availability of surfactant replacement therapy has been linked to a decrease in respiratory distress syndrome mortality among premature infants over the past 10 years.

Despite advancements in neonatal survival rates, a notable percentage (5–25%) of infants continue to experience long-term respiratory issues and even mortality. Pulmonary problems are often linked to factors like oxygen toxicity, barotrauma, underdevelopment, and nutritional deficiencies. However, research suggests that genetic factors also play a role in determining respiratory outcomes. Family history, ethnicity, and inherited surfactant protein B deficiency are all indicators of genetic risk for respiratory distress in infants. Unlike respiratory issues caused by environmental factors, genetic disorders can lead to both acute and chronic respiratory failure. Identifying genetic markers associated with respiratory distress could help develop preventative and therapeutic measures to mitigate the high medical and economic costs associated with these conditions. Variations in surfactant protein genes and other extrapulmonary genes have shown promise in identifying individuals at risk for respiratory issues. There are two main groups of genetic markers: those linked to respiratory distress risk and those causing surfactant function loss.

8.1.1. Surfactant Protein A

Three genes make up the human surfactant protein A locus: SP-A1, SP-A2, and a pseudogene. Four coding exons are present in each of the two functional genes, which regulate the synthesis of two different primary translation products. One ($1A^0$) of the more than 15 SP-A2 gene alleles that have been found so far has recently been found to occur much more frequently in unrelated premature white infants who are over 28 weeks gestation and experiencing respiratory distress. Low levels of surfactant protein A transcript have also been linked to this allele in human lung tissue from unrelated people. In a recent study, distinct surfactant protein A alleles were associated with both susceptibility and protective effects in 88 infants with respiratory distress syndrome and 88 control subjects from the genetically homogeneous Finnish population.

Surfactant protein A, along with surfactant protein D, mannose-binding protein, and conglutinin, is a member of the collectin subgroup of mammalian C-type lectins. Research suggests that low levels of surfactant protein A may increase the risk of respiratory distress and infection in humans. However, no infants lacking surfactant protein A have been found, and the effects of certain genetic variations, such as the SP-A2 $1A^0$ allele, on respiratory health are still not fully understood. The complexity of how surfactant protein A impacts respiratory distress and infection risk in infants means that current knowledge of its genetic contributions is promising but not yet useful for predicting individual risk.

8.1.2. Surfactant Protein B

Unlike surfactant protein A, disruption of surfactant protein B expression results in a clear respiratory issue in newborns. The surfactant protein B gene has been fully sequenced and its regulatory regions studied. The gene is around 10 kilobases long with 11 exons. These exons produce a 2-kilobase transcript that codes for a 381-amino acid preproprotein, which is modified before becoming part of pulmonary surfactant. The mature 8-kilodalton protein is the result of exons 6 and 7. Mutations and single nucleotide polymorphisms can be found throughout the surfactant protein B gene (Figure 8.1).

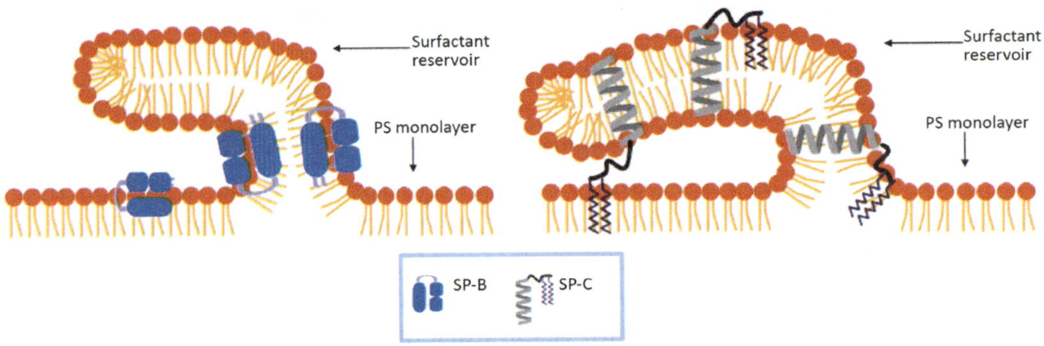

Figure 8.1. *Representation of the squeeze-out and folding of the pulmonary surfactant monolayer into a multilayered surfactant reservoir during expiration-induced compression, including proteins SP-B and SP-C.*

Source: *Dziura M, Mansour B, DiPasquale M, Chandrasekera PC, Gauld JW, Marquardt D. Simulated Breathing: Application of Molecular Dynamics Simulations to Pulmonary Lung Surfactant. Symmetry. 2021; 13(7):1259. https://doi.org/10.3390/sym13071259.*

The first documented genetic cause of infantile respiratory distress syndrome was a deficiency of surfactant protein B. The mutation that caused the affected infants in the first type involved a 3-bp insertion and a 1-bp deletion at codon 121 in exon 4 of the surfactant protein B gene (121ins2). This mutation causes a frameshift and an early translation stop signal at codon 214, which explains why tracheal effluent and immunohistochemical staining both show no protein. Using the nuclei from the lungs of the affected infants, nuclear run-on assays reveal that although the mutated gene is transcribed normally, the transcript is unstable. The mutation makes a new *Sfu* I restriction site, which makes it easier to identify it quickly. Additionally, affected infants with genetically engineered abrogation of surfactant protein B synthesis have been shown to exhibit pro-surfactant protein C peptides with aberrant mobility on SDS-PAGE and with increased abundance by immunohistochemical staining and Western blot analysis. The altered mobility of pro-surfactant protein C is most likely due to abnormal processing. It is unknown what mechanism leads to enhanced accumulation. When a baby is homozygous for this mutation, the clinical phenotype is consistent: full-term babies experience respiratory distress in the first 12 to 24 hours of life and pass away in the first 1–6 months of life if they do not receive a lung transplant. This result is not reversible with surfactant replacement therapy, corticosteroid treatment, or mechanical ventilator support. Lung transplants are the only available treatment for these infants. These family studies suggested that infants with irreversible respiratory distress syndrome are caused by a loss-of-function mutation in a single gene. Correlating biochemical and clinical phenotype with genotype requires investigations involving animals, humans, and populations in order to make this genetic marker applicable for individual risk assessment.

According to genetic and biochemical research on compound heterozygote infants and adults with targeted disruption of the surfactant protein B gene, about half of the normal synthesis of surfactant protein B may be enough for normal pulmonary function at birth. It is unknown how much surfactant protein B must be produced at a minimum for human lung function and surfactant metabolism to be normal. Due to various loss-of-function mutations on each chromosome, the newborn produced only 8–10% of the normal amount of surfactant protein B, resulting in both acute and chronic respiratory distress from birth and respiratory death at 9–5 months of age. A homozygous mutation in exon 5 (479G T) resulting in an alternative donor splice site and decreased surfactant protein B caused long-term respiratory distress in two other unrelated children. One of them needed a lung transplant, while the other suffered from chronic respiratory insufficiency.

Population-based studies assessing genotype-phenotype correlation were required to ascertain whether microsatellite markers would help predict the genetic risk of respiratory distress. Among the 1260 individuals analyzed, polymorphic tandem-repeat sequences in intron 4 and intergenic microsatellite markers have been associated with a risk of respiratory distress. However, the use of these markers in clinical practice or parental counseling has been hampered by small control populations.

In two sizable population-based cohorts, we employed clinical and molecular ascertainment techniques to ascertain the frequency of the 121ins2 mutation. By using molecular ascertainment, we discovered one 121ins2 allele for every 3300 individuals from a New York cohort, and by using clinical ascertainment, we discovered one 121ins2 allele for every 1000 individuals from a Missouri cohort. Parents of fetuses or infants homozygous for the 121ins2 mutation can receive clear counseling regarding the course of the disease, prognosis, and available treatments due to the mutation's uncommon population frequency, homozygous infants' consistent phenotype, and the lack of biologic redundancy for surfactant protein B function. The 121ins2 mutation, which was present on about 60% of chromosomes, was the most commonly discovered mutation in a cohort of infants with hereditary surfactant protein B deficiency. In the surfactant protein B gene, we, and other researchers have found 27 mutations or single-nucleotide polymorphisms. Some loss-of-function mutations seem to be familial in nature and cause respiratory distress, though they can also cause respiratory failure that progresses more gradually. These results enable the prediction of respiratory distress, either acute or chronic, in infants with any loss-of-function mutations on both alleles.

8.1.3. Surfactant Protein C

Hydrophobic surfactant protein C is produced by proteolytic cleavage from a precursor consisting of 191 or 197 amino acids, contingent on the primary transcript's differential splicing. Remarkably, pro-surfactant protein C has hydrophobic domains but lacks an N-terminal signal peptide. Mature surfactant protein C is present in both lamellar bodies and airways, and it has 35 amino acid residues.

Furthermore, no known human respiratory illness that affects newborns and is brought on by mutations that cause the surfactant protein C gene to lose its function has been found. A recent report, however, details a family that developed chronic interstitial lung disease in members of the affected family due to a splice site mutation at the first base of intron 4 of the surfactant protein C gene. The inheritance pattern of this family is autosomal dominant. According to this report and the surfactant protein C knockout lineage results, chronic respiratory disease rather than acute respiratory distress syndrome of infancy is caused by genetic variation in the surfactant protein C gene.

8.1.4. Surfactant Protein D

Surfactant protein D is expressed in extrapulmonary tissues and belongs to the collectin family. One of its roles is to recognize the carbohydrate domain on the surface of pathogens. At birth, there are no respiratory abnormalities in mouse lineages where the surfactant protein D gene has been specifically ablationed. During the first eight weeks of life, there was a progressive extracellular accumulation of surfactant lipids and surfactant proteins A and B, as well as activation of alveolar macrophages and peribronchiolar-perivascular inflammation and the development of emphysema. There has never been a human baby or elderly person found to have respiratory distress and a mutation in the surfactant protein D gene. Surfactant protein D's genomic and cDNA sequences differ, but there hasn't been much research done on the genetic variation in humans for this gene. There are two known biallelic polymorphisms in the surfactant protein D gene. A change in an amino acid in this region may have a greater effect on function because the amino-terminal region plays a crucial role in the multimerization of dodecamers that are essential for many of the functions of surfactant protein D. Further research is necessary to determine how sequence variants in the surfactant protein D gene contribute to respiratory distress syndrome in infants.

8.1.5. Extrapulmonary Gene Products

Pulmonary alveolar proteinosis was caused by targeted disruption of the genes encoding granulocyte-macrophage colony-stimulating factor (GM-CSF/IL-3/IL-5 receptor common β-chain) or its receptor. These findings illustrated the critical role extrapulmonary gene products play in the synthesis and functionality of surfactants. Later, it was discovered that patients with acquired alveolar proteinosis were either negative for the GM-CSF/IL-3/IL-5 receptor common β-chain or had neutralizing antibodies of the IgG isotype against the colony-stimulating factor of granulocyte-macrophage in bronchoalveolar lavage. When granulocyte-macrophage colony-stimulating factor or its receptor expression is disrupted and surfactant homeostasis is restored, either by aerosolizing the granulocyte-macrophage colony-stimulating factor or by transplanting wild-type bone marrow cells into the bone marrow, new approaches to treating respiratory distress syndrome in infants are suggested. Nevertheless, to allow the use of these genetic markers for individual family counseling, studies of newborns and informative kindreds, genotype-phenotype studies, and population studies have not yet been carried out.

The identification of infants homozygous for the 121ins2 mutation in the surfactant protein B gene, whether antenatally or postnatally, enables clear counseling regarding the infants' lethal prognosis and available treatment options. Identification of mutations in this gene that cause loss of function allows for reliable prediction of the development of acute or chronic respiratory distress. Genetic testing for these mutations should be considered if there is a family history of neonatal or infant mortality due to unexplained respiratory distress. To estimate the contribution of mutations in surfactant protein genes and extrapulmonary genes to the incidence of respiratory distress syndrome and subsequent pulmonary disease, more population-based analyses of genotype-phenotype correlations are needed. These analyses should address both respiratory distress in the neonatal period and long-term respiratory morbidity. For instance, the frequencies of mutations leading to decreased production of surfactant protein B have not been evaluated, even though the 121ins2 mutation is rare in the general population. Such frequency estimation is feasible through molecular amplification and high-throughput analysis techniques, which allow identification of genetic variation in DNA samples from large populations without sequencing the DNA of each individual.

Because of factors like ethnic stratification, environmental selection, or genotype-phenotype heterogeneity, population-based studies are essential to preventing the overestimation or underestimation of the contribution of particular mutations or polymorphisms to respiratory distress syndrome in infants. DNA samples can be anonymously linked to databases of birth and infant death certificates that have clinical data or enough identifiers to assess respiratory phenotype. These databases are made available through ongoing state programs for the detection of inherited diseases. Once found, these mutations will make it possible to create more sensible treatment plans for hereditary lung diseases of infancy and to provide families whose children are genetically predisposed to respiratory distress at birth or in early childhood with more accurate counseling (Whitsett et al., 2015; Griese, 2017; Liszewski et al., 2017; Goetz and Ren, 2019).

8.2. Acute Respiratory Distress

Preterm infants are expected to experience acute respiratory distress during the neonatal period, which is characterized by hypoxemia and retractions, because of immature lung development. However, surfactant deficiency or dysfunction should be taken into consideration if these signs and symptoms occur in a full-term infant, or if they do so to a greater extent than would be expected from prematurity alone. Disorders characterized by surfactant dysfunction arise due to irregular synthesis or transportation of the proteins and phospholipids that make up the pulmonary surfactant complex. Alveolar type II epithelial cells produce surfactant before birth, which is necessary to lower the surface tension in the alveolar space. Hypoxemia and hypercapnia are caused by alveolar collapse and inadequate gas exchange, which are brought on by abnormal surfactant quantity or quality. Signs of respiratory distress are frequently seen in infants with surfactant dysfunction, which can result in respiratory failure in the newborn nursery.

Neonatals can sometimes be healthy enough to be sent home after delivery, but they still exhibit retractions, persistent tachypnea, and poor growth. These babies frequently have crackles on examination and are hypoxemic. In less severe cases, symptoms may gradually appear over time, sometimes even into adulthood. Dyspnea and exercise intolerance, along with related digital clubbing, are symptoms. It is possible that these patients were diagnosed with pulmonary fibrosis or interstitial lung disease. On physical examination, crackles or wheezing may be audible, and patients may present with recurrent respiratory infections (i.e., infectious exacerbations of the underlying surfactant dysfunction). Low lung volumes and diffuse homogenous granular opacities are common findings on chest X-rays. In older patients, chest computed tomography (CT) findings include atelectasis, fibrosis, cysts, and ground glass opacities. Common non-genetic causes of respiratory failure in a full-term newborn include infection, meconium aspiration, or aspiration due to an anatomical defect. These should be considered before genetic testing. Genetic causes of respiratory failure in newborns can include surfactant deficiencies related to mutations in genes such as ABCA3, SFTPB, SFTPC, and NKX2-1. Pulmonary alveolar proteinosis (PAP) is another condition that affects surfactant homeostasis and may have a genetic component, although it does not typically present in the newborn period. Figure 8.2 illustrates the cellular pathology of surfactant dysfunction and the corresponding genetic mutations.

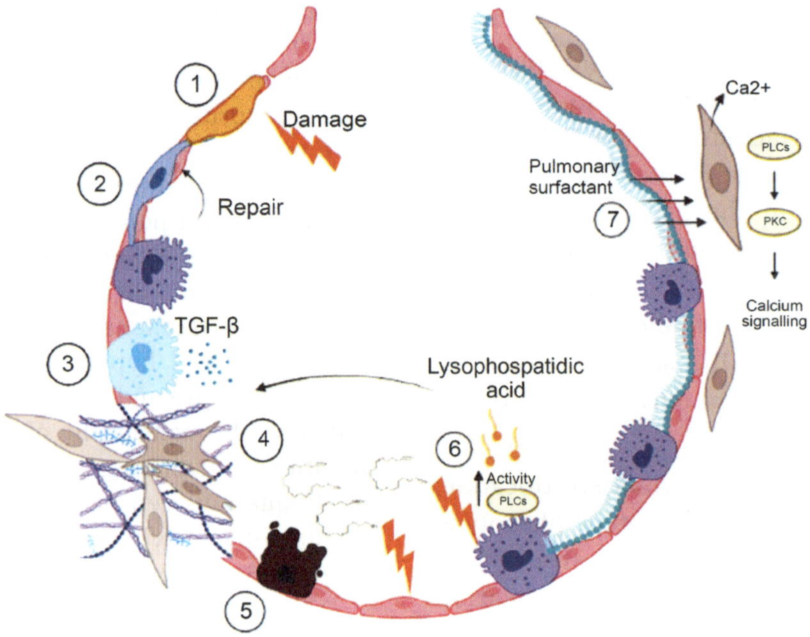

Figure 8.2. *During IPF, damage occurs in the epithelium (1); normally, when there is a lesion, the ATII cells recover the epithelium (2). In IPF, the ATII cells respond in an aberrant manner which means that they secrete cytokines (3) that provoke migration, proliferation, and differentiation of fibroblasts (4). These fibroblasts secrete extracellular matrix and change the architecture of the alveolus, causing it to lose its function. The damage to the ATII cells is progressive, and there is a change in the metabolism of PLs. During this process, fatty acids such as arachidonic acid are released, which decreases the viability of epithelial cells (5), and also increases the activity of phospholipases which produces palmitic acid that mediates scarring in the fibrotic process, prevents the regeneration of the epithelium and increases the recruitment of fibroblasts resistant to apoptosis (6). PS is important for maintaining alveolar homeostasis and inducing apoptosis of cells such as fibroblasts in which PS induces a calcium signal (7).*

Source: Tlatelpa-Romero B, Cázares-Ordoñez V, Oyarzábal LF, Vázquez-de-Lara LG. The Role of Pulmonary Surfactant Phospholipids in Fibrotic Lung Diseases. International Journal of Molecular Sciences. 2023; 24(1):326. https://doi.org/10.3390/ijms24010326.

PIG (pulmonary interstitial glycogenosis) and neuroendocrine hyperplasia of infancy (NEHI) are two additional causes of neonatal interstitial lung disease that need to be taken into account.

While NKX2-1 mutations have been reported in a small percentage of NEHI cases, no genetic mutations have been linked to PIG; more investigation is required to determine whether these diseases have a common genetic predisposition. Surfactant abnormalities are also a feature of some immunodeficiencies, namely GATA2-deficiency and 22q11.2 microdeletion syndrome, commonly referred to as DiGeorge syndrome.

In addition to primary ciliary dyskinesia (PCD) and alveolar capillary dysplasia with misalignment of pulmonary veins (ACD/MPV), other genetic conditions can lead to respiratory distress in full-term neonates. One example is loss-of-function mutations in the FLNA gene, which produces filamin A, a crucial protein for cell shape and movement. These mutations can cause lobar hyperinflation and respiratory failure in young infants, as well as pulmonary hypertension and pneumothorax in older age groups.

8.2.1. Surfactant Dysfunction Disorders

The most common causes of surfactant dysfunction are mutations in the SFTPC, SFTPB, or ABCA3 genes. Depending on the underlying genetic defect, different inheritance patterns and clinical presentations are linked to surfactant dysfunction. Surfactant dysfunction linked to SFTPC is inherited in an autosomal dominant pattern, whereas deficiencies related to ABCA3 and SFTPB are inherited in an autosomal recessive pattern.

Mutations in the ABCA3 gene, responsible for surfactant production and transport, are the most common genetic cause of surfactant dysfunction. This dysfunction can manifest in infancy, childhood, or rarely in adulthood. Lung biopsy may reveal conditions such as PAP and desquamative interstitial pneumonitis in infants, and nonspecific interstitial pneumonitis in older children. Abnormal lamellar bodies can be seen on electron microscopy. Loss of function or null mutations in ABCA3 can lead to a complete absence of protein production, resulting in a more severe clinical presentation with lung transplantation or death within the first year of life. On the other hand, missense variants and other mutation types are associated with a more variable disease progression.

The clinical course of individuals with pathogenic alterations in the SFTPB gene, which encodes surfactant protein B, can resemble that of those with mutations in the ABCA3 gene; these individuals usually experience acute respiratory failure and death during the neonatal period. Additionally, PAP desquamative interstitial pneumonitis is seen on lung biopsy; however, electron microscopy reveals no lamellar bodies.

The SFTPC gene, which produces the surfactant protein C, is linked to decreased penetrance, variable severity, and autosomal dominant inheritance. People with SFTPC mutations typically present with interstitial lung disease at varying ages of onset, though they can also show signs of newborn respiratory distress. Lamellar bodies on electron microscopy may be normal or disorganized, and lung biopsy reveals varying degrees of PAP, fibrosis, and desquamative interstitial pneumonitis. Some SFTPC mutations are inherited, frequently from parents who are not affected or only slightly affected, but the majority arise as de novo mutations. While most missense variants of SFTPC result in the production of an aberrant protein product that disrupts function, other mutations cause the protein to lose its function.

8.2.2. Brain-Lung-Thyroid Syndrome

Neonatal or childhood-onset interstitial lung disease is also linked to mutations in the NKX2-1 gene, formerly known as the thyroid transcription factor-1 (TTF1) gene. However, individuals with NKX2-1 mutations frequently present with additional clinical features resulting from disruption of thyroid and brain development, unlike those with ABCA3, SFTPB, and SFTPC-related surfactant deficiencies. All three organ systems are involved in about half of the cases, with the other half displaying any combination of the related characteristics. One of the main characteristics of the disease is the onset of chorea in childhood, although most people have some neurological involvement. Aside from these conditions, patients may also experience myoclonus, dystonia, ataxia, sensorineural hearing loss, intention tremor, dysarthria, facial apraxia, hypotonia, motor delay, and learning disabilities. Hypoplasia or aplasia, compensated hypothyroidism, and congenital hypothyroidism are examples of thyroid issues.

The primary cause of death for individuals with brain-lung-thyroid syndrome is lung disease. Although the clinical presentation and age at which lung disease onset vary, about 50% of people with NKX2-1 mutations have some degree of pulmonary dysfunction. While some patients may present at any age with interstitial lung disease or pulmonary fibrosis, respiratory distress can also occur in the neonatal period. Patients with lung disease may have mild to diffuse ground-glass opacities, atelectasis, fibrosis, and cysts on their CT scans. There is little information available from lung biopsies in these patients, although these biopsies may show signs of surfactant dysfunction disorders. Rare cases of NEHI, a type of interstitial lung disease marked by tachypnea, retractions, crackles, and hypoxemia in infancy, have been linked to NKX2-1 mutations. The majority of NEHI cases lack a distinct genetic cause; lung biopsies or standard CT patterns are used to make the diagnosis. A few cases of pulmonary carcinoma have also been reported in people with NKX2-1 mutations; however, it is still unknown whether NKX2-1-related disorders are linked to cancer.

Reduced hormone production in the thyroid gland, altered expression of surfactant genes in the lungs, and dysregulation of neuron development and migration in the brain are the causes of brain-lung-thyroid syndrome. The homeobox gene NKX2-1, which codes for the transcription factor Nkx-2.1, is partially responsible for all of these functions. Brain-lung-thyroid disease and other disorders related to NKX2-1, like benign hereditary chorea, are linked to mutations in the NKX2-1 gene that cause decreased protein synthesis or aberrant protein function. There have also been reports of complete NKX2-1 gene deletions. Affected individuals' expressivity varies significantly, and NKX2-1-related conditions are inherited in an autosomal dominant pattern.

8.2.3. Pulmonary Alveolar Proteinosis

The homeostasis of surfactants is also disturbed by PAP. Instead of a lack of surfactant, PAP typically manifests as an accumulation of surfactant in the alveolar space in adolescents or adults. PAP patients may experience symptoms of interstitial lung disease, such as dyspnea, intolerance to exercise, and dry cough. Additionally, they may exhibit crackles during physical examination and a "crazy paving" pattern on chest CT scans. A lung biopsy reveals an amorphous periodic acid-Schiff-positive fluid filled in the alveolar space, while bronchoalveolar lavage reveals copious frothy liquid.

The most common cause of PAP is autoimmune PAP, which is caused by autoantibodies that target granulocyte-macrophage colony-stimulating factors (GM-CSF), though PAP can also result from exposure to toxins or infections. Although rare, genetic causes of PAP should be taken into account, particularly in young children. Autosomal recessive PAP with decreased penetrance has been linked to mutations in the genes that encode the GM-CSF target receptors, CSF2RA and CSF2RB (Whitsett et al., 2015; Griese, 2017; Liszewski et al., 2017; Goetz and Ren, 2019).

8.3. Bronchiectasis

Irreversible bronchial lumen dilatation resulting in decreased mucus clearance is known as bronchiectasis. There are two types of bronchiectasis: focal and isolated and progressive and diffuse. Chronic aspiration, allergic hypersensitivity, severe lung infection, and inhalation injury are examples of nongenetic causes of bronchiectasis. Inflammation and infection are more common in bronchiectasis-affected lung regions. Cough, sputum production, recurrent respiratory infections, and occasionally hemoptysis are among the clinical features. When treating pediatric patients with bronchiectasis, genetic causes such as immune defects, PCD, cystic fibrosis (CF), and pseudo hypoaldosteronism should be taken into account.

8.3.1. Cystic Fibrosis

One of the most prevalent genetic disorders in children is cystic fibrosis (CF), which is characterized by obstructive lung disease and pancreatic insufficiency. Cystic fibrosis transmembrane conductance regulator (CFTR), an epithelial chloride ion channel, is encoded by the CFR gene. Mutations in this gene cause the autosomal recessive disorder. Atypical chloride transport brought on by CFTR expression loss obstructs mucus flow in the lungs and pancreatic ducts.

These patients may experience dyspnea, bronchiectasis, sputum production, hemoptysis, airway obstruction, and pneumothorax as a result of recurrent infections. Due to the accumulation of significant lung damage, people with CF eventually experience respiratory failure, which is the main cause of death in this patient population. Bronchiectasis linked to cystic fibrosis typically manifests in the initial years of life and is a progressive condition. It typically affects both sides and has a saccular or cystic appearance. The CF population is prone to infections caused by different strains of *Haemophilus influenzae*, *Staphylococcus aureus*, and *Pseudomonas*. Other signs and symptoms include diabetes, sinusitis, gastrointestinal issues, and infertility in men due to congenital vas deferens absence.

As part of the newborn screening program, all Americans are now routinely checked for CF; however, since this screening does not identify everyone who is affected, further diagnostic work-up should be guided by clinical suspicion. A certified cystic fibrosis center should perform the pilocarpine iontophoresis ("sweat test") to quantify sweat chloride in response to a positive newborn screen or a high degree of clinical suspicion at any age. A clinical diagnostic laboratory should perform complete gene sequencing, including deletion and duplication analysis, on any individual whose sweat chloride levels are found to be elevated (>60 mmol/L).

Based on how they cause disease, pathogenic variants in the CTR are divided into five classes. These mutation classes are linked to symptoms that express themselves in different ways. More severe mutations cause the classical multisystemic presentation, whereas milder mutations can be found in asymptomatic individuals or are linked to isolated congenital absence of the vas deferens.

All ethnic groups can have patients with cystic fibrosis (CF), but Caucasians are the most likely to have the disease, with carrier rates of roughly 1:28 among those with Northern European ancestry. Thanks to advancements in treatment, the life expectancy of patients with cystic fibrosis (CF) has steadily increased, rising from 28 years in 1986 to 47.7 years in 2016. A significant advancement in the management of CF patients has been the development of CFTR modulators, which in patients with certain mutations can partially restore the function of the chloride channel. This is especially true with the recent launch of elexacaftor-tezacaftor-ivacaftor combination therapy, which is recommended for almost 90% of patients. In the upcoming years, these medications and other treatments in development ought to have a significant effect on these patients' overall life expectancy and quality of life.

The terms "CF-related metabolic syndrome," "CF screen positive inconclusive diagnosis," and "CF-related disorders" are used to characterize people who do not fully fit the criteria for cystic fibrosis. These people may show no symptoms at all, or they may develop specific symptoms of cystic fibrosis (CF), such as bronchiectasis, sinusitis, or lack of vas deferens. With one or no CF-causing mutation, their sweat chloride level may be intermediate (30–59 mmol/L), or they may have two CFTR mutations but still have a normal sweat chloride level (<30 mmol/L). Even though some mutation combinations have genotype-phenotype predictions available, disease expression can also be influenced by genetic modifiers and environmental factors. As a result, this data cannot be used to predict a patient's clinical course on an individual basis, and patients with minor mutations should nevertheless undergo routine monitoring for CF symptoms.

8.3.2. Primary Ciliary Dyskinesia

PCD is one of a group of genetic conditions known as ciliopathies, which are characterized by ciliary dysfunction. It was formerly known as immotile cilia syndrome or, if combined with situs inversus, Kartagener's syndrome. PCD arises from anomalies in the composition or operation of motile cilia, which border the respiratory tract, the Fallopian tubes, and the ventricles of the central nervous system, and are necessary for the motility of sperm. The most prevalent ultrastructure abnormalities in PCD patients are either absent or shortened cilia dynein arms, which are necessary for a healthy beating. Mucus retention brought on by insufficient mucociliary clearance is the root cause of PCD's pulmonary symptoms, which also include bronchiectasis and recurrent respiratory tract infections.

Though the diagnosis of PCD is rarely made in infancy, people with the condition frequently present as full-term neonates needing supplemental oxygen due to respiratory distress and nasal congestion during the newborn period. The symptoms of PCD-associated respiratory distress include atelectasis, hypoxemia, lobar collapse, and tachypnea. The majority of people get bronchiectasis, which affects the lower and middle lobes of the right brain. These patients also exhibit recurrent infections, obstructive lung disease, digital clubbing, and a chronic cough.

Recurrent sinusitis and persistent otitis media, which can cause conductive hearing loss if they are severe, are examples of extrapulmonary features. Heterotaxy with or without polysplenia, situs inversus totalis, and congenital heart defects are among the laterality defects reported to affect about 50% of people with PCD. The high clinical suspicion for PCD when these laterality defects are found, however, may introduce ascertainment bias into these reported rates. In people with consistent sino-pulmonary features, PCD should therefore still be taken into consideration even in the absence of laterality defects. Except for those with CCDC114 mutations, the majority of affected males are infertile as a result of anomalies in sperm flagellar structure. Though cilia play a part in egg transport, females can have problems even though they are normally fertile.

Guidelines for PCD diagnosis were recently released by the American Thoracic Society. When possible, it is advised to use nasal nitric oxide (nNO) as the initial testing method before moving on to ciliary biopsies and/or genetic testing to confirm the diagnosis. Gene panel testing is advised as the initial diagnostic investigation when nNO is not feasible. Remarkably, a negative gene panel does not completely rule out PCD because about 30% of people with a high clinical suspicion have results from genetic testing that are negative or equivocal. As a primary research method, transmission electron microscopy analysis of ciliary ultrastructure—obtained by taking a sample of the nasal or carinal epithelium—is not advised because many PCD patients have subtle structural changes, and ciliary biopsies may even seem unremarkable. On the other hand, ciliary ultrastructure analysis can help clarify a diagnosis, especially when the results of genetic testing are unclear.

The most common causes of PCD are biallelic pathogenic alterations in the DNAI1, DNAH5, and DNAH11 genes. PCD is normally inherited in an autosomal recessive pattern. Two genes, RPGR, and OFD1, are linked to recessive syndromic X-linked forms of Parkinson's disease. More than 40 genes have been linked to PCD to date.

8.3.3. Primary Immunodeficiencies

Primary immunodeficiencies (PID) comprise more than 180 monogenic disorders resulting in an inherent immune system defect. Different clinical severity or infection tendencies can be present in PID patients. While milder types can cause minimal symptoms or be subclinical, the most severe types are fatal in infancy or early childhood. PID patients may experience inflammatory-mediated interstitial lung disease or recurrent, persistent infections brought on by microorganisms that are rarely contagious in the general population. These disorders can have pulmonary phenotypes (bronchiectasis, asthma, chronic cough, and dyspnea) that are comparable to those seen in patients with CF and PCD.

Life-threatening infections first appear in infants with severe combined immunodeficiency (SCID), a rare severe condition that affects both cellular and humoral immunity. T lymphocytes are absent, and B and natural killer cell function is variable. The IL2RG gene is mutated in the most prevalent type of SCID, which is inherited in an X-linked recessive pattern. The ADA, CD3D, DCLRE1C, JAK3, RAG1, and RAG2 genes are mutated in the majority of autosomal recessive causes of SCID. Due to its deadly nature in the absence of a bone marrow transplant, sickle cell disease (SCID) is included in the national newborn screening program in the United States and many other nations.

One of the most common PIDs, common-variable immune deficiency (CVID), is characterized by B cell dysfunction leading to low immunoglobulin levels. Many times, CVID is mild, and it might not be identified until adulthood. Most cases of CVID are found in people who do not appear to have a family history of the condition, and the inheritance pattern may be complex. The most frequently mutated gene when a genetic cause is found is TNFRSF13B (formerly known as TACI). There are two possible inheritance patterns for TNFRSF13B-associated CVID: autosomal dominant and recessive.

Most pediatric-onset PID is inherited in autosomal recessive or X-linked recessive patterns; however, underlying genetic causes are unknown in a significant number of individuals with suspected immune deficiencies. Furthermore, it is noteworthy that many syndromic genetic conditions are linked to immunodeficiency, such as trisomy 21,

DiGeorge syndrome, Noonan syndrome, ataxia-telangiectasia, and Wiskott-Aldrich syndrome. Recurrent infections in these patient populations may necessitate additional immune testing and treatment.

When a child's unusual pathogens or recurrent/severe infections are identified, an immune evaluation should be initiated. This evaluation should include measurements of complement function, neutrophil function, immunoglobulin levels (including response to immunizations), mitogen, and antigen responses, and immune cell populations using flow cytometry. The evaluation should be guided by the clinical suspicion of the underlying immune defect.

8.3.4. Autosomal Recessive Pseudo hypoaldosteronism-Type 1

Salt wasting that results in hyponatremia, hyperkalemia, and severe dehydration is a characteristic of autosomal recessive pseudo hypoaldosteronism-type 1 (PHA1). In the first two weeks of life, systemic PHA1 frequently manifests itself, albeit to differing degrees. Muscle weakness, nausea, vomiting, exhaustion, and failure to thrive are among the symptoms. Plasma levels of renin and aldosterone are elevated in those with autosomal recessive PHA1. Skin eruptions, cholelithiasis, cardiac arrhythmias, and short stature are additional characteristics. While salt supplementation is usually required for life, the frequency and severity of episodes of salt waste tend to diminish with time.

Similar to cystic fibrosis (CF), autosomal recessive PHA1 causes respiratory symptoms such as coughing, chest congestion, thickened mucus in the airways, and recurrent lower respiratory infections. Furthermore, sweat chloride testing results in a positive result in PHA1 patients, which may result in a misdiagnosis of CF. But unlike the progressive clinical course of CF, PHA1 patients' respiratory symptoms usually get better with time.

Autosomal recessive PHA1 is caused by mutations in the genes SCNN1A, SCNN1B, and SCNN1G, which encode the alpha, beta, and gamma subunits of the epithelial sodium channel, respectively. The epithelial sodium channel, which is present in the kidneys, lungs, and sweat glands, functions less or not at all when these genes are not functioning, which results in a decreased stimulatory response to aldosterone. The PHA1 autosomal dominant form is exclusive to the renal symptoms (Whitsett et al., 2015; Griese, 2017; Liszewski et al., 2017; Goetz and Ren, 2019).

8.4. Pulmonary Fibrosis

Pulmonary fibrosis should be taken into consideration for patients who present with hypoxia, desaturation with activity, or exercise intolerance. Auscultation of the lungs reveals crackles, and pulmonary function testing reveals restrictive patterns with a reduced capacity for diffusion. Patchy peripheral reticular abnormalities with intralobular linear opacities, subpleural honeycombing, irregular septal thickening, and traction bronchiectasis are seen on chest CT scans. While pulmonary fibrosis in adults can arise from a complex interplay of genetic and environmental risk factors, it is incredibly uncommon in children and has well-established underlying causes, including genetic disorders like Hermansky-Pudlak syndrome and short telomere syndromes. In addition to the conditions already mentioned, pulmonary fibrosis has also been linked to Marfan syndrome, brain-lung-thyroid syndrome, and surfactant deficiencies.

8.4.1. Short Telomere Syndromes

Telomeres are repetitive sequences found at the ends of eukaryotic chromosomes that safeguard the chromosome's integrity and coding DNA. Telomere length typically decreases by a small amount with each mitotic cell division. Cell death happens when telomeres are sufficiently shortened. Although this is a normal aspect of aging, people who have telomeres that are abnormally short for their age can exhibit a variety of clinical symptoms that impact different organ systems. Defects in telomere elongation or maintenance lead to a marked decrease in telomere length, which is the cause of short telomere syndromes. Shorter telomere lengths are generally associated with more severe disease states, which disproportionately affect tissue types like immune cells, skin, and bone marrow that have high rates of cell proliferation.

Variable expressivity is seen in short telomere syndromes, encompassing a broad spectrum of clinical characteristics and onset ages. On the more severe end of the spectrum is a syndromic condition known as dyskeratosis congenita (DC), which manifests in childhood. The diagnostic triad of reticulated pigmentation, nail dystrophy, and oral leukoplakia are among the symptoms. There may also be signs of lymphopenia, dental abnormalities, short stature, developmental delay, early graying or loss of hair, esophageal stricture or narrowing, hyperhidrosis, brain abnormalities, intrauterine growth restriction, and genitourinary abnormalities. Epiphora is an excessive watering of the eyes caused by blockage of the lacrimal duct. Pulmonary arteriovenous malformations, or AVMs, have been documented in a small number of cases.

While children with DC can exhibit pulmonary fibrosis, pulmonary fibrosis in children with short telomere syndromes is uncommon in other cases. However, adult-onset pulmonary fibrosis, which frequently co-occurs with aplastic anemia or liver cirrhosis, maybe the first potentially fatal sign of short telomere syndromes. Evaluation of family members' genetic makeup may be taken into consideration if a family member exhibits signs of short telomere syndrome.

When a child exhibits clinical signs of DC, genetic testing can verify the diagnosis. In situations where an underlying genetic mutation cannot be found, the diagnosis of short telomere syndromes can be confirmed by measuring the leukocyte telomere length using automated multicolor flow cytometry fluorescence in situ hybridization. The primary enzyme involved in telomere elongation, telomerase, exhibits decreased activity in the most prevalent genetic defects that cause short telomere syndromes. The most commonly reported mutations are those encoding the proteins that comprise the major subunits of the telomerase complex, TERT, DKC1, and TERC. Rare causes of short telomere syndromes have also been found, including mutations in the TNIF2, RTEL1, CTC1, ACD, NOP10, NHP2, PARN, USB1, and WRAP53 genes.

Genetic anticipation indicates that the severity of the clinical presentation may increase with each successive generation in families with TERT- and TRC-related autosomal dominant forms of the disease. The higher degree of illness is thought to be caused by the compounding effect of inheriting a mutation that shortens telomeres along with cells that have shorter telomeres on average from an affected parent.

8.4.2. Hermansky-Pudlak Syndrome

HPS is an autosomal recessive disease characterized by oculocutaneous albinism combined with a deficiency of platelet delta granules, resulting in a bleeding diathesis. Compared to other family members, people with HPS typically have lighter skin, hair, and eyes. They also have ocular abnormalities like nystagmus, photophobia, decreased visual acuity, and lack of visual attention. Easy bruising, epistaxis, prolonged bleeding following minor procedures, postpartum hemorrhage, colonic bleeding, gingival bleeding, and prolonged menstruation are other symptoms that can be experienced by people with HPS. HPS is linked to pathogenic variants in the AP3B1, AP3D1, BLOC1S3, BLOC1S6, DTNBP1, HPS1, HPS3, HPS4, HPS5, and HPS6 genes. Proteins involved in the biogenesis of lysosome-related organelle complexes (BLOCs) are encoded by these genes. Melanosomes and platelet dense granules are examples of lysosome-related organelles that are transported by BLOCs. Improper trafficking of these organelles due to defective BLOC function causes bleeding diathesis and albinism.

There are certain HPS subtypes that are linked to particular clinical traits. The development of early-onset pulmonary fibrosis, which usually manifests in the third decade of life and can resemble idiopathic pulmonary fibrosis, is associated with the HPS1, HPS4, and AP3B1 genes. Granulomatous colitis is also linked to the HPS1 and HPS4 genes, whereas immunodeficiencies, severe neutropenia, and increased neurological involvement are linked to the AP3B1 and AP3D1 genes. While HPS affects people of all ethnicities, people of northwest Puerto Rican descent have a higher incidence of HPS1 and HPS3-related disease because of founder mutations in that population (Whitsett et al., 2015; Griese, 2017; Liszewski et al., 2017; Goetz and Ren, 2019).

8.5. Abnormalities of the Pulmonary Vasculature

When there is severe hypoxemia or dyspnea without accompanying pulmonary parenchymal or cardiac structural abnormalities, genetic disorders linked to anomalies of the pulmonary vasculature should be taken into consideration. The structure and function of the pulmonary veins and arteries may be altered by genetic causes of pulmonary vascular disease, which are frequently linked to anomalies of the vasculature in other body parts or additional syndromic features. While ACD, PAH, and HHT (hereditary hemorrhagic telangiectasia) are mentioned, pediatric pulmonary patients can also be affected by numerous other genetic syndromes linked to vascular anomalies.

8.5.1. Alveolar Capillary Dysplasia with Misalignment of Pulmonary Veins

ACD/MVP typically results in death in the newborn stage. Infants experience severe hypoxemia and respiratory distress shortly after birth, and these conditions are unresponsive to conventional therapies like mechanical ventilation and extra oxygen. An echocardiography reveals chronic pulmonary hypertension that does not go better when nitric oxide is inhaled. The majority of ACD/MVP patients have extrapulmonary involvement. Malformations related to the heart, stomach, and genitourinary system have been identified. These include omphalocele, intestinal malrotation, Hirschsprung's disease, imperforate anus, duodenal atresia, and atrial septal defects. There have been rare reports of the disease developing later in life with a milder phenotype.

The main cause of respiratory problems is malpositioned alveolar capillaries, which impair the flow of oxygen from the alveoli to the bloodstream. Histologically, lung tissue is typified by pulmonary veins that are not in the right place, reduced, and misaligned alveolar wall capillaries, inadequate pulmonary lobular development, and thickening of the small pulmonary arteries' muscle walls, which may indicate pulmonary lymphangiectasis.

Autosomal dominant ACD/MVP is caused by mutations in the FOXF1 gene. Numerous genes, including those involved in the development of the pulmonary mesenchyme, are impacted by the transcription factor encoded by FOXF1.

The FOXF1 gene stops functioning as a result of the majority of pathogenic mutations. Due to de novo mutations, nearly all instances of FOXF1-related ACD/MPV affect people who have never had the condition in their family. A potential imprinting effect has been suggested by the discovery that variations in FOXF1 were inherited from an unaffected mother in a small number of documented cases. Some people's FOXF1 genes are mutated, while others have the complete FOXF1 gene lost due to a microdeletion at position 16q24.1. Microdeletions in this area may affect adjacent genes and be linked to extra characteristics like cardiac abnormalities.

8.5.2. Heritable PAH

Individuals should be assessed for hereditary PAH if they exhibit dyspnea, exhaustion, syncope, leg edema, chest pain, palpitations, and an echocardiogram or electrocardiogram reveals evidence of pulmonary hypertension. Increased pulmonary arterial pressure and right ventricular overload are the outcomes of PAH, which is caused by the narrowing and obstruction of the pulmonary arterioles. It can strike at any age, and the average survival time after diagnosis is 2–8 years. It is frequently linked to a sharp decline in health.

The majority of hereditary PAH cases are inherited in an autosomal dominant pattern and are brought on by mutations in the BMPR2 gene. The most frequent cause of hereditary PAH is variation that results in loss of function of the BMPR2 gene, which results in an absent or shortened protein product. The bone morphogenetic protein receptor type 2, or BMPR2, is involved in the development of bone and cartilage. It is not yet known, though, how pathogenic variants in this gene cause PAH.

Rarely, harmful variations in different genes have been found in PAH patients. ACVRL1, BMPR1B, CAV1, CBLN2, EIF2AK4, ENG, KCNA5, KCNK3, and SMA9 are some of these genes. HHT is also linked to the ACVRL1 and ENG genes, which are discussed in more detail below. Other genetic syndromes linked to PAH include sickle cell anemia, pulmonary veno-occlusive disease, Gaucher disease, and FLNA-associated periventricular heterotopia.

Variable expressivity and a significant reduction in penetrance of about 20% are characteristics of hereditary PAH. Males are less likely to be affected than females, but affected males typically experience a more severe course of the disease. Pregnancy can be risky and is linked to a high death rate in people with hereditary PAH.

8.5.3. Hereditary Hemorrhagic Telangiectasia

As with PAH, patients who experience dyspnea or hypoxemia during exertion should consider HHT. Recurrent, potentially severe epistaxis that typically starts in childhood and the existence of telangiectasias are characteristics that set HHT apart. The mucocutaneous surfaces of the body, including the lips, mouth cavity, fingers, face, and chest, are prone to telangiectasias. They can cause gastrointestinal bleeding, which is a frequent consequence of HHT, when they are present in the gastrointestinal mucosa.

Larger AVMs that develop in the brain, liver, or lungs can be fatal. While only 30 to 50% of people with HHT develop pulmonary AVMs, the majority of those who do have HHT. The size of pulmonary AVMs typically grows over time, and major side effects include transient ischemic attacks from paradoxical emboli, stroke, and brain abscesses. Every now and then, they burst, resulting in hemoptysis, and some people with pulmonary AVMs get PAH. When IV contrast is added, CT imaging of the chest shows well-circumscribed regions of increased blood supply. Occasionally, a feeding vessel can be seen. In people with HHT, hepatic AVMs are also common, though they are often asymptomatic. Roughly 10% of people have cerebral AVMs, which are typically present from birth and can cause bleeding.

The most common cause of HHT, which is inherited in an autosomal dominant pattern, is pathogenic variants in the ENG, SMADL4, and ACVRL1 genes. GDF2 mutations are an uncommon cause of HHT. Juvenile polyposis syndrome, which is marked by a propensity to develop hamartomatous polyps in the gastrointestinal tract and an increased risk of gastrointestinal cancers, coexists with HHT in SMADL4-related cases. Many people fit the clinical criteria for an HHT diagnosis but do not have detectable mutations in any of these genes, indicating that there may be other genetic etiologies for HHT that are not yet known about or that these people may have a different syndrome with overlapping features.

The ENG and ACVRL1 genes encode proteins that are relevant to the development of smooth muscle cells in growing vessels as well as the differentiation of blood vessels into veins and arteries. The transforming growth factor-β pathway's signaling protein is encoded by the Smad4 gene. Although the precise mechanism by which Smad4 mutations cause HHT with juvenile polyposis is unclear, it serves as both a transcription factor and tumor suppressor (Whitsett et al., 2015; Griese, 2017; Liszewski et al., 2017; Goetz and Ren, 2019).

8.6. Pneumothorax

Pneumothorax can occur spontaneously or as a result of trauma, but if it occurs frequently, especially in the presence of a family history of the condition, it may have a genetic basis, such as a connective tissue disease or Birt-Hogg-Dubé (BHD). Genetic testing should also be prompted by other clinical manifestations, such as joint laxity, skin anomalies, dysmorphic facial features, or the presence of lung blebs or cysts on chest imaging.

Although recurrent pneumothorax may prompt genetic evaluation, it is typically not a life-threatening condition. However, extrapulmonary complications such as vascular issues in connective tissue disorders and renal cancer in BHD are associated with high mortality rates if not detected early. Therefore, accurate diagnosis is crucial for effective screening and treatment. Since most of the genetic conditions mentioned have autosomal dominant inheritance and potentially life-threatening extrapulmonary symptoms, it is important to consider the impact of these diagnoses on family members who may also require genetic testing and clinical monitoring.

8.6.1. Connective Tissue Disorders

A broad, genetically diverse group of illnesses known as connective tissue disorders are linked to anomalies in the cutaneous, skeletal, and vascular systems. They are usually caused by mutations in genes related to the structure or function of the main proteins—collagen, elastin, and glycosaminoglycans—that make up connective tissues. The onset of pneumothorax is linked to a subset of connective tissue disorders.

8.6.1.1. Marfan Syndrome

Mutations in the FBN1 gene cause Marfan syndrome, an autosomal dominant condition. This gene encodes the fibrillin protein, which is a structural component of microfibrils. Microfibrils are found in elastic fibers in skin, ligaments, and blood vessels, as well as providing support in tissues like bone. Although the characteristics of Marfan syndrome can vary, they typically include distinctive phenotypic alterations in the skeletal, ocular, and cardiovascular systems. People who have Marfan syndrome frequently have longer limbs, arachnodactyly, pectus deformities, scoliosis, and lax joints than their unaffected family members. Myopia, retinal detachment, and ectopia lentis are examples of ocular manifestations. Aortic dilatation, mitral valve prolapse, tricuspid valve prolapse, and potentially fatal pulmonary artery root enlargement are examples of cardiovascular complications.

Pneumothorax affects 5–10% of people with Marfan syndrome. Different people have different underlying causes for this condition, such as the existence of apical pulmonary blebs or bullae, abnormalities in the lung parenchyma's connective tissue, and mechanical stress from tall habitus on the lung apices. Other pulmonary manifestations that can occur in people with Marfan syndrome include cystic changes, emphysema, bronchiectasis, congenital malformations, and fibrosis.

8.6.1.1. Ehlers-Danlos Syndromes

13 disorders collectively known as Ehlers-Danlos syndromes (EDS) are typified by hypermobile joints, hyperextensible skin, and fragile tissues. The majority of cases of spontaneous pneumothorax that have been reported involve individuals with the vascular subtype of EDS, an autosomal dominant disorder brought on by mutations in the COL3A1 gene. Type III collagen, which is present in the skin, lungs, intestinal walls, and vascular walls, is encoded by the gene COL3A1. The vascular form of Ehlers-Danlos syndrome (vEDS) is characterized by tissue fragility, thin, translucent skin, easy bruising, and distinctive facial features. The high death rate linked to ventilator-associated endocarditis (vEDS) is caused by gastrointestinal perforations, organ ruptures, and artery ruptures or dissections. Although they have not yet been linked to pneumothorax, a number of other forms of EDS may share similarities with vEDS and have genetic causes.

Pneumothorax in vEDS may occur spontaneously or repeatedly, and it may manifest in childhood or adulthood. There have been reports of hemopneumothorax and hemomothorax in vEDS patients, and these conditions are frequently linked to lung nodules, cystic legions, or pulmonary blebs. Hemostases and severe recurrent hemoptysis are other possible conditions.

8.6.1.2. Loeys-Dietz Syndrome

An autosomal dominant disorder with vascular, skeletal, craniofacial, and cutaneous characteristics is called Loeys-Dietz syndrome (LDS). Arachnodactyly, talipes equinovarus, scoliosis, pectus deformities, and joint laxity are examples of skeletal manifestations. Aortic dilatation, which can result in aortic dissection and is observed in over 95% of people with LDS, is one of the vascular complications. Other organs may also exhibit tortuosity and arterial aneurysms. Hypertelorism, bifid uvula, cleft palate, and craniosynostosis are examples of craniofacial features. On the skin, there is velvety, translucent skin, easy bruising, and dystrophic scarring. It is unknown how common restrictive lung disease and pneumothorax are in LDS patients. The majority of LDS cases are caused by mutations in the TGFBR1 and TGFBR2 genes; rarer causes include mutations in the SMD2, SMAD3, TGFB2, and TGFB3 genes.

8.6.1.3. Cutis Laxa

Skin that is loose, saggy, and inclastic—especially around the neck, armpits, and groyne—is a hallmark of cutis laxa. Cutis laxa patients may also have visceral diverticula, joint hypermobility, developmental problems, inguinal, umbilical, and diaphragmatic hernia, and cardiovascular involvement. Neonatal or childhood-onset emphysema is one of the pulmonary manifestations that can cause pneumothorax, laryngomalacia, tracheomalacia, bronchomalacia, bronchiolitis, and pulmonary hypertension. It can also be severe and progressive. The onset of emphysema and cutis laxa are linked to the EFN5, EFEMP2, LTBP4, and ELAN genes. Autosomal recessive cutis laxa is linked to LTBP4 and EFEMP2, while mutations in FLLN5 can have either an autosomal dominant or recessive inheritance pattern. Autosomal dominant cutis laxa may result from mutations in the ERN gene. Notably, deletion of the ELAN gene may also result in Williams syndrome, a microdeletion at 7q11.23-associated disorder characterized by distinct facial features, intellectual disability, and unique personality traits. This deletion may lead to complications related to connective tissue, such as pneumothorax or emphysema.

8.6.2. Birt-Hogg-Dubé Syndrome

BHD syndrome is caused by mutations in the FLCN gene, which is believed to encode the folliculin protein. While the specific role of folliculin is not fully understood, it may act as a tumor suppressor. This syndrome primarily impacts the skin, lungs, and kidneys, with the gene being expressed in various organs including the brain, heart, and testes. BHD is known to have high penetrance, but the presentation and severity of symptoms can vary greatly, leading to the belief that it is often underdiagnosed.

Acrochordons, trichodiscomas, and fibrofolliculomas are examples of cutaneous hamartomas that are frequently present but usually harmless. The most common skin condition, fibrofolliculomas, usually develop in adulthood and show up on the face, neck, and upper trunk. Most people with BHD have bilateral multifocal medial or basal lung cysts. Although these lung cysts don't cause any symptoms at first, patients are highly susceptible to recurring pneumothoraces. Pneumothoraces can be the initial symptom of BHD and typically happen in adolescence or adulthood. A kidney screen should be performed as soon as a BHD diagnosis is made because people with BHD have a 15% to 30% lifetime risk of developing renal tumors. Renal oncocytomas, chromophobe renal cell carcinoma, and oncocytic hybrid tumors are the most frequently found tumors in BHD patients. Papillary and clear cell renal cell carcinomas have also been documented. Although the kidney tumors associated with BHD typically grow slowly, it is crucial to detect them early in this high-risk group to prevent cancer. Renal cysts are frequently discovered on imaging in people with BHD (Whitsett et al., 2015; Griese, 2017; Liszewski et al., 2017; Goetz and Ren, 2019).

8.7. Congenital Central Hypoventilation Syndrome

A condition affecting the respiratory and autonomic nervous systems is known as congenital central hypoventilation syndrome (CCHS). When CCHS first manifests in the newborn stage, episodes of alveolar hypoventilation during non-rapid eye movement sleep are more common. In severe situations, babies may experience hypoventilation when awake and total apnea when they sleep. In people with CCHS, hypoventilation frequently leads to hypoxemia and hypercapnia, necessitating the implantation of a diaphragmatic pacemaker or mechanical ventilation. Some people need mechanical ventilation assistance around the clock. Even though CCHS-related respiratory problems can be fatal, prognosis, and quality of life can be greatly enhanced by prompt diagnosis and aggressive treatment.

Additional complications of autonomic nervous system dysfunction affecting multiple body systems are present in individuals with CCHS. Reduced heart rate variability, dysrhythmias, syncope, gastrointestinal problems, altered pain perception, ophthalmological abnormalities, dysregulation of sweating and body temperature, and urinary problems are among the symptoms. Furthermore, some people have altered neural crest-derived structure development, which can result in neural origin tumors or Hirschsprung's disease. Although later onset has been documented, the majority of cases occur during the newborn stage. The phenotype of patients with later-onset disease is typically milder.

8.7.1. Genetic Condition

The PHOX2B gene is mutated in CCHS, which is inherited autosomally dominantly. The majority of PHOX2B mutations are expansions of exon 3's polyalanine repeat region. The amino acid alanine is encoded by 20 repeats of three nucleotides in an individual. People are impacted by CCHS when this region grows to 25 alanine repeats or more. Some people with 25 repeats and those with 24 repeats may exhibit a mild clinical presentation. These mutations can be challenging to find using conventional sequencing techniques because the polyalanine region is repetitive. To characterize these variations, targeted fragment length analysis might be required. Some people with CCHS have different kinds of PHOX2B gene mutations, mostly frameshift variations.

While most repeat expansions are the result of de novo mutations, some parents who do not exhibit symptoms have somatic mosaicism for the polyalanine repeat variations that have been found in their offspring. Although somatic mosaicism can be challenging to diagnose, this is a significant discovery because it implies that, in contrast to most other conditions primarily caused by de novo mutations that are rarely known to recur in families, the recurrence risk of CCHS in the offspring of these individuals may not be insignificant. A homeobox domain transcription factor, encoded by PHOX2B, is expressed during embryonic development and is necessary for the appropriate development of the central and peripheral autonomic nervous systems. PHOX2B is required for the maturation of neural crest cells and hindbrain motor neurons.

Table 8.1. *Eligibility for Genomic Testing for Familial Pulmonary Fibrosis as Per the Latest Version of UK National Genomic Test Directory for Rare and Inherited Disease*

UK NHS National Genomic Test Directory – Testing Criteria for Rare and Inherited Disease, version 5.1, May 2023
R421 Pulmonary Fibrosis Familial testing criteria: ILD and ONE of the following:
ILD, no identifiable cause or association, and age < 50 years.
Family history of ILD regardless of identifiable cause or association.
For suspected telomerase complex mutations, testing to be considered in the absence of 1. and 2. above if one or more of the following are present in addition to ILD: – Unexplained hematological abnormalities including macrocytosis, anemia, thrombocytopenia, leukopenia and/or lymphopenia; premature greying, Or unexplained liver function abnormalities. – Consideration of lung transplantation.

Source: Stanel SC, Callum J and Rivera-Ortega P (2023) Genetic and environmental factors in interstitial lung diseases: current and future perspectives on early diagnosis of high-risk cohorts. Front. Med. 10:1232655. doi: 10.3389/fmed.2023.1232655.

Pathogenic mutations in PHOX2B are thought to cause disease via a dominant-negative effect, although most PHOX2B mutations are repeated expansion variations or frameshift variants, which typically have a loss-of-function impact on gene function. It is believed that the aberrant protein product from the mutated allele dimerizes with the (wild-type allele) normal protein product, impairing its function and causing the dominant-negative effect (Whitsett et al., 2015; Griese, 2017; Liszewski et al., 2017; Goetz and Ren, 2019) (Table 8.1).

An increasing number of pediatric pulmonary diseases have been found to have genetic causes. The cost of genetic testing has decreased and recent technological advancements have made genetic evaluation a standard part of the diagnostic work-up. Pediatric pulmonologists should be knowledgeable about the most recent advancements in pulmonary genetic disease and the most efficient way to obtain genetic testing.

The initial stage of providing care for a patient with a genetic condition involves genetic evaluation and diagnosis. Patients who have a genetic condition that has been confirmed should be linked to the relevant registries and treated according to guidelines. Genetic therapies will eventually be accessible for a growing number of these illnesses. In conclusion, genetics is an essential part of pediatric pulmonary medicine, and it is becoming standard practice to recognize and appropriately incorporate genetic evaluation in the pulmonary clinic (Whitsett et al., 2015; Griese, 2017; Liszewski et al., 2017; Goetz and Ren, 2019).

A Closer Look

A Genomics First Approach towards Better Understanding of Pediatric PAH

It has been suggested that identifying the molecular subtypes of PAH will enhance risk assessment, management, and results. Compared to adults, children need more thorough genetic testing to receive a genetic diagnosis. Children should be assessed genome-wide for rare de novo and inherited variants using trio (parental and child) exome sequencing/chromosome microarray or genome sequencing if testing for a panel of genes known to be associated with PAH is not diagnostic. To provide more individualized care for each genetically defined group, information about the causal gene can be used to refine the natural history, penetrance, and response to treatment for that particular genetic subtype of PAH. One can then compare individuals with different genes in the same biological pathway to determine the similarities and differences between them.

To obtain sufficient sample sizes given the limited number of pediatric PAH patients at individual sites, collaboration among national and international clinical PH centers is essential. PPHNet is a pediatric-specific PAH consortium recruiting patients at 13 clinical sites across North America. Other large-scale PAH cohorts include PVDomics, a US multicenter study started in 2014, and PAH-ICON, a new international initiative. The definition of PAH has been updated to include mPAP levels of 20–25 mmHg in both adults and children, alongside the previous cutoff of ≥25 mmHg. Pediatric PAH is characterized by elevated mPAP after 3 months of age, combined with an indexed PVRI ≥3 Woods units/m2. Classification of PAH subtypes aims to enhance clinical management and research, typically following the World Symposium on Pulmonary Hypertension (WSPH) guidelines updated in 2018. In children, a pediatric-specific classification system developed by the PVRI Pediatric Task Force in Panama offers a more precise categorization of developmental and complex phenotypes.

It is preferable to use biological trios consisting of two unaffected parents and an affected child for pediatric studies on PAH, as this helps identify both inherited and de novo variants that may be causing the disease. However, as the availability of ethnically matched genomic data in public databases increases, the necessity for trios may decrease. DNA can be easily obtained from small blood or saliva samples. In a large national autism study, we have developed methods to collect saliva from pediatric patients and their parents at home, with instructional videos to assist clinical sites with remote biospecimen collection. Biological samples can then be sent to a central biorepository for DNA extraction, processing, and sequencing using a single genetic platform.

Currently, there is limited added value in analyzing genome sequencing compared to exome sequencing data, as annotation tools for noncoding variants and the yield of structural variants from genome sequencing are still in development. After thorough quality control, filtering, and annotation, sequencing data is screened for rare deleterious variants in known candidate genes, and undergo trio analysis for de novo variants, or association analysis for inherited variants. Candidate genes identified through these methods are further evaluated by mapping variant locations to protein structures, assessing expression levels in PAH-relevant tissues and cell types, investigating variant function *in vitro*, and studying the effects of pathogenic variants in model organisms *in vivo*. Human mutations can be introduced into cells and PAH-sensitized mice using CRISPR technology, allowing for the assessment of phenotypic "rescue" through the delivery of normal proteins to support the causation of the disease.

When genetic subtypes are identified, cases with variations in the same gene or pathway can be compared based on demographic information, clinical phenotypes, and imaging data (lung biopsies, chest X-ray or CT scans, chest/cardiac MRI, and pulmonary vascular angiography). For focused clinical evaluations, pertinent cases can be called back or interviewed virtually to see if there are any commonalities between cases having uncommon variants in the same gene or pathway.

Large sequencing centers, clinical diagnostic laboratories, and GeneMatcher can be used to identify additional cases, thereby increasing rigor and allowing assessment of the full phenotypic spectrum of the new genetic subtypes. Both retrospectively and prospectively, longitudinal phenotypes of the genetic subtypes can be evaluated. These phenotypes include lung function changes, response to medication, death or transplant, and other medical diagnoses. When it comes to inherited variants, penetrance by age and sex can be determined by combining clinical evaluation of "unaffected" individuals who carry the relevant genetic variant with cascade genetic testing of family members. "Virtual" family meetings can be arranged to provide families with updates on new research related to their conditions and to create communities for each of the rare endophenotypes to support families who have received a genetic diagnosis.

A genetic diagnosis has three benefits for families: it can be used to identify additional associated features, identify family members who are at risk of developing PAH, and clarify reproductive risks and offer family planning options. For pulmonary veno-occlusive disease/ pulmonary capillary hemangiomatosis, which can be challenging to diagnose clinically without a lung biopsy, biallelic mutations in EIF2AK4 are diagnostic. Patients may benefit from being placed for transplant earlier in the course of the disease, potentially improving outcomes. As previously indicated, carriers of the TBX4 variant should be evaluated for related orthopedic (hips, knees, and feet) and developmental problems (lung, heart). Patients with ENG/ACVRL1 variant carriers need to have regular MRI surveillance because they are susceptible to arteriovenous malformations in the liver, lungs, intestine, and brain. To identify those at risk who might benefit from yearly surveillance and early diagnosis/treatment, additional family members of a patient with PAH can be screened for the family variant following the patient's genetic diagnosis. Additionally, young adults with diagnoses are capable of making well-informed decisions about family planning.

Summary

- Respiratory distress syndrome in newborn infants is the most frequent respiratory cause of death and morbidity in children <1 y of age in the United States. It is also predictive of risk for chronic pulmonary diseases in childhood.
- The human surfactant protein A locus consists of two functional genes (SP-A1 and SP-A2) and a pseudogene. Each of the two functional genes contains four coding exons and directs the synthesis of a distinct primary translation product.
- In contrast to surfactant protein A, genetic disruption of surfactant protein B expression causes an unambiguous neonatal respiratory phenotype in human infants. The surfactant protein B gene has been sequenced and its regulatory regions characterized.
- Surfactant protein C is a hydrophobic protein that is synthesized from a precursor of either 191 or 197 amino acids (depending on differential splicing of the primary transcript) and proteolytically cleaved.
- Surfactant protein D is a member of the collectin family and is expressed in extrapulmonary tissues. Its functions include carbohydrate domain recognition on the surface of pathogens.
- Targeted disruption of the genes that encode either granulocyte-macrophage colony-stimulating factor or its receptor (GM-CSF/IL-3/IL-5 receptor common β-chain) resulted in pulmonary alveolar proteinosis.
- Acute respiratory distress during the neonatal period, as characterized by hypoxemia and retractions, is expected in preterm infants due to immature lung development.
- Surfactant dysfunction most often results from mutations in the *ABCA3*, *SFTPB*, or *SFTPC* genes. Surfactant dysfunction is associated with various inheritance patterns and clinical presentations depending on the underlying genetic defect. *ABCA3* and *SFTPB*-related surfactant deficiencies are inherited in an autosomal recessive pattern, while *SFTPC*-related surfactant dysfunction is inherited in an autosomal dominant pattern.
- Mutations in the *NKX2-1* gene, previously known as the thyroid transcription factor-1 (*TTF1*) gene, are also associated with neonatal or childhood-onset interstitial lung disease.
- Bronchiectasis is irreversible dilation of the bronchial lumen, with resulting reduced mucus clearance. Bronchiectasis can be focal and isolated, or it can be progressive and become diffuse. Nongenetic causes of bronchiectasis can include chronic aspiration, allergic hypersensitivity, severe lung infection, and inhalation injury.
- Primary Ciliary Dyskinesia (PCD), previously known as immotile cilia syndrome or, if in conjunction with situs inversus, Kartagener's syndrome, is one of a group of genetic conditions known as ciliopathies that are characterized by ciliary dysfunction.
- Primary immunodeficiencies (PID) encompass over 180 monogenic disorders that cause an intrinsic defect in the immune system. PID can present with varying clinical severity or infection tendencies. The most severe types are lethal in infancy or early childhood, while milder types can cause minimal symptoms or be subclinical.
- Patients presenting with exercise intolerance, hypoxia, or desaturation with activity should prompt the consideration of pulmonary fibrosis. Crackles can be heard on auscultation of

the lungs, and pulmonary function testing reflects restrictive patterns with a decreased diffusion capacity.

- Genetic conditions associated with abnormalities of the pulmonary vasculature should be considered when there is significant shortness of breath or hypoxemia without underlying pulmonary parenchymal or cardiac structural abnormalities.
- Although pneumothorax may develop spontaneously or following trauma, repeated occurrences of pneumothorax should prompt suspicion of an underlying genetic etiology, such as a connective tissue disorder or Birt-Hogg-Dubé (BHD), especially if there is a family history of pneumothorax.
- Congenital central hypoventilation syndrome (CCHS) is a disorder of the respiratory and autonomic nervous systems. CCHS classically presents in the newborn period with alveolar hypoventilation with increased episodes during non-rapid eye movement sleep.

References

1. Carre, A., Szinnai, G., Castanet, M., et al. (2009). Five new TTF1/NKX2.1 mutations in brain-lung-thyroid syndrome: Rescue by PAX8 synergism in one case. *Human Molecular Genetics, 18*(12), 2266–2276.
2. Carrington, J. M., & Hershberger, D. M. (2018). *Pulmonary Alveolar Proteinosis.* Treasure Island, FL: StatPearls.
3. Cutz, E., Chami, R., Dell, S., Langer, J., & Manson, D. (2017). Pulmonary interstitial glycogenosis associated with a spectrum of neonatal pulmonary disorders. *Human Pathology, 68*, 154–165.
4. de Gusmao, C. M., Kok, F., Casella, E. B., & Waugh, J. L. (2016). Benign hereditary chorea related to NKX2-1 with ataxia and dystonia. *Neurology Genetics, 2*(1), e40.
5. Doan, M. L., Guillerman, R. P., Dishop, M. K., et al. (2008). Clinical, radiological and pathological features of ABCA3 mutations in children. *Thorax, 63*(4), 366–373.
6. Dyhdalo, K., & Farver, C. (2011). Pulmonary histologic changes in Marfan syndrome: A case series and literature review. *American Journal of Clinical Pathology, 136*(6), 857–863.
7. Farrell, P. M., White, T. B., Ren, C. L., et al. (2017). Diagnosis of cystic fibrosis: Consensus guidelines from the Cystic Fibrosis Foundation. *Journal of Pediatrics, 181S*, S4.e1–S15.e1.
8. Galambos, C., Levy, H., Cannon, C. L., et al. (2010). Pulmonary pathology in thyroid transcription factor-1 deficiency syndrome. *American Journal of Respiratory and Critical Care Medicine, 182*(4), 549–554.
9. Goetz, D., & Ren, C. L. (2019). Review of cystic fibrosis. *Pediatric Annals, 48*(4), e154–e161.
10. Gomes, V. C., Silva, M. C., Maia Filho, J. H., et al. (2013). Diagnostic criteria and follow-up in neuroendocrine cell hyperplasia of infancy: A case series. *Jornal Brasileiro de Pneumologia, 39*(5), 569–578.
11. Gras, D., Jonard, L., Roze, E., et al. (2012). Benign hereditary chorea: Phenotype, prognosis, therapeutic outcome and long-term follow-up in a large series with new mutations in the TTF1/NKX2-1 gene. *Journal of Neurology, Neurosurgery & Psychiatry, 83*(10), 956–962.
12. Griese, M. (2017). Pulmonary alveolar proteinosis: A comprehensive clinical perspective. *Pediatrics, 140*(2), e20170610.

13. Guillot, L., Carré, A., Szinnai, G., et al. (2010). NKX2-1 mutations leading to surfactant protein promoter dysregulation cause interstitial lung disease in "brain-lung-thyroid syndrome." *Human Mutation*, *31*(2), E1146–E1162.
14. Hamvas, A., Deterding, R. R., Wert, S. E., et al. (2013). Heterogeneous pulmonary phenotypes associated with mutations in the thyroid transcription factor gene NKX2-1. *Chest*, *144*(3), 794–804.
15. Kremer, T. M., Lindsay, M. E., Kinane, T. B., Hawley, M. H., Little, B. P., & Mino-Kenudson, M. (2019). Case 28-2019: A 22-year-old woman with dyspnea and chest pain. *New England Journal of Medicine*, *381*(11), 1059–1067.
16. Kröner, C., Reu, S., Teusch, V., et al. (2015). Genotype alone does not predict the clinical course of SFTPC deficiency in pediatric patients. *European Respiratory Journal*, *46*(1), 197–206.
17. Kröner, C., Wittmann, T., Reu, S., et al. (2017). Lung disease caused by ABCA3 mutations. *Thorax*, *72*(3), 213–220.
18. Liszewski, M. C., Stanescu, A. L., Phillips, G. S., & Lee, E. Y. (2017). Respiratory distress in neonates: Underlying causes and current imaging assessment. *Radiologic Clinics of North America*, *55*(4), 629–644.
19. Middleton, P. G., Mall, M. A., Dřevínek, P., et al. (2019). Elexacaftor-tezacaftor-ivacaftor for cystic fibrosis with a single Phe508del allele. *New England Journal of Medicine*, *381*(19), 1809–1819.
20. Milliron, B., Henry, T. S., Veeraraghavan, S., & Little, B. P. (2015). Bronchiectasis: Mechanisms and imaging clues of associated common and uncommon diseases. *Radiographics*, *35*(4), 1011–1030.
21. Nathan, N., Borensztajn, K., & Clement, A. (2018). Genetic causes and clinical management of pediatric interstitial lung diseases. *Current Opinion in Pulmonary Medicine*, *24*(3), 253–259.
22. Nattes, E., Lejeune, S., Carsin, A., et al. (2017). Heterogeneity of lung disease associated with NK2 homeobox 1 mutations. *Respiratory Medicine*, *129*, 16–23.
23. Nettore, I. C., Mirra, P., Ferrara, A. M., et al. (2013). Identification and functional characterization of a novel mutation in the NKX2-1 gene: Comparison with the data in the literature. *Thyroid*, *23*(6), 675–682.
24. Nevel, R. J., Garnett, E. T., Worrell, J. A., et al. (2016). Persistent lung disease in adults with NKX2.1 mutation and familial neuroendocrine cell hyperplasia of infancy. *Annals of the American Thoracic Society*, *13*(8), 1299–1304.
25. Pelizzo, G., Collura, M., Puglisi, A., et al. (2019). Congenital emphysematous lung disease associated with a novel filamin A mutation: Case report and literature review. *BMC Pediatrics*, *19*(1), 86.
26. Ren, C. L., Morgan, R. L., Oermann, C., et al. (2018). Cystic fibrosis foundation pulmonary guidelines: Use of cystic fibrosis transmembrane conductance regulator modulator therapy in patients with cystic fibrosis. *Annals of the American Thoracic Society*, *15*(3), 271–280.
27. Schafer, J., Griese, M., Chandrasekaran, R., Chotirmall, S. H., & Hartl, D. (2018). Pathogenesis, imaging, and clinical characteristics of CF and non-CF bronchiectasis. *BMC Pulmonary Medicine*, *18*(1), 79.

28. Thurm, T., Kaltenborn, E., Kern, S., Griese, M., & Zarbock, R. (2013). SFTPC mutations cause sp-c degradation and aggregate formation without increasing ER stress. *European Journal of Clinical Investigation*, *43*(8), 791–800.

29. Trapnell, B. C., Whitsett, J. A., & Nakata, K. (2003). Pulmonary alveolar proteinosis. *New England Journal of Medicine*, *349*(26), 2527–2539.

30. Turcu, S., Ashton, E., Jenkins, L., Gupta, A., & Mok, Q. (2013). Genetic testing in children with surfactant dysfunction. *Archives of Disease in Childhood*, *98*(7), 490–495.

31. Whitsett, J. A., Wert, S. E., & Weaver, T. E. (2015). Diseases of pulmonary surfactant homeostasis. *Annual Review of Pathology*, *10*, 371–393.

32. Willemsen, M. A., Breedveld, G. J., Wouda, S., et al. (2005). Brain-thyroid-lung syndrome: A patient with a severe multi-system disorder due to a de novo mutation in the thyroid transcription factor 1 gene. *European Journal of Pediatrics*, *164*(1), 28–30.

33. Young, L. R., Deutsch, G. H., Bokulic, R. E., Brody, A. S., & Nogee, L. M. (2013). A mutation in TTF1/NKX2.1 is associated with familial neuroendocrine cell hyperplasia of infancy. *Chest*, *144*(4), 1199–1206.

34. Zeitlin, P. L. (2000). Pharmacologic restoration of delta F508 CFTR-mediated chloride current. *Kidney International*, *57*(3), 832–837.

35. Zvereff, V. V., Faruki, H., Edwards, M., & Friedman, K. J. (2014). Cystic fibrosis carrier screening in a North American population. *Genetics in Medicine*, *16*(7), 539–546.

Chapter

9

LUNG DISEASE ASSOCIATED WITH SYSTEMIC DISORDERS

Contents

Introduction

A collection of respiratory conditions known as lung diseases associated with systemic disorders are linked to underlying systemic or whole-body diseases. These illnesses cover a wide range of ailments that either directly or indirectly affect the lungs, from metabolic syndromes to autoimmune diseases. It is necessary to comprehend both the pulmonary pathology and the systemic mechanisms that cause or exacerbate lung involvement to comprehend these diseases. The main systemic disorders linked to lung manifestations are autoimmune diseases, such as scleroderma, rheumatoid arthritis, and systemic lupus erythematosus (SLE). Under these circumstances, the immune system of the body inadvertently targets healthy tissues, causing inflammation and harm to multiple organs, including the lungs. The lung tissue fibrosis and inflammation that characterize interstitial lung disease (ILD) are frequently caused by autoimmune disorders. It may cause the lungs to gradually scar, which would make it harder for them to function normally and cause symptoms like coughing and shortness of breath.

Apart from autoimmune diseases, another category of systemic disorders that can impact the lungs are systemic vasculitis syndromes. Vasculitis is characterized by inflammation of all blood vessels in the body, including the lungs. Respiratory symptoms such as cough, hemoptysis (coughing up blood), and pulmonary infiltrates can result from conditions like granulomatosis with polyangiitis (GPA) and eosinophilic granulomatosis with polyangiitis (EGPA), which can cause pulmonary vasculitis. Lung problems are also linked to metabolic syndromes like obesity and diabetes mellitus. For example, diabetes can exacerbate lung function, put a person at risk for respiratory infections, and raise the possibility of developing asthma and chronic obstructive pulmonary disease (COPD). Similarly, excess adipose tissue reduces lung volumes, which is a mechanical factor in obesity. It also causes systemic inflammation, which aggravates respiratory conditions like obstructive sleep apnea (OSA) and asthma.

Sarcoidosis is one example of a systemic disease that affects the connective tissue and can have a significant impact on lung health. The development of granulomas, or tiny inflammatory nodules, in many organs, including the lungs, is a hallmark of sarcoidosis. These granulomas can cause complications like pulmonary fibrosis and restrictive lung disease in addition to respiratory symptoms like cough, chest pain, and dyspnea (difficulty breathing). Liver disorders can also affect pulmonary function, especially those that result in portal hypertension. Hepatopulmonary syndrome (HPS) and portopulmonary hypertension (PPH) are disorders that can arise from portal hypertension, which is frequently observed in diseases such as cirrhosis. While HPS is characterized by abnormal gas exchange due to dilated pulmonary vessels, resulting in hypoxemia (low blood oxygen levels), PPH is associated with increased blood pressure in the pulmonary arteries, causing symptoms like dyspnea and fatigue.

Orientation and Directional Terms

Term	Definition	Illustration
Interstitial lung disease	An umbrella term used for a large group of diseases that cause scarring (fibrosis) of the lungs. The scarring causes stiffness in the lungs which makes it difficult to breathe and get oxygen to the bloodstream.	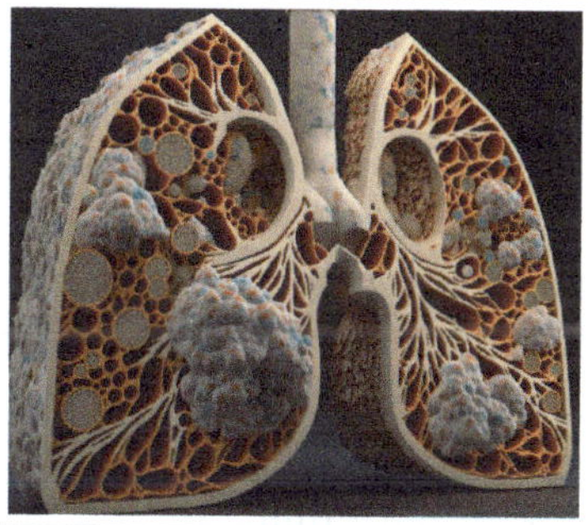
Portopulmonary hypertension	Portopulmonary hypertension is defined by the coexistence of portal and pulmonary hypertension. PPH is a serious complication of liver disease, present in 0.25 to 4% of all patients with cirrhosis.	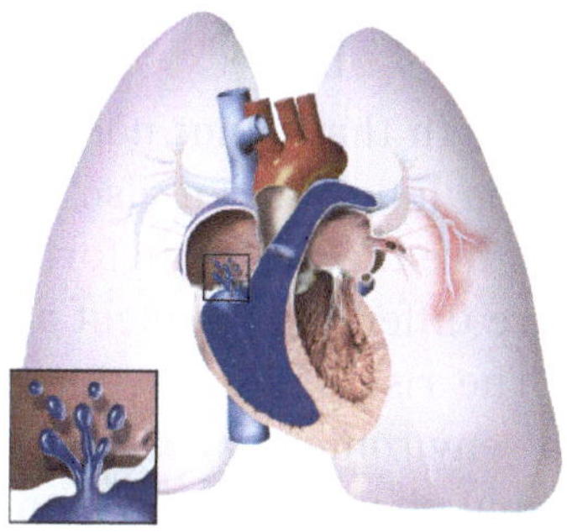
Endocrine disorders	Encompass a wide range of conditions that affect the endocrine system, which consists of glands that produce hormones responsible for regulating various bodily functions. These disorders can disrupt hormone production, secretion, or action, leading to a multitude of symptoms and complications.	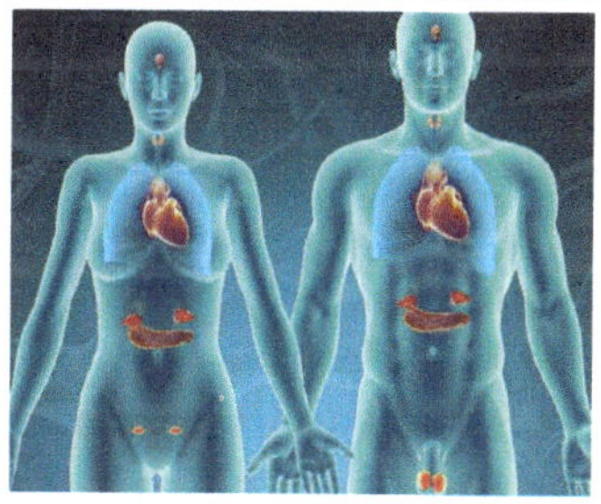
Drug therapy	Defined as medical treatment that utilizes one or more pharmaceutical drugs to improve ongoing symptoms, treat the underlying condition, or act as prevention for other diseases.	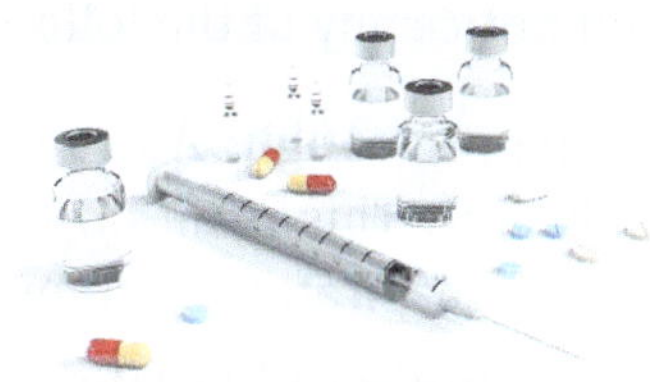
Cystic fibrosis	An inherited disorder that causes severe damage to the lungs, digestive system and other organs in the body.	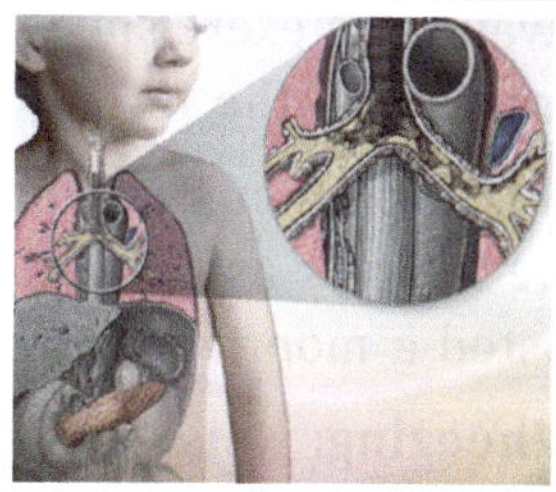

9.1. Lung Disease

The term "lung disease" covers a wide range of illnesses or conditions that impair lung function. Both pulmonary function, or how well the lungs function, and respiratory function, or the capacity to breathe, can be impacted by lung disease. Lung diseases come in a wide variety, and some of them are brought on by fungal, viral, or bacterial infections. Lung diseases such as lung cancer, mesothelioma, and asthma are linked to environmental factors. Emphysema, chronic bronchitis, and chronic obstructive pulmonary disease (COPD) are among the conditions collectively referred to as chronic lower respiratory diseases. In the US, the collective term for chronic lower respiratory diseases is the primary cause of death. Airway narrowing or blockage is a contributing factor to respiratory diseases like asthma and COPD, which decrease airflow. The lungs' capacity to hold air is diminished in other lung diseases like pneumonia, a bacterial or viral infection that causes air sacs to fill with fluid, and pulmonary fibrosis, a scarring of the lung tissue that can be brought on by a variety of factors.

Cell growth that is not normal is the cause of lung cancer. Even though lung cancer typically begins in the lungs, it can also spread to other parts of the body. Small cell and non-small cell lung cancer are the two main forms, and each has a unique growth and dissemination pattern that may require different treatment approaches. The primary cause of lung cancer overall is cigarette smoking. The risk of contracting the illness can also rise from breathing in secondhand smoke. Additional environmental factors associated with lung disease include air pollution, radon gas, asbestos, and chemicals like arsenic, vinyl chloride, beryllium, and uranium.

9.1.1. Warning Signs

Even though a minor cough or wheeze may not seem like much during our hectic days, it is vital to take notice of any symptoms, no matter how minor. Some people mistakenly believe that breathing difficulties are a natural part of aging. These symptoms should be closely monitored, as they may indicate the onset of lung diseases such as COPD, asthma, and lung cancer. It can be beneficial to recognize the early indicators of lung disease so that you can start treatment before the condition worsens or even becomes life-threatening. Schedule a visit with your healthcare provider right away if you notice any of the following warning indicators. Early identification might prevent death.

- **Chronic cough:** A cough that you have had for eight weeks or longer is considered chronic. This is an important early symptom that tells you something is wrong with your respiratory system.
- **Shortness of breath:** It's not normal to experience shortness of breath that doesn't go away after exercising, or that you have after little or no exertion. Labored or difficult breathing—the feeling that it is hard to breathe in out—is also a warning sign.
- **Chronic mucus production:** Mucus, also called sputum or phlegm, is produced by the airways as a defense against infections or irritants. If your mucus production has lasted a month or longer, this could indicate lung disease.
- **Wheezing:** Noisy breathing or wheezing is a sign that something unusual is blocking your lungs' airways or making them too narrow.
- **Coughing up blood:** If you are coughing up blood, it may be coming from your lungs

or upper respiratory tract. Wherever it's coming from, it signals a health problem.

- **Chronic chest pain:** Unexplained chest pain that lasts for a month or more—especially if it gets worse when you breathe in or cough—also is a warning sign.

Prepare for a visit to your healthcare provider by following these steps:

- Take a copy of your medical records with you. Or, see if your previous healthcare provider can send a copy. If you are unable to obtain your medical records, you can also write a short note about your health problems, when they occurred and the healthcare provider(s) that took care of you.
- Make a list of all the medicines that you are using now. This means prescribed and over-the-counter medicines, as well as herbs and supplements and any non-traditional methods you use to treat your condition.
- Make a list of all the healthcare providers you see and why you see them.
- Make a list of the symptoms you are having and note which ones bother you the most. Write down when they started and what you have done (if anything) to make them better.

9.1.2. Lung Diseases Affecting the Airways

Among the most prevalent medical conditions worldwide are lung diseases. The United States has tens of millions of lung disease sufferers. Most lung diseases are caused by genes, smoking, and infections. As a component of an intricate system, your lungs expand and contract thousands of times a day to take in oxygen and expel carbon dioxide. Any issue with any component of this system can lead to lung disease. The trachea, your windpipe, divides into bronchi, which are smaller tubes that spread throughout your lungs. These airways can be affected by the following diseases:

- **Asthma.** Your airways are constantly inflamed and may spasm, causing wheezing and shortness of breath. Allergies, infections, or pollution can trigger asthma symptoms.
- **Chronic obstructive pulmonary disease (COPD).** With this lung condition, you can't exhale the way you usually would, which causes trouble breathing.
- **Chronic bronchitis.** This form of COPD brings a long-term wet cough.
- **Emphysema.** Lung damage allows air to be trapped in your lungs in this form of COPD. Trouble blowing air out is its hallmark.
- **Acute bronchitis.** This sudden infection of your airways is usually caused by a virus.
- **Cystic fibrosis.** With this condition, you have trouble clearing mucus out of your bronchi. This leads to repeated lung infections.

9.1.3. Lung Diseases Affecting the Air Sacs (Alveoli)

Your airways branch into tiny tubes (bronchioles) that end in clusters of air sacs called alveoli. These air sacs make up most of your lung tissue. Lung diseases affecting your alveoli include:

- **Pneumonia.** An infection of your

alveoli, usually by bacteria or viruses, including the coronavirus that causes COVID-19.

- **Tuberculosis** Pneumonia that slowly gets worse, caused by the bacteria *Mycobacterium tuberculosis.*
- **Emphysema.** This happens when the fragile links between alveoli are damaged. Smoking is the usual cause. (Emphysema also limits airflow, affecting your airways).
- **Pulmonary edema.** Fluid leaks out of the small blood vessels of your lung into the air sacs and the area around them. One form is caused by heart failure and back pressure in your lungs' blood vessels. In another form, injury to your lung causes the leak of fluid.
- **Lung cancer.** It has many forms and may start in any part of your lungs. It most often happens in the main part of your lung, in or near the air sacs.
- **Acute respiratory distress syndrome (ARDS).** This is a severe, sudden injury to the lungs from a serious illness. COVID-19 is one example. Many people who have ARDS need help breathing from a machine called a ventilator until their lungs recover.
- **Pneumoconiosis.** This is a category of conditions caused by inhaling something that injures your lungs. Examples include black lung disease from coal dust and asbestosis from asbestos dust (Oppedal et al., 2007; Laghi et al., 2009; Spagnolo et al., 2015; Dursunoglu et al., 2016; Farag, 2017).

9.1.4. Lung Diseases Affecting the Interstitium

The interstitium is the thin, delicate lining between your alveoli. Tiny blood vessels run through the interstitium and let gas transfer between the alveoli and your blood. Various lung diseases affect the interstitium:

- **Interstitial lung disease (ILD).** This is a group of lung conditions that includes sarcoidosis, idiopathic pulmonary fibrosis, and autoimmune disease.
- **Pneumonia** and **pulmonary edema** can also affect your interstitium.

9.1.5. Lung Diseases Affecting Blood Vessels

The right side of your heart gets low-oxygen blood from your veins. It pumps blood into your lungs through the pulmonary arteries. These blood vessels can have diseases, as well.

- **Pulmonary embolism(PE).** A blood clot breaks off, travels to your heart, and is pumped into your lungs. This condition is known as deep vein thrombosis and typically occurs in a deep leg vein. Low blood oxygen levels and shortness of breath are frequently the results of the clot becoming lodged in a pulmonary artery.
- **Pulmonary hypertension.** Your pulmonary arteries can become hypertensive due to a variety of medical conditions. Chest pain and dyspnea may result from this. Your doctor will refer to it as idiopathic pulmonary arterial hypertension if they are unable to identify the cause.

9.1.6. Lung Diseases Affecting the Pleura

The thin lining that lines the inside of your chest wall and encircles your lung is called the pleura. With every breath, a thin film of fluid allows the pleura on the surface of your lung to move along the chest wall. Pleural lung diseases include:

- **Pleural effusion.** The area between your lung and chest wall becomes clogged with fluid. Usually, this is brought on by heart failure or pneumonia. Breathing difficulties may arise from large pleural effusions, which may require draining.
- **Pneumothorax.** Air may get into the space between your chest wall and the lung, collapsing the lung.
- **Mesothelioma.** This is a rare form of cancer that forms on the pleura. Mesothelioma tends to happen several decades after you come into contact with asbestos.

9.1.7. Lung Diseases Affecting the Chest Wall

Breathing also heavily relies on your chest wall. Your chest expands because of the muscles that hold your ribs together. With every breath, your diaphragm descends and your chest expands. Conditions that impact your chest wall consist of:

- **Obesity hypoventilation syndrome.** Extra weight on your chest and belly can make it hard for your chest to expand. This may cause serious breathing problems.
- **Neuromuscular disorders.** When the nerves that regulate your respiratory muscles malfunction, it can be difficult for you to breathe.

Neuromuscular lung diseases include myasthenia gravis and amyotrophic lateral sclerosis.

9.2. Pulmonary Complications of Endocrine Diseases

Common endocrine disorders can have a range of effects on the respiratory system, including upper airway compression in patients with goiter and an increased risk of certain infections in patients with diabetes. Numerous studies on the pulmonary physiology of patients with endocrine disorders have been conducted, and some of these studies have identified functional abnormalities that are clinically significant. Physiologic abnormalities have contributed to our understanding of lung parenchymal growth and development, response to extrathoracic influences, and possibly even aging, but in other studies, they have not translated into clinical dysfunction.

9.2.1. Diabetes Mellitus

Diabetes is becoming more and more common; in 2012, 29.8 million Americans, or 9.3% of the population, had the disease. The significant rise in type 2 diabetes prevalence in recent decades—the most prevalent subtype of diabetes mellitus—seems to have been primarily caused by the obesity epidemic. Insulin resistance and type 2 diabetes are linked to active cigarette smoking in addition to genetic predisposition, obesity, and other variables like diet and inflammatory mediators. Although pancreatic islet cells express nicotinic acetylcholine receptors, and nicotine exposure has been linked to increased beta cell apoptosis and beta cell dysfunction, the exact mechanism underlying this association remains to be determined. The incidence of type 1 diabetes mellitus has increased both globally and in the United States, albeit less dramatically. In genetically predisposed individuals, type 1 diabetes is caused by the autoimmune destruction of pancreatic beta cells, which is most likely brought on by environmental factors. Now that the genetic basis of autoimmune type 1 diabetes has been largely established, certain genetic associations with traits associated with atopy have been identified.

It's unclear how diabetes and asthma are related. Since the 1990s, the prevalence of common, complex disorders like obesity, diabetes, and asthma among young people has increased. In a large observational trial, the prevalence of asthma varied by race/ethnicity, with 10% of youth with type 1 diabetes under 20 years old and 16 points 1% of youth with type 2 diabetes having the condition. Particularly in the group with type 1 diabetes, young people with asthma were more likely to have higher body mass index (BMI) values and worse glycemic control. More than 90% of the type 2 diabetes group was overweight or obese, which could explain why there was no correlation between BMI and asthma in this group. The Framingham Heart Study's Offspring Cohort found no link between diabetes diagnosis and chronic obstructive pulmonary disease (COPD), nor did diabetes appear to hasten the disease's onset in smokers. Nonetheless, comorbid conditions, such as diabetes mellitus, are highly prevalent in patients hospitalized for COPD exacerbations; in a large multicenter study, 35.7% of patients hospitalized for COPD had diabetes. With the caveat that diabetes mellitus prevalence increases with age, the use of inhaled corticosteroids was linked to an increased risk of needing initial drug therapy for diabetes and an increased risk of requiring insulin in patients previously treated with oral antidiabetics over the 5-year observation period in a large population-based cohort study involving over 350,000 patients with COPD or asthma. Inhaled corticosteroids are a mainstay of treatment for asthma, but they should only be prescribed when absolutely necessary for patients with COPD who have more severe disease or frequent exacerbations.

Table 9.1. *Potential Mechanisms of the Links Between COPD and T2DM*

Obesity that is associated with increased adipose and systemic inflammation and reduced insulin sensitivity. Cigarette smoke that directly impairs insulin action and reduces peripheral glucose uptake. Oxidative stress from both environmental and cellular sources that promotes insulin resistance and alters energy production. Decrease in endogenous antioxidants. Lung inflammation that induces insulin resistance by blocking signaling through the insulin receptor of proinflammatory cytokines. Chronic low-grade inflammation. Activation of the innate immune system. Impaired adaptive responses to hypoxia due to insufficient activation of hypoxia-inducible factors signaling. Low lung function values that have a higher risk of developing insulin resistance. High glucose concentrations that increase the responsiveness of ASM to contractile agents. Microangiopathy of lung vasculature. Glucotoxicity that activates nonenzymatic glycosylation of lung collagen and elastin by AGEs resulting in reduced lung elasticity. Insulin that induces ASM contraction.

AGEs, advanced glycosylation end products; ASM, airway smooth muscle.

Source: Cazzola M, Rogliani P, Ora J, Calzetta L, Lauro D, Matera MG. Hyperglycaemia and Chronic Obstructive Pulmonary Disease. Diagnostics. 2023; 13(21):3362. https://doi.org/10.3390/diagnostics13213362.

Regarding the results regarding pulmonary function, a meta-analysis that included information from over 3000 individuals who had never had pulmonary disease before discovered that having diabetes was linked to a mild to moderate impairment in pulmonary function (Table 9.1). The pattern was restrictive, with a slight reduction in carbon monoxide diffusing capacity, and it held true regardless of BMI, smoking status, length of diabetes, or HbA1c levels. Sub analyses revealed that type 2 diabetes showed a stronger correlation than type 1 diabetes. These mild functional abnormalities, which are typically well within 80% of the reference value, have been linked to early lung aging in a manner akin to the development of microangiopathic changes and nonenzymatic protein glycosylation in many affected organs in diabetes patients. In conclusion, routine pulmonary function testing in patients with diabetes is not necessary because diabetes mellitus (in the absence of cystic fibrosis) does not appear to cause clinically significant pulmonary impairment, although it may cause a mild decline in pulmonary function measurements.

Patients with diabetes associated with cystic fibrosis had higher rates of treatment failure and pulmonary infection with multiple antibiotic-resistant Pseudomonas aeruginosa than patients with cystic fibrosis alone. Because research results have been inconsistent, it is unclear whether diabetes related to cystic fibrosis is linked to a higher rate of decline in pulmonary function when compared to cystic fibrosis subjects without diabetes. Diabetes's chronic metabolic disturbances lead to the development of cardiovascular and end-organ dysfunction in many of its patients. In patients with diabetes, cardiovascular factors seem to be more responsible for reduced physical performance than pulmonary factors. Patients with diabetes not only have a higher risk of cardiovascular events, but they also experience heart failure more frequently, for reasons unrelated to high blood pressure or coronary artery disease. Patients with insulin-dependent diabetes appear to have a higher incidence of left ventricular systolic and diastolic dysfunction with exercise than do people without the disease. Furthermore, patients with diabetes are more likely to experience pleural effusions and exercise limitation in comparison to patients with comparable levels of left ventricular dysfunction. Type 2 diabetes is more likely to develop in people who actively smoke cigarettes. In terms of lowering one's risk for a wide range of complications, including cardiovascular events, quitting smoking has significant health benefits. However, quitting smoking often results in weight gain—4 to 5 kg in the first year following cessation. Subjects who had recently stopped smoking had more significant increases in weight, waist circumference, and fasting glucose levels, as well as a higher risk of developing type 2 diabetes, compared to those who had never smoked in a large prospective multisite cohort study of individuals without diabetes at baseline. The greater risk for diabetes peaked three years after quitting, and these metabolic alterations were more prevalent in older men who had smoked heavily before quitting. Patients who stopped smoking saw a decrease in overall cardiovascular events even though they gained weight after quitting. In conclusion, there is a correlation between an elevated risk for type 2 diabetes and both active smoking and the post-cessation period. For patients who are at higher risk, it may be necessary to target the immediate post-quit period with more aggressive weight management and lifestyle modifications. One complication of diabetic ketoacidosis that has been documented is acute respiratory distress syndrome (ARDS). However, compared to patients without diabetes, diabetes mellitus—apart from diabetic ketoacidosis—is not linked to an increased risk of developing ARDS and may even be protective. Idiopathic pulmonary fibrosis has been linked to an increased risk of developing in people with diabetes.

Macrosomia and preterm delivery are risks that newborns of diabetic mothers face; the greatest risk is associated with mothers who do not take good care of themselves. Nonetheless, the majority of diabetic pregnant women can deliver their babies at or near term without experiencing the related respiratory distress syndrome if they have adequate maternal metabolic control and precise gestational age estimates. Obesity increases the risk of developing type 2 diabetes and obstructive sleep apnea. According to reports, the prevalence of obstructive sleep apnea in patients with type 2 diabetes ranges from 23 to 36%, and it can reach up to 70% in those with a BMI of more than 35 kg/m2. In diabetic patients with obstructive sleep apnea, higher apnea-hypopnea indices are linked to worse glucose regulation. Furthermore, oxygen desaturation is specifically linked to insulin resistance in patients who are extremely obese. Obstructive sleep apnea may also impose stress that increases sympathetic neural output during sleep, which in turn contributes to insulin resistance. Obstructive sleep apnea may raise the risk of diabetic peripheral neuropathy in diabetic patients, possibly as a result of elevated oxidative stress and compromised microvascular control. In the short term at least, weight loss may be necessary for continuous positive airway pressure therapy to improve metabolic control in diabetic patients with obstructive sleep apnea.

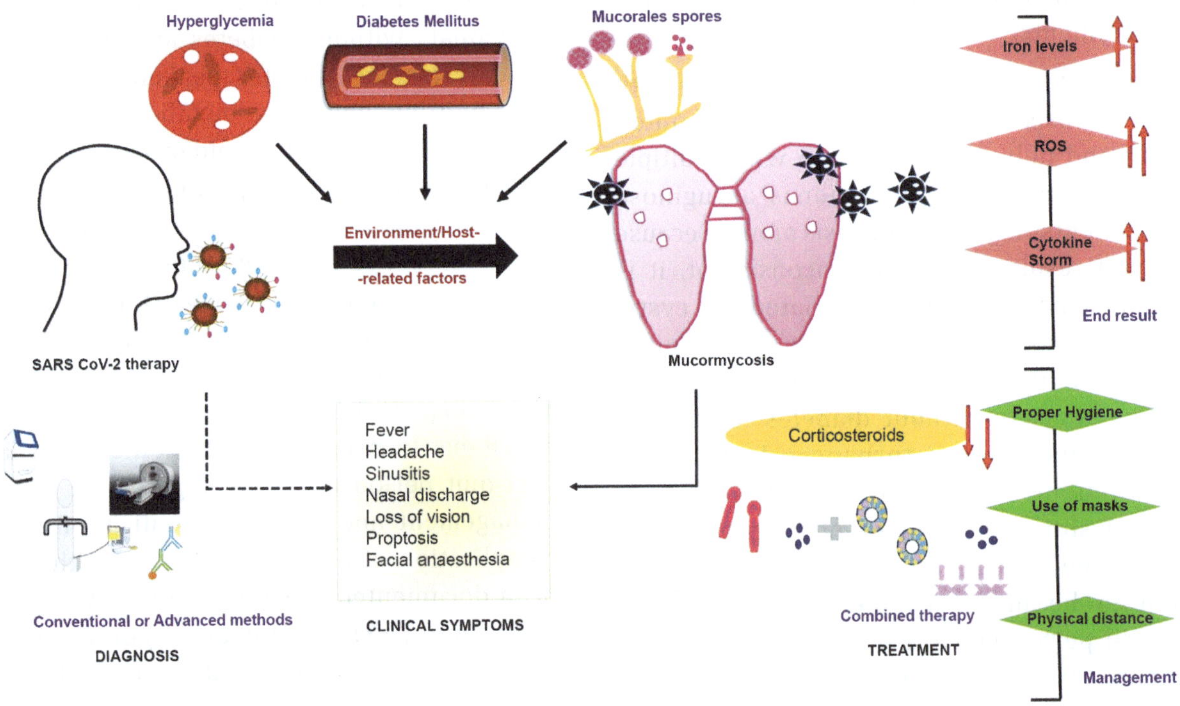

Figure 9.1. *Mucormycosis.*

Source: Girdhar D, Manocha E. A Comprehensive Review on the Management of COVID-19-Associated Mucormycosis (CAM): The New Basics. BioMed. 2022; 2(2):181-198. https://doi.org/10.3390/biomed2020017.

Similar to invasive aspergillosis, pulmonary mucormycosis is primarily observed in patients receiving organ transplants, hematologic malignancies, diabetes, or glucocorticoid or deferoxamine therapy. Mold spores inhaled can cause thrombosis and ischemia by penetrating bronchiole walls and invading arterioles (Figure 9.1). Fever, pleuritic chest pain, and nonspecific cough appear. One-fourth of cases may develop hemoptysis, which can be quite severe. Consolidation is the most typical pattern on chest radiographs; cavitation is observed in approximately one-third of cases; adenopathy and pleural effusions are less common but may also occur. Diabetes patients seem to be more susceptible to endobronchial disease; however, sputum culture seems to have a very low diagnostic yield. Histopathologic examination seems to be more sensitive than fungal cultures for specimens taken during bronchoscopy. Antifungal medication and, if localized, surgical resection are necessary for treatment. One possible consequence is bronchial stenosis.

Drug-sensitive and multidrug-resistant tuberculosis is associated with diabetes mellitus as an independent risk factor. Studies on diabetic adults in Brazil and children in South Africa have supported the association between diabetes mellitus and an increased risk of tuberculosis (relative risk, 3.11; 95% CI 2.27–4.26) which was found after a review of 13 observational studies. In comparison to patients with tuberculosis alone, those with diabetes and tuberculosis tended to be older, had a higher death rate, and were more likely to produce positive smears for acid-fast bacteria. The tuberculosis radiographic site in diabetes. Patients with diabetes and tuberculosis seem to have a higher rate of cavitation; the case series determines the lobe predilection (upper or lower). Currently, treating latent tuberculosis in diabetic patients who have a positive purified protein derivative skin test with more than 10 mm of induration or a positive interferon-gamma release assay is advised.

Patients with diabetes may or may not experience bacterial pneumonia more frequently. In a study involving over 4000 senior citizens in a single township, diabetes mellitus was not found to be a separate risk factor for pneumonia acquired in the community. The results of studies on whether diabetes predicts a worse prognosis for people who develop pneumonia are conflicting. It doesn't seem that diabetes is a separate risk factor for ventilator-associated pneumonia or pneumonia linked to medical care. Almost everyone with diabetes should receive a pneumococcal vaccination due to the vaccine's proven effectiveness and the rising incidence of penicillin resistance in pneumococcal strains. Diabetes is linked to a high mortality rate among those who contract Legionella pneumonia and appears to be a risk factor for the illness. Aspiration pneumonia may be more likely in individuals with diabetes due to pharyngeal dysfunction and diabetic gastroparesis. Diabetes raises the risk of periodontitis and caries, two chronic oral infections that can increase the risk of aspiration pneumonia. During seasonal influenza outbreaks, there is a higher risk of bacterial pneumonia and the corresponding death in patients with diabetes. For patients with diabetes who are older than six months old, influenza vaccination is advised following the guidelines set forth by the Advisory Committee on Immunization Practices. About 60% of patients with documented diabetes have received yearly influenza vaccinations, but only 49% have reached the recommended level of pneumococcal vaccination. Preexisting diabetes has been linked to a higher death rate in patients with severe acute respiratory syndrome, similar to other pathogens.

9.2.2. Thyroid Disorders

Although the routine use of iodized salt is reducing the incidence of multinodular goiter in the United States, neglected goiters are still found. Even massive goiters may not result in tracheal impingement because of the thyroid's ease of expansion in the anterior space, where it is only constrained by skin, thin muscle, and connective tissue. But certain goiters can also result in airway compression, tracheal deviation, unilateral or uneven lobe enlargement, wheezing, coughing, and dyspnea. Should the goiter extend posteriorly to the trachea, the likelihood of compression or concentric narrowing of the trachea increases (Figure 9.2). Sometimes patients present with acute respiratory distress, necessitating urgent intubation or semiurgent surgery, even though goiters usually grow slowly.

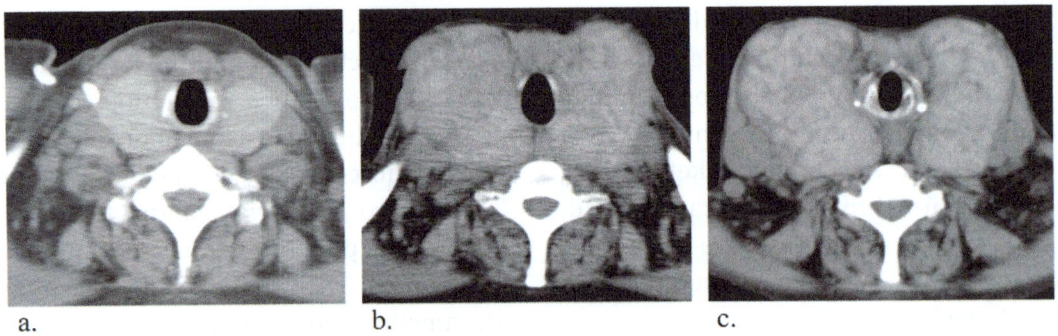

Figure 9.2. *Thyroid goiter. Computed tomography imaging course of thyroid gland enlargement. (**a**) At 45 years of age. (**b**) At 52 years of age. (**c**) At 54 years of age. The thyroid gland gradually was enlarged.*

Source: Nishiura K, Nakazato K, Yokokawa T, Suzuki Y, Kurosawa Y, Wada K, Shimizu T, Oikawa M, Kobayashi A, Sugimoto K, et al. A Case of Giant Goiter Associated with Airway Stenosis Caused by Long-Term Intravenous Epoprostenol Therapy for Idiopathic Pulmonary Arterial Hypertension. Journal of Clinical Medicine. 2023; 12(19):6359. https://doi.org/10.3390/jcm12196359.

Some goiters are substernal and/or intrathoracic. There is variability in the definition of "intrathoracic goiter"; most experts concur that some portion of the goiter is permanently retrosternal (below the sternal notch), even when the neck is retroflexed. Bulky and/or substernal goiters may cause orthopnea because of airflow limitation in the supine position. In these patients, flow-volume loops in the recumbent position may demonstrate upper airway obstruction not apparent in upright testing. CT scanning and magnetic resonance imaging generally are the most useful diagnostic imaging studies and can estimate the degree of tracheal compression.

Specifically, because it can cause hyperthyroidism and prevent thyroid nuclear imaging for several weeks, CT scanning with iodinated contrast media should generally be avoided. Compressive symptoms are typically relieved by surgically resecting substernal goiters. It seems that postoperative tracheomalacia is uncommon. For certain patients with large goiters, such as those with intrathoracic extension who are not candidates for surgery due to comorbid conditions, iodine-131 is an alternate treatment option. In the week after treatment, patients with baseline tracheal compression frequently experience additional airway compromise and transient goiter enlargement due to edema. Nevertheless, most patients respond well to glucocorticoid prophylaxis and experience goiter shrinkage as a result. As an alternative, compressive benign or malignant nonoperable thyroid disease can cause significant airway obstruction that can be relieved by bronchoscopic tracheal stent insertion. Obstructive sleep apnea can also be brought on by large, multinodular goiters with retrolaryngopharyngeal extension, and this condition can resolve following a thyroidectomy. One percent of all newly diagnosed cancers is thyroid carcinoma, of which papillary thyroid carcinoma is the most prevalent type. 10 to 15% of these will go on to form metastases, the majority of which are located in the thoracic cavity. Larger nodules, a miliary pattern of metastases, and even localized pulmonary opacities are visible (Figure 9.3). Dyspnea may or may not be present, depending on the lung cancer burden. The trachea may also be directly invaded by thyroid cancer. Resection associated with tracheal reconstruction has proven successful in patients who are otherwise excellent candidates for surgery.

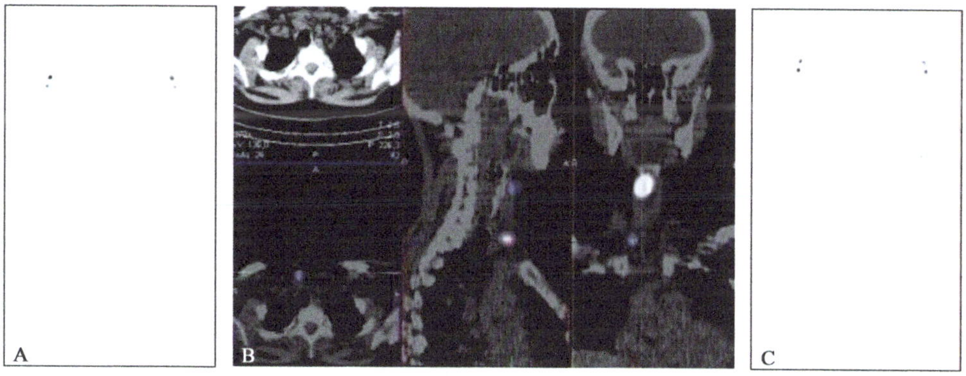

Figure 9.3. *40 years old female, with multifocal papillary microcarcinoma (left lobe 7 mm and 2 foci of 1 mm in the right lobe (pT1a(m)N0). TSH 67.83 mIU/L, Tg 11.83 μg/L (<2 μg/L), and TgA 2.2 kIU/L (<4.5 kIU/L). Diagnostic WBS and SPECT/CT (A, B) performed after application of 74 MBq of [^{131}I] show two focuses of [^{131}I] uptake—larger in the right upper part of the region VI and small focus lower in the region VI, right paratracheal. The patient was treated with 1665 MBq (45 mCi) of [^{131}I]. Post-treatment [^{131}I] WBS (C) shows an accumulation of the [^{131}I] in the same two focuses.*

Source: Giovanella L, Deandreis D, Vrachimis A, Campenni A, Petranovic Ovcaricek P. Molecular Imaging and Theragnostics of Thyroid Cancers. Cancers. 2022; 14(5):1272. https://doi.org/10.3390/cancers14051272.

Smoking is a risk factor for hyperthyroidism, including Graves disease, toxic nodular goiter, and autoimmune hypothyroidism (Hashimoto thyroiditis), especially in women. Smoking increases the risk of Graves ophthalmopathy beyond the risk associated with hyperthyroidism alone (Oppedal et al., 2007; Laghi et al., 2009; Spagnolo et al., 2015; Dursunoglu et al., 2016; Farag, 2017).

9.2.2.1. Hyperthyroidism

Both resting and exertional dyspnea are common complaints among hyperthyroidism patients. Six percent of patients with newly diagnosed hyperthyroidism present with congestive heart failure, which likely explains some of these complaints. Some patients with hyperthyroidism have reduced vital capacity, weaker respiratory muscles, and elevated resting minute ventilation that increases with exercise (possibly because of an increased central ventilatory drive). Vital capacity and respiratory muscle strength improve with treatment, though persistent dyspnea persists in some patients. If β-blocker agents are used to control hyperthyroidism symptoms, patients with concomitant asthma and thyrotoxicosis may experience worsening asthma control. Asthma, Graves' disease, and atopic disease might all be related. Serum levels of immunoglobulin E (IgE) are elevated in about 30% of patients with hyperthyroid Graves' disease, and this subset of patients is more likely to have a personal or family history of atopy.

Many reports have indicated a connection between pulmonary hypertension and hyperthyroidism, particularly Graves' disease, where treatment for hyperthyroidism can improve or even return pulmonary artery pressures to normal. There are a few possible explanations for this association: a generalized autoimmune state; changes in the metabolism of the vasodilators and vasoconstrictors in the pulmonary vasculature; decreased production and function of surfactants; or excessive stimulation of the cardiovascular system by the sympathoadrenal system. To relieve the pulmonary vascular system of the additional burden of cardiovascular stress, hyperthyroidism must be treated. Rarely, placental transfer of maternal thyrotropin receptor-stimulating antibodies causes mothers with hyperthyroidism from Graves' disease to give birth to infants with hyperthyroidism. Newborns with neonatal Graves' disease have persistent pulmonary hypertension in addition to a range of metabolic and developmental issues. Remarkably, individuals suffering from primary pulmonary hypertension might also have a higher incidence of hypothyroidism. In addition, studies on patients with Graves disease receiving propylthiouracil have shown an increase in antinuclear cytoplasmic antibodies and even granulomatosis with polyangiitis, also known as Wegener granulomatosis. Alveolar hemorrhage and nonspecific interstitial pneumonia induced by propylthiouracil have also been documented.

9.2.2.2. Hypothyroidism

Pleural effusions, respiratory failure, obstructive, and central sleep apnea, dyspnea upon exertion, and alveolar hypoventilation have all been linked to hypothyroidism. In mixed populations of obese and nonobese hypothyroid patients, lung volumes are usually normal or slightly reduced. Weight loss and/or thyroid replacement therapy usually result in improved lung volumes, though not always. A diminished ability to diffuse carbon monoxide is observed in certain hypothyroid, non-obese individuals with normal arterial blood gases and lung volumes, which recover to almost normal following replacement medication. According to maximal inspiratory and expiratory pressures, hypothyroidism is linked to general respiratory muscle weakness. The degree of impairment is directly correlated with the degree of hypothyroidism before treatment. Diaphragmatic muscle weakness in hypothyroid patients, whether obese or not, can vary in severity from mild impairment that restricts exercise tolerance to severe dysfunction characterized by marked dyspnea at rest and persistent hypercarbia. Respiratory muscle strength can be enhanced by thyroid replacement therapy. The ventilatory response to hypoxia and hypercapnia is significantly blunted in some nonobese and obese hypothyroid patients. This often gets better within weeks of starting thyroid hormone replacement therapy. There may be a primary cause for the aberrant ventilatory response as this improvement is not correlated with alterations in maximal voluntary ventilation or spirometric function. Hypothyroidism may result in respiratory failure requiring continuous mechanical ventilation.

The majority of hypothyroidism patients also have congestive heart failure, even though up to 25% of them show radiographic signs of a pleural effusion (Figure 9.4). A tiny portion of hypothyroid patients do not have any other underlying medical conditions that could account for the effusion. The hypothyroid-related effusions in these patients are usually non-inflammatory, transudates or exudates, unilateral or bilateral, serous or serosanguineous, and small—less than one-third of the pleural space. Treatment for hypothyroidism usually resolves hypothyroid-related effusions.

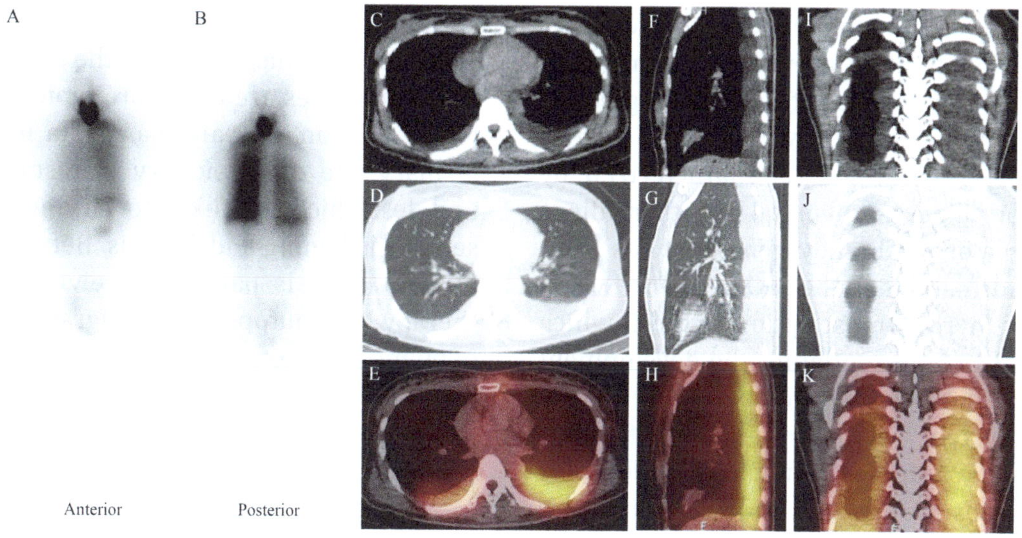

Figure 9.4. *Whole-body scan ((A), anterior view; (B), posterior view) on day 3 post ^{131}I administration, showing ^{131}I distribution in left thyroid lobe and chest. SPECT/CT images of chest ((C–E), transaxial; (F–H), sagittal; and (I–K), coronal) showing bilateral pleural effusion, predominantly in the left side. Neither abnormal uptake nor lesion was found in either lung.*

Source: Qiu X, Wang P, Sa R, Cheng L, Jin Y, Song H, Chen L. Diagnosis and Treatment of Acute Pleural Effusion following Radioiodine Remnant Ablation Post Lobectomy for Thyroid Cancer. Diagnostics. 2022; 12(12):2982. https://doi.org/10.3390/diagnostics12122982.

Patients with hypothyroidism may be at risk for developing sleep apnea due to weight gain, abnormal ventilatory control, mucopolysaccharide, and protein deposition in the tongue and oropharynx, and/or narrowing of the upper airway. Patients with sleep apnea may have neurocognitive impairment, which may be exacerbated by hypothyroidism. In a particular case series, hypothyroidism was discovered in only 31.1% of patients with obstructive sleep apnea; in contrast, obstructive sleep apnea was discovered in 25% of newly diagnosed hypothyroid patients. The strongest indicators of concomitant obstructive sleep apnea were age and body weight. The ventilatory responses to hypoxia and hypercapnia are weakened in hypothyroid patients with obstructive sleep apnea. Thyroid replacement therapy has been shown to improve the sleep respiratory disturbance index and the awake ventilatory response to hypoxia and hypercapnia in certain studies; however, in other studies, the treatment showed little to no improvement in sleep apnea. Patients with hypothyroidism may also exhibit central sleep apnea, and thyroid replacement therapy may improve the hypoxic ventilatory response.

The maturation of the lung's surfactant system and the growth and development of the lung are both significantly influenced by thyroid hormones. Prolonged hypothyroxinemia and respiratory distress syndrome are prevalent in premature babies. On the other hand, a large multicenter trial found that giving maternal antenatal thyrotropin-releasing hormone, which raises fetal thyroid hormone levels, had no effect on reducing the frequency or severity of respiratory distress syndrome in premature babies. Additionally, there was no reduction in the prevalence of respiratory distress syndrome, the need for surfactant therapy, or the overall developmental outcome at 24 months after treating premature infants with thyroxine. 119A rare type of neonatal progressive respiratory failure known as the "brain-thyroid-lung syndrome" is characterized by respiratory illness, congenital hypothyroidism, and chorea or cerebral dysgenesis. It has to do with abnormalities in the NKX2-1 gene, which codes for thyroid transcription factor-1, which is thought to be essential for the development and function of the thyroid, lungs, and central nervous system. Thyroid transcription factor-1 deficiency syndrome disrupts the production of surfactant protein-A in the lung, causing a range of symptoms from moderate to severe and ultimately fatal respiratory failure (Oppedal et al., 2007; Laghi et al., 2009; Spagnolo et al., 2015; Dursunoglu et al., 2016; Farag, 2017).

In patients with end-stage renal disease, hyperparathyroidism—typically secondary hyperparathyroidism—can result in diffuse metastatic calcification in the lungs. Whereas dystrophic calcification refers to the calcification of diseased or aberrant tissue, such as granulomatous processes, metastatic calcification is the deposition of calcium salts in previously normal tissue. Patients with renal failure are susceptible to metastatic calcification even with hemodialysis, phosphate binders, and dietary restriction. This risk is heightened when the product of calcium-phosphorus concentration rises above 70 mg^2/dL^2. In alkaline environments, precipitation of calcium salts is common. In fact, the apical regions of the lungs are more likely to experience metastatic calcification , the stomach, and the kidneys—all tissues that have a relative alkalinity as a result of excretion of hydrogen ions or removal of carbon dioxide. The estimated pH at the lung apex is 7.5, while the pH at the base is 7.3. This difference can be attributed to the lower carbon dioxide concentration and the higher ventilation-perfusion ratio at the apex. The skin and soft tissues are two more typical locations for deposition. The alveolar septa may be the primary site of pulmonary metastatic calcific nodules, which are linked to varying degrees of septal thickening and fibrosis. Between 60 and 80% of dialysis patients receiving long-term therapy have autopsy or scintigraphic evidence of pulmonary metastatic calcification, suggesting that this phenomenon is widespread.

The majority of patients with metastatic pulmonary calcification and end-stage renal disease are asymptomatic, with normal pulmonary function and chest radiographs. Patients who have a high concentration of calcific nodules, however, may experience dyspnea and a productive cough, and respiratory failure is not always a possibility. Patients with more extensive calcification usually show up radiographically as many nodules, ranging in size from 3 to 10 mm, which are easier to see on CT scans than on standard chest radiographs. Patchy consolidation and ground-glass attenuation may be observed in addition to the nodular densities. The small size of the calcium deposits may make the calcific nature of the nodules invisible on plain radiography or even CT images. Nonetheless, radionuclide bone scans typically show significant uptake in the lungs and other organs that are impacted. Patients with extensive metastatic calcification may exhibit low carbon monoxide diffusing capacity and ventilatory restriction with hypoxemia on pulmonary function tests. Reduce the calcium-phosphorus double product, reverse abnormalities in bone scans, reverse organ deposition, and potentially improve pulmonary function with parathyroidectomy or vitamin D analog treatment (Table 9.2; Figure 9.5).

Table 9.2. *Main Types of Calcification Found in Thyroid Lesions*

	Localization	Type of Lesion	Description
Microcalcification ≤1 mm			
Psammoma bodies (PBs)	Inside lymph vessels or in the papillae axis	True PBs Classical PTC	50–70 μm round-shaped, concentrically laminated, calcified concretions with a glassy appearance
Inspissated colloid calcified	Inside follicles	False PBs Benign nodules	Thick colloid (colloid crystals) can present microcalcifications over inspissated colloid and lead to focal hyperechogenic foci; can potentially be confused with PBs
Stromal microcalcification	Around follicles	False PBs	Spherical crystalline bodies with a diameter of 0.1–2.5 μm. Usually too small to be detected by light microscopy and apparently arise within basal laminae as a result of concentric deposition of calcium salts or calcifications of membrane-bound vesicles. Calcified collagen fibrils can rarely be observed.
Bone calcification	Connective tissue	False PBs	Bone formation is considered when there is both bone matrix and osteocytes in the connective tissue of a thyroid nodule, regardless of being neoplastic or not.
Macrocalcification >1 mm			
Eggshell, annular, or rim-like calcifications		Benign and malignant lesions	Annular or rim-like peripheral calcification, defined in US as curvilinear hyperechoic structures parallel to the margin of the nodule.
Coarse calcifications	Stroma	Benign and malignant lesions	An irregularly shaped focus of calcification (can comprise micro- and macrocalcifications).

Source: Ferreira LB, Gimba E, Vinagre J, Sobrinho-Simões M, Soares P. Molecular Aspects of Thyroid Calcification. International Journal of Molecular Sciences. 2020; 21(20):7718. https://doi.org/10.3390/ijms21207718.

Bronchial and pulmonary artery wall calcification is also linked to hyperparathyroidism. Notably, pulmonary hypertension affects approximately one-third of end-stage renal disease patients receiving long-term hemodialysis via arteriovenous access; however, pulmonary hypertension does not appear to be correlated with parathyroid hormone levels or the presence or severity of pulmonary artery calcification. Rarely, vocal cord impingement and hoarseness, tracheal compression with stridor, or both, can result from enlarged mediastinal parathyroid cysts. The preferred course of treatment is surgical excision. A common complication of hyperparathyroidism is fatigue and weakness in the muscles. Additionally, there may be effects on respiratory muscle function. Improvements in forced vital capacity and forced expiratory volume in one second following a parathyroidectomy be correlated with preoperative serum calcium and preoperative parathyroid hormone levels.

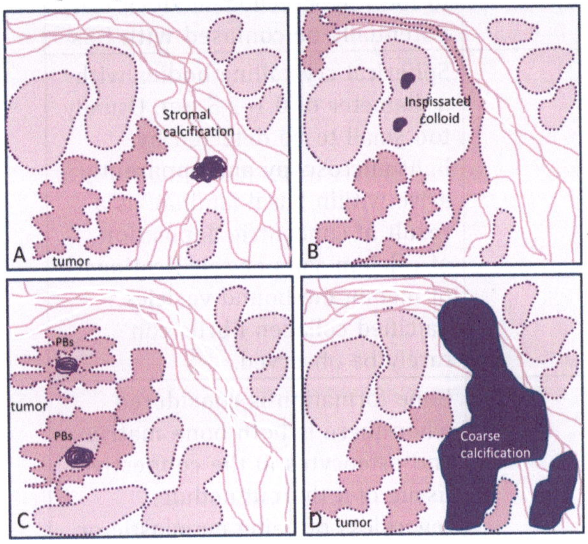

Figure 9.5. *Graphical representation of the different types of calcification in thyroid tissue sections: (A) focus of stromal calcification (in purple color) in the tumor stroma, (B) inspissated colloid calcified, (C) psammoma bodies (PBs) (in purple color) located in the papillary thyroid carcinoma present inside lymphatic vessels or in the stalk of the papillae, and (D) coarse macrocalcification (in purple color). Shapes in pink correspond to non-tumor thyroid; shapes in deeper pink correspond to tumor thyroid.*

Source: Ferreira LB, Gimba E, Vinagre J, Sobrinho-Simões M, Soares P. Molecular Aspects of Thyroid Calcification. International Journal of Molecular Sciences. 2020; 21(20):7718. https://doi.org/10.3390/ijms21207718.

Bone integrity and skeletal muscle strength can be impacted by vitamin D deficiency and metabolic bone disease, which can have a negative impact on lung function. A vitamin D deficiency has been linked, unrelated to skeletal effects, to a higher severity of asthma and a higher risk of asthma exacerbations in children. Adults with low vitamin D levels have been shown to have worsening lung function, and smokers' lung function declines more quickly. Exacerbations of COPD have not been linked to vitamin D deficiency, and taking high-dose vitamin D supplements does not prevent exacerbations of COPD in the future. Osteomalacia or rickets can result from hyperphosphatasia caused by mutations in the gene encoding the tissue-nonspecific isozyme of alkaline phosphatase. Babies with severe cases may develop a progressive chest deformity leading to fatal respiratory insufficiency. Improved results on skeletal radiographs as well as enhanced pulmonary and physical function in afflicted children are linked to enzyme replacement therapy.

9.2.3. Adrenal Diseases

Cushing syndrome endogenous (i. e, not from the administration of glucocorticoids) can be brought on by adrenal neoplasia, pituitary Cushing disease, ectopic production of adrenocorticotropic hormone from small-cell lung cancer, or carcinoids originating from a variety of organs, particularly the lung, including pulmonary carcinoid tumorlets. Compared to pituitary Cushing disease, cortisol levels are typically significantly higher in conditions involving ectopic production of adrenocorticotropic hormone and adrenal neoplasia, which increases the risk of infection. Patients with hypercortisolism are especially vulnerable to opportunistic lung infections and fungal infections of the mucocutaneous tract. The most frequent causes of lung infections are Mycobacterium tuberculosis, *Aspergillus*,

Nocardia, Pneumocystis, and Cryptococcus. *Pneumocystis jirovecii* pneumonia is more common in patients whose morning cortisol levels are particularly elevated. Reversing hypercortisolism is a crucial side effect of antibiotic treatment. A hypercoagulable state and a rise in clinically significant thromboembolic events are also linked to Cushing syndrome.

Increased stress and significantly elevated cortisol levels at presentation seem to be independent predictors of poorer outcomes in community-acquired pneumonia, even in patients without baseline hypercortisolism.

Adrenal insufficiency can result from secondary adrenal insufficiency or primary adrenal failure (Addison disease). Most frequently, hypothalamic-pituitary axis diseases or the cessation of exogenous glucocorticoid therapy are the causes of secondary adrenal insufficiency. While tuberculosis continues to be the most common cause of Addison disease in resource-poor nations, autoimmune diseases account for 70–80% of cases of the disease in industrialized nations. Since adrenal calcification can be caused by tuberculosis and histoplasmosis, CT scanning can be useful in diagnosing Addison's disease. Stressed, very low birth weight babies may exhibit adrenal insufficiency through hypothalamic-pituitary axis dysfunction, which may increase their risk of developing bronchopulmonary dysplasia.

9.2.4. Acromegaly

Adults with an excess of growth hormone secreted, known as acromegaly, typically have a benign pituitary adenoma. Excess growth hormone-releasing factor, which promotes excess growth hormone secretion, is sporadically produced by bronchial carcinoid or small-cell lung cancer. Clinically, acromegaly is characterized by coarsening of facial features, hypertrophy of soft tissues, and excessive bone growth. Growth hormone and insulin-like growth factor I (IGF-I), which is secreted in response to growth hormone, appear to be the cause of these changes; the overall effect is an increase in somatic growth and metabolic disturbances. Although controlling acromegaly can significantly reduce coronary heart disease risk factors, particularly in patients whose IGF-I levels are normalized, the primary cause of mortality in acromegaly is cardiovascular disease. Acromegaly patients may experience vocal cord constriction and edema, oropharyngeal airway narrowing, nasal polyps, and macroglossia. Furthermore, coincidental goiter is a common condition that can exacerbate upper airway narrowing. Acromegaly can cause respiratory symptoms such as vocal cord dysfunction, sleep apnea, extrathoracic airway obstruction, and challenging intubation.

It has been estimated that between 20 and 60% of people have sleep apnea. A narrowed upper airway from osseous enlargement, hypertrophy of oropharyngeal tissues, inspiratory collapse of the hypopharynx, and macroglossia may be the cause of increased rates of obstructive sleep apnea. The development of sleep apnea in acromegaly can be predicted by the circumference of the fingers and neck, but not by BMI. Acromegaly can be treated with pituitary ablation or somatostatin analogs to treat obstructive sleep apnea, although results vary greatly. It's possible that irreversible upper airway remodeling is the reason why obstructive sleep apnea persists after treatment. Furthermore typical is central sleep apnea. Compared to acromegalic patients with obstructive sleep apnea, patients with central sleep apnea and acromegaly have higher levels of growth hormone and IGF-I as well as higher ventilatory responses to carbon dioxide. Therefore, altered ventilatory control may be the cause of central sleep apnea in these patients.

When comparing patients with acromegaly to controls, total lung capacity and vital capacity are generally higher, and they seem to be correlated with the length of the acromegaly and the level of IGF-I. The hypertrophy or enlargement of a single alveolar or an increase in the total number of alveoli are two possible explanations for the increased lung volumes in these patients. The ability to diffuse carbon monoxide may be high or within normal ranges. Patients with acromegaly have a barrel chest due to changes in rib morphology and vertebrae morphology. Acromegaly also causes a decrease in respiratory muscle force, which may exacerbate dyspnea and make exercise exhausting. 30 to 50% of patients with acromegaly show evidence of variable extrathoracic airway obstruction on flow-volume loops. As mentioned, vocal cord fixation, vocal cord edema, prolapse of an enlarged tongue, and soft tissue thickening of the oropharynx may make intubation more challenging for patients with acromegaly. Somatostatin analog preoperative therapy may reduce soft tissue edema and facilitate simpler intubation (Oppedal et al., 2007; Laghi et al., 2009; Spagnolo et al., 2015; Dursunoglu et al., 2016; Farag, 2017).

9.3. Metabolic Disorders in Chronic Lung Diseases

Chronic lung diseases, such as asthma, interstitial lung diseases (ILDs), and chronic obstructive pulmonary disease (COPD), are complicated conditions that have a significant financial and medical burden in addition to a steadily rising incidence and mortality. Therefore, a thorough, individualized, multidisciplinary approach is needed for their management, which includes comorbid condition assessment. As a result of recent data supporting the involvement of endocrine system dysfunction in the pathogenesis of chronic lung diseases, physicians have included metabolic disorders in the Venn diagram of chronic lung disease comorbidities (Figure 9.6). Specifically, metabolic comorbidities have a significant effect on patients' mortality and quality of life. The metabolic comorbidities that are most frequently reported in patients with chronic lung disease are diabetes mellitus, dyslipidemia, osteoporosis, and thyroid disorders (hypothyroidism and hyperthyroidism). In respiratory diseases, there has been a growing body of scientific research on the three pillars of cellular metabolism: genes, age, and nutrition. In addition to reporting future perspectives on their role in disease management, this section aims to summarize the most common metabolic comorbidities and their impact on chronic lung diseases.

The primary metabolic comorbidities of long-term lung conditions are shown above. Chronic lung diseases serve as models for how harmful environmental factors and genetic predisposition interact. In patients with chronic obstructive lung diseases, insulin resistance may result from the release of reactive oxygen species and pro-inflammatory mediators (IL1, 6, TNFa, NF-κB, leptin, adiponectin, and resistin) into the bloodstream. Long-term exogenous corticosteroid treatment may worsen insulin resistance and reduce insulin production, which would further impact the glycemic status. Adipokine dysregulation, the lipotoxic state, and the abdominal obesity of children with asthma may indicate a possible causal relationship between asthma and dyslipidemia. In the context of lung fibrosis, thyroid metabolism seems to have an impact on alveolar epithelial cell homeostasis. Patients with IPF who have hypothyroidism typically have poorer clinical outcomes. Patients with IPF lung disease also have elevated levels of type 2 iodothyronine deiodinase (DIO2). By improving mitochondrial function and requiring the survival of the PTEN-induced putative kinase (PINK1) and peroxisome proliferator-activated receptor gamma coactivator 1-alpha (PPARGC1A) signaling pathways, aerosolized thyroid hormone administration mitigates experimental lung fibrosis in two murine models. It is currently unknown how vitamin D contributes to chronic lung inflammation. It's unclear if this is an underlying factor causing lung fibrogenesis or merely an epiphenomenon associated with other comorbidities. Clinical data indicates that vitamin D deficiency was more common in patients with asthma and higher levels of sputum eosinophilia or exhaled nitric oxide.

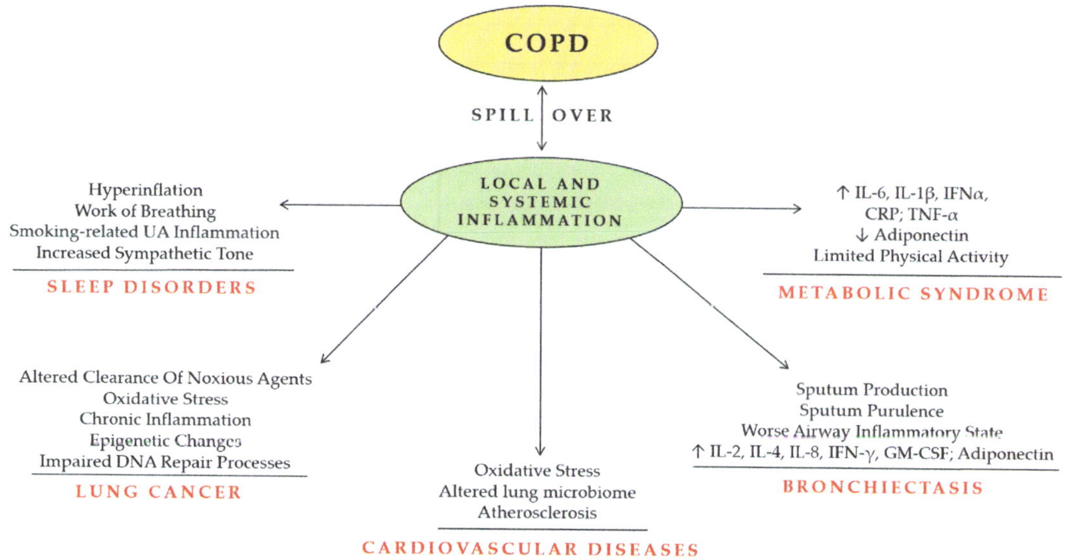

Figure 9.6. *Chronic obstructive pulmonary disease (COPD) and comorbidities. COPD: Chronic obstructive pulmonary disease; IL-6: Interleukin 6; IL-1β: Interleukin-1beta; IFNα: Interferon alfa; CRP: C-reactive protein; TNFα: Tumor Necrosis Factor alfa; IL-2: Interleukin 2; IL-4: Interleukin 4; IL-8: Interleukin 8; GM-CSF: granulocyte–macrophage colony-stimulating factor (GM-CSF); increased expression; reduced expression*

Source: Mariniello DF, D'Agnano V, Cennamo D, Conte S, Quarcio G, Notizia L, Pagliaro R, Schiattarella A, Salvi R, Bianco A, et al. Comorbidities in COPD: Current and Future Treatment Challenges. Journal of Clinical Medicine. 2024; 13(3):743. https://doi.org/10.3390/jcm13030743.

9.3.1. Metabolic Disorders and COPD

There is strong evidence that COPD is a lung condition that involves more than just remodeling and inflammation of the airways. Although well known, extrapulmonary comorbidities such as metabolic disorders remain poorly understood. Current pathogenetic theories postulate a relationship between the effects of age-related comorbid conditions that affect the lungs and the systemic diffusion of local inflammation (Table 9.3).

The most common metabolic COPD comorbidity is osteoporosis. 31% (69–35%) of COPD patients have bone disease. According to epidemiological studies, patients with COPD had a twofold higher risk of osteoporosis than controls. The following are risk factors for osteoporosis in COPD patients: low body mass index, age, use of corticosteroids, hypogonadism, and conditions unique to COPD. The latter's comprise the COPD phenotype (emphysematous versus non-emphysematous) as determined by computed tomography scan, respiratory failure, dyspnea severity, and COPD functional stage. Prospective studies are desperately needed because it is unclear from a therapeutic perspective whether managing osteoporosis may improve the course of the disease.

Table 9.3. *Clinical Evaluation Recommended in the Acute Care Setting for a Patient with AECOPD and/or HF*

Laboratory Tests	Imaging
Blood cell count Plasma electrolytes	Chest radiography
ESR	Lung sonography with assessment of diaphragmatic excursion and pleural effusion
CRP	Chest computed tomography scan
D-dimer	**Diagnostic tests**
	Electrocardiography
hs-cardiac troponin	Pulse oximetry
Glycemia	Blood gas analysis
Eosinophilic and neutrophilic pattern	
NT-proBNP (recommended both as a diagnostic/prognostic test for heart overload or HF or to exclude them)	

ESR: erythrocyte sedimentation rate; CRP: C-reactive protein; hs-troponin: high-sensitivity troponin; NT-proBNP: N-terminal prohormone of brain natriuretic peptide; HF: heart failure.

Source: *Bianco A, Canepa M, Catapano GA, Marvisi M, Oliva F, Passantino A, Sarzani R, Tarsia P, Versace AG. Implementation of the Care Bundle for the Management of Chronic Obstructive Pulmonary Disease with/without Heart Failure. Journal of Clinical Medicine. 2024; 13(6):1621. https://doi.org/10.3390/jcm13061621.*

Abdominal obesity, elevated triglycerides, atherogenic dyslipidemia, elevated blood pressure, high blood glucose and/or insulin resistance are clinical indicators of metabolic syndrome, a complex disorder. When systemic inflammation coexists with COPD, patients are often confronted with metabolic syndrome. Diabetes prevalence in people with COPD varies from 10 to 18%. According to a study involving 103,614 women, individuals with COPD had a 1.8 relative risk of developing diabetes. It has also been demonstrated that diabetes and reduced lung function are related. Many pathogenetic similarities between diabetes and COPD have been proposed, but there is still a lack of information. Increased lung collagen synthesis and deposition, which is mediated by higher levels of advanced glycation products, may result from the spillover of pro-inflammatory mediators and reactive oxygen species (IL1, 6, TNFa, NF-κB, leptin, adiponectin, and resistin) into the circulation. Insulin resistance may also be caused. Prolonged exogenous corticosteroid administration may worsen the vicious cycle of dysglycemia, systemic inflammation, and COPD by reducing insulin synthesis and raising insulin resistance as a result of increased muscle catabolism, lipolysis, and free fatty acid production. By releasing multiple pro-inflammatory mediators into the bloodstream, coexisting obesity may also exacerbate insulin resistance and systemic inflammation, perpetuating both local and systemic inflammation.

Although abnormalities in lipoprotein metabolism have been linked to COPD, there is currently a dearth of relative mechanistic information. Dyslipidemia was found in 31.7% of controls and 48.3% of COPD patients, according to a recent study. The correlation between COPD and dyslipidemia is underscored by the therapeutic criterion that statins account for 36% of the decrease in the death rate of COPD patients. In this context, more research should be done on the pleiotropic effects of statins, such as their immunomodulatory and anti-inflammatory capabilities. There has been a recent resurgence of interest in the role thyroid dysfunctions play in COPD patients. Strong data revealed that many traits common to COPD patients may raise their chance of developing hypo- or hyperthyroidism. Subclinical or overt hypothyroidism may be caused, in particular, by the degree of airway obstruction, hypoxemia, and systemic inflammation. Reduced respiratory muscle function, decreased exercise tolerance, and an increased risk of sleep-related breathing disorders that cause inspiratory and expiratory weakness in COPD patients have all been linked to hypothyroidism. Reduced myosin heavy chain expression, phrenic nerve neuropathy, or reduced neuromuscular transmission could be the causes of this weakness. In COPD patients, hyperthyroidism has also been linked to a decreased ability to exercise and contract respiratory muscles. Restoring physiologic thyroid signaling may have therapeutic benefits for COPD patients, it is important to note, given the reported significant drop in oxygen levels accompanied by carbon dioxide retention (Oppedal et al., 2007; Laghi et al., 2009; Spagnolo et al., 2015; Dursunoglu et al., 2016; Farag, 2017).

9.3.2. Metabolic Disorders and Asthma

Asthma is among the most common chronic diseases worldwide. The disease is poorly controlled despite available therapeutic regimens in a substantial minority of patients. Among factors impairing the control of symptoms and treatment response are comorbid conditions including metabolic disorders.

According to recent data, the most prevalent metabolic dysfunction was dyslipidemia, which affected 18% of patients with asthma. Conversely, 84% of patients with asthma had either type 1 or type 2 diabetes mellitus. It has been shown that in both children and young adults with asthma, there is a correlation between metabolic syndrome and functional indices. Children with asthma were more likely to have acanthosis nigricans, a sign of insulin resistance that eventually leads to diabetes and elevated triglycerides. The complex effects of insulin and insulin receptors on the lung and airways may be suppressed in metabolic syndrome-induced lung impairment in asthma; however, the precise mechanism by which these receptors may affect the developing lung is still unknown. There is currently a lack of evidence to support the theory that asthma and dyslipidemia are related to circulating levels of fatty acids and the lipotoxic state, which triggers innate immune responses through a variety of inflammatory mechanisms like pattern recognition receptor activation or intracellular signaling pathways. Another important component of the metabolic syndrome, abdominal obesity, has been linked to asthmatic lung function impairment. Obesity was a risk factor for severe asthma, and in obese subjects, the incidence of asthma nearly doubled. Experimental evidence indicated that visceral fat of obese asthmatic patients expressed more inflammatory markers and adipokines; consequently, adipokine dysregulation was proposed as a potential mechanism underlying obesity-mediated asthmatic airway abnormalities.

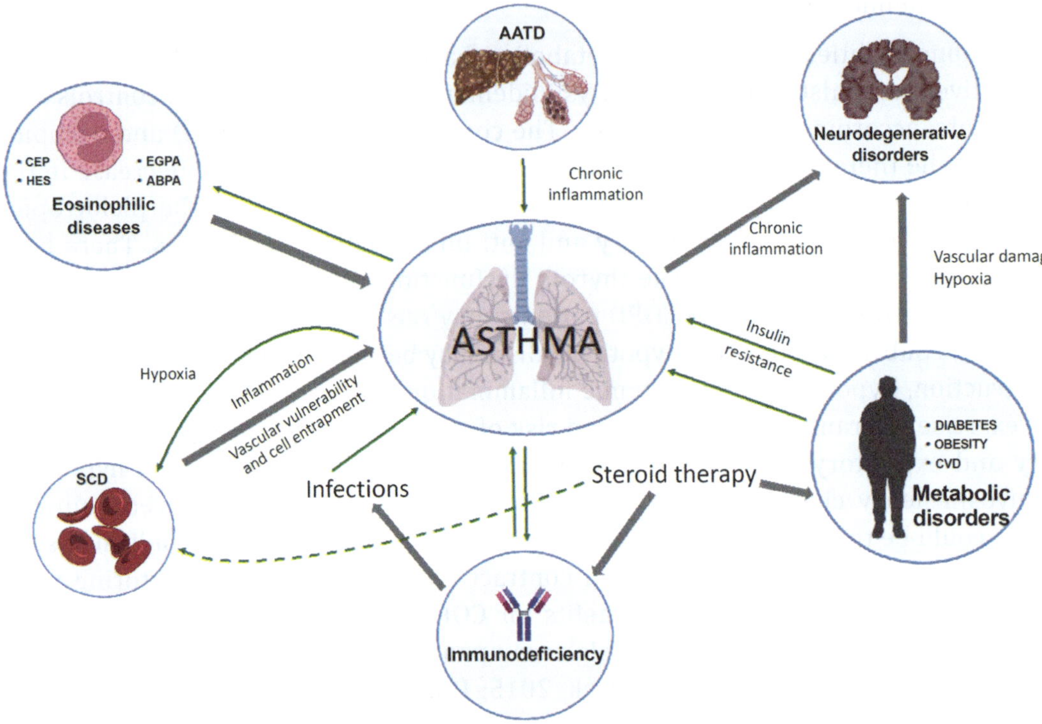

Figure 9.7. *Overview of different conditions potentially coexisting and interacting with bronchial asthma. Grey, thick arrows indicate a pathobiological contribution in the development of the disease; green, thin arrows highlight a negative impact on the disease control, burden, and evolution. AATD: α1-Antitrypsin deficiency; ABPA: allergic bronchopulmonary aspergillosis; EGPA: eosinophilic granulomatosis with polyangiitis; CEP: Chronic Eosinophilic Pneumonia; CVD: cardiovascular Disease; HES: Hyper-eosinophilic Syndrome; SCD: Sickle Cell Disease.*

Source: Maule M, Olivieri B, Guarnieri G, De Franceschi L, Martinelli N, Vaia R, Argentino G, Vianello A, Senna G, Caminati M. Hidden Comorbidities in Asthma: A Perspective for a Personalized Approach. Journal of Clinical Medicine. 2023; 12(6):2294. https://doi.org/10.3390/jcm12062294.

Chronic corticosteroid therapy has also been associated with osteoporosis in cases of asthma; however, the effects of inhaled corticosteroids on musculoskeletal disorders are highly controversial. Even though this result was not consistent, studies have reported lower bone mineral density in adult asthmatic patients using inhaled glucocorticoids when compared to untreated controls. There is substantial evidence to support the dose-response association between oral glucocorticoid use and asthmatic patients' fracture risk.

It has been reported that there is an epidemiologic and mechanistic interaction between vitamin D deficiency and exacerbations of asthma. Lower serum 25-hydroxyvitamin D levels have been linked to higher hospitalization and prevalence rates, as well as lower lung function and more airway hyperresponsiveness in children with asthma. Research revealed that among children with asthma, the prevalence of vitamin D deficiency was 53.3%, while in adults with asthma, it was 17%. While vitamin D deficiency was strongly linked to sputum eosinophilia, higher levels of exhaled nitric oxide, and impairment of lung function, other studies found no differences in the mean levels of the vitamin between asthmatics and healthy controls. These data suggest that in patients who are already at risk of developing the disease, low vitamin D levels may possibly exacerbate asthma. Mechanistically, vitamin D deficiency has been associated with increased contractility of smooth muscle in the airways, especially in steroid-refractory asthma and asthma exacerbations. Through suppression of the Th2 immunologic response, vitamin D, a steroid hormone, has also been linked to a possible anti-inflammatory role.

To achieve this, treatment approaches involving supplements have been used on sizable patient cohorts with positive outcomes. A recent Cochrane meta-analysis of two studies involving 658 adults and seven trials involving 435 children found that taking an oral vitamin D supplement decreased the risk of hospitalization for severe asthma exacerbations from 6% in the control group to 3% in the treatment arm. The aforementioned data primarily stem from three trials, and it is currently unknown whether this therapeutic effect can be expanded to all asthmatic patients or in those with low baseline levels of vitamin D. Despite the encouraging therapeutic efficacy, there is still much to be learned (Oppedal et al., 2007; Laghi et al., 2009; Spagnolo et al., 2015; Dursunoglu et al., 2016; Farag, 2017).

9.3.3. Metabolic Disorders and ILDs

Diffuse parenchymal lung disorders, or interstitial lung diseases, are linked to significant morbidity and mortality. Sarcoidosis and idiopathic pulmonary fibrosis (IPF) are two of the most prevalent ILDs. The recent resurgence of the role of metabolic disorders in ILDs has prompted research into potential targets for treatment for ILD patients.

Diabetes mellitus represents the most frequently encountered endocrine comorbidity in patients with IPF. The prevalence of diabetes in patients with IPF ranged from 10 to 39%. A potential association between IPF and diabetes could be attributed to complications from chronic corticosteroid therapy. The impact of diabetes on disease mortality still remains elusive and controversial.

Recently, there has been evidence linking thyroid disorders to a common comorbid condition among IPF patients. Two recent studies showed that patients with IPF were more likely to have hypothyroidism (16.8% of IPF subjects and 7.1%) compared to control subjects. Remarkably, the affected percentages were 28% for women and 13% for men. One noteworthy finding was that individuals with IPF who also had hypothyroidism had worse outcomes. It's interesting to note that our research team discovered that type 2 iodothyronine deiodinase (DIO2), the enzyme responsible for converting T4 to active T3, was elevated in the lungs of IPF patients, especially in the metabolically active alveolar epithelial cells of the lung. Given that DIO2 knockout mice displayed enhanced fibrotic responses to bleomycin, DIO2 induction may have represented a compensatory response to boost local conversion of T4 to T3, improving the metabolic state of alveolar epithelial cells under stress. Interestingly, research results demonstrated that the administration of aerosolized thyroid hormone had anti-fibrotic effects in two experimental models of lung fibrosis, via a mechanism involving enhanced mitophagy and mitochondrial function. The same outcomes were noted with sobetirome, a thyroid-mimetic drug that selectively binds to the thyroid hormone receptor to activate thyroid hormone signaling. We eagerly await more research examining the impact of thyroid hormone administration in IPF patients.

The reported prevalence of dyslipidemia in patients with IPF varies from 11.7 to 21.7%. It is still unknown how precisely dyslipidemia, high fatty acid levels, and oxidative stress from Nicotinamide Adenine Dinucleotide Phosphate Oxidase Activation contribute to the pathophysiology of pulmonary fibrosis. The inflammatory disease sarcoidosis affects multiple systems and is distinguished by the presence of non-caseating granulomas in the afflicted organs. In excess of 90% of sarcoidosis patients have lung involvement. There is a dearth of information on the effects of metabolic comorbidities in sarcoidosis, most of which have concentrated on calcium metabolism. Specifically, 5% of patients with osteoporosis, 7% of patients with diabetes, and 13% of patients with sarcoidosis also had a thyroid disease diagnosis. The two main risk factors for metabolic comorbidities were age and the multiorgan involvement of sarcoidosis. Lastly, a possible correlation between autoimmune thyroid disorders and sarcoidosis was proposed by a case-control study involving 111 sarcoidosis patients.

Only a small but significant percentage of sarcoidosis patients experience hypercalcemia and hypercalciuria, but when they do, it's an indication for treatment. Recent data indicates that the true prevalence of hypercalcemia in sarcoidosis patients is between 10 and 15%, despite previous studies reporting that it was present in 2–63% of cases. Increased levels of 1,25-dihydroxyvitamin D3 (calcitriol), the hormonally active metabolite of vitamin D that causes hypercalcemia, have been linked to increased activity of the 1-alpha hydroxylase enzyme of tissue macrophages. Since then, a great deal of knowledge has been gained regarding the best therapeutic approach for treating hypercalcemia brought on by sarcoidosis. Glucocorticoids have been the first-line treatment for hypercalcemia linked to sarcoidosis; however, they have serious side effects that need to be handled carefully. Methotrexate and azathioprine are two examples of steroid-sparing medications that are frequently used in cases of advanced disease or steroid resistance with debatable outcomes. Lastly, research is currently being done to determine how biphosphonates, particularly zoledronic acid, contribute to sarcoid hypercalcemia.

9.3.4. Metabolomics in Chronic Lung Diseases

Cellular bioenergetics and metabolism have drawn a lot of attention in recent years due to their potential role in the etiology of chronic lung diseases. The systematic study of metabolic pathways (metabolome) and biochemical substances produced in a living system at a particular timepoint, known as metabolites, is referred to as "metabolomics." Currently, nuclear magnetic resonance spectroscopy (NMR) and mass spectrometry are the two methods used to quantify the metabolites of a biological system. Urine, due to its rich chemical composition, low cell and protein content, and ease of collection, is the most promising biological specimen for studying metabolomics among lung tissue, plasma, and urine. The metabolome of the airway lining fluid can be studied using exhaled breath condensate, an accessible biomarker tool. However, it has significant limitations because it is influenced by several confounding factors, including age, sex, smoking, temperature, humidity, and oral cavity contamination. Asthma and COPD are examples of heterogeneous syndromes with complex underlying pathogenesis that may be reliably diagnosed using a urine metabolomics profile. Of particular importance is the ability to distinguish between the two conditions based on their respective metabolomic profiles. Leukotrienes from exhaled breath condensate have been used to differentiate asthmatic patients from controls. Patients with COPD have abnormal muscular bioenergetics and impaired metabolites related to the microbiome, as demonstrated by elevated levels of branched-chain amino acids in plasma and formate and hippurate in urine, respectively. The metabolomics profile has also been utilized to differentiate between COPD patients with varying phenotypes according to the degree of functional impairment and the existence of cachexia and emphysema.

Major events of impaired mitochondrial metabolism in patients with COPD and IPF have been identified as disrupted glycolysis, enhanced fatty acid accumulation, increased production of lactic acid and lactate dehydrogenase, and haem degradation. Additionally, the glutathione synthesis pathway was disrupted in IPF lungs, which led to an increase in oxidant burden. It has also been observed that IPF lungs produce more proline, a crucial substrate for collagen biosynthesis, from ornithine by activating ornithine aminotransferase. It's interesting to note that functional indices of disease severity, such as FVC, have a negative correlation with elevated levels of ornithine aminotransferase. Lactic acid is one of the intermediate metabolites of glycolysis that has been demonstrated to trigger the TGF-β pathway, thereby inducing the differentiation of myofibroblasts. Recent research has linked the Warburg effect, which is observed in cancer cells, to the differentiation of fibroblasts into myofibroblasts through glycolytic reprogramming. In experimental lung fibrosis, inhibition of glycolysis produced therapeutic effects by reorienting important cellular constituents' metabolic requirements toward oxidative phosphorylation, thereby exposing a novel therapeutic area. A recent study demonstrating that downregulated levels of PINK1, the master transcription factor of mitophagy, result in damaged and dysfunctional mitochondria in the alveolar epithelial cells of IPF lungs, highlights the role of impaired mitochondrial metabolism in the pathogenesis of lung fibrosis. As previously reported, a recent publication from our study group highlights the critical role that mitochondrial metabolism plays in alveolar epithelial cell apoptosis in the context of lung fibrosis. This publication also demonstrates the therapeutic effects of aerosolized hormone administration in experimental lung fibrosis through the enhancement of mitochondrial bioenergetics. It's interesting to note that lung macrophages and fibroblasts have recently been linked, albeit in a cell-specific way, to impaired mitophagy-mediated lung fibrosis. Given the importance to humans, the aforementioned results also demonstrate that products of fibroblasts' mitochondrial metabolism, such as mitochondrial DNA (mtDNA), have been demonstrated to function as prognosticators of IPF mortality in recent studies. The preclinical studies mentioned above emphasize the significance of using circulating metabolites as biomarkers of treatment response and disease prognosis, as well as the therapeutic restoration of the disrupted metabolome.

9.4. Pulmonary Manifestations of Systemic Diseases

The hallmarks of systemic diseases are their common occurrences in multiple organ systems. Sarcoidosis, connective tissue disease, and vasculitis are among the most prevalent systemic diseases that impact the lungs. Computed tomography, in particular, is crucial for imaging in many ways, including: (1) diagnosing a patient; (2) identifying the type of injury that is present; and (3) serially evaluating patients who exhibit acute or progressive symptoms. Analyzing the distinctive clinical presentations of systemic diseases in various organ systems is necessary for diagnosis. Radiologic findings, histopathology, and serologic abnormalities are frequently correlated with clinical features. Numerous different thoracic compartments, such as the heart, vessels, lymph nodes, pericardium, lungs, and pleura, can be impacted by systemic diseases. Although their extrapulmonary manifestations frequently offer crucial diagnostic hints, they will also be discussed in light of the lung manifestations that are the main focus of this discussion. Lung involvement is not always present in all systemic diseases; for example, it is a common feature in sarcoidosis and granulomatosis with polyangiitis (GPA, formerly Wegener's granulomatosis), but it is rare in other diseases like Henoch-Schönlein purpura.

Depending on the particular illness, imaging plays a different role in systemic diseases. To establish a diagnosis, radiology, and specifically computed tomography (CT), may be crucial. For instance, typical CT findings are frequently essential in establishing an accurate diagnosis of sarcoidosis. Conversely, the diagnosis of connective tissue disease typically relies primarily on clinical and serologic findings, meaning that imaging plays a somewhat limited role in the process. In clinical practice, however, it is also observed that certain findings on CT, such as indications of lung fibrosis (particularly the NSIP pattern), catalyze further investigation to determine whether an underlying systemic disease is present. Even in cases where imaging is not a major diagnostic tool, it remains valuable for determining the presence, course, and extent of lung disease, all of which influence treatment choices. Imaging plays a significant role in the evaluation of patients with acute or worsening symptoms as well as in the serial follow-up of lung abnormalities over time. The more prevalent systemic illnesses—such as sarcoidosis, connective tissue diseases, and vasculitis—that lead to pulmonary abnormalities will be discussed in the sections that follow. Although it is not feasible to conduct a thorough examination of all systemic diseases' lung manifestations, a few uncommon conditions will be touched on, such as amyloidosis, inflammatory bowel disease, Erdheim-Chester disease, and IgG4-related sclerosing disease.

9.4.1. Sarcoidosis

The cause of the systemic disease sarcoidosis is unknown. Familial clustering observations suggest a genetic susceptibility to sarcoidosis. Noncaseating epithelioid cell granulomas in several organs are the hallmark of sarcoidosis; however, pulmonary manifestations, which affect more than 90% of patients, are closely associated with morbidity and mortality. Pulmonary sarcoidosis has a very variable CT appearance, and it is known to mimic many other diffuse infiltrative lung diseases; on the other hand, several diseases can mimic classical sarcoidosis. The histology of pulmonary sarcoidosis is characterized by noncaseating granulomas that may resolve or induce fibrosis, and a rim of lymphocytes and fibroblasts distributed perilymphatically. Although the disease can strike anyone at any age, it primarily strikes those in the 20–40 age range and very infrequently strikes those over 65. The prognosis is generally favorable, with mortality falling between 1% and 5% and disease resolution frequently taking place in less than two years. The presence of noncaseating granulomas, the exclusion of other diseases, and typical clinical and radiological manifestations are the three criteria for diagnosis. Each criterion's weight varies depending on the presentation of the patient. For example, in certain patients with suspected sarcoidosis, standard chest radiograph findings may be sufficient if done in the right setting (i.e., uveitis, erythema nodosum), in certain patients a classic nodular pattern on CT is required to establish the diagnosis, and in the final subgroup of patients, histological confirmation is required due to equivocal or nonspecific clinical and radiological findings (e.g., skin lesion biopsy, transbronchial needle aspiration guided by endobronchial ultrasound for mediastinal or hilar lymphadenopathy).

CT scans of the lungs reveal small, clearly defined nodules in a typical perilymphatic distribution concerning the subpleural surface, along thickened interlobular septa, adjacent to vessels in the lobular core, and beside major fissures. Although the nodules can be evenly distributed in both lungs, with the upper and middle lung zones predominating, they can also be clustered in the perihilar and peribronchovascular regions, sparing the lung periphery in relative terms, or they can be grouped in small areas. The confluence of granulomas causes poorly defined opacities (ground glass or consolidations, up to 10 cm, alveolar sarcoidosis) or larger nodules (1–4 cm, nodular sarcoid, galaxy sign). Usually, lymphadenopathy presents with a symmetric hilar distribution, right paratracheal, aortopulmonary, and subcarinal distribution. An eggshell or amorphous cloudlike ("icing sugar") pattern is observed in lymph nodes with advanced-stage CT calcifications.

A quarter or more of patients progress to stage IV irreversible pulmonary fibrosis, which is characterized by architectural distortion, interlobular septa displacement, traction bronchiectasis, honeycombing, and bullae. Conglomerate masses, found primarily in perihilar regions, are indicative of fibrosis regions exhibiting traction bronchiectasis. Septemberal displacement and hilar retraction are linked to upper lobe volume loss. Airway anomalies include traction bronchiectasis brought on by surrounding fibrosis and airway compression brought on by surrounding lymphadenopathy. The large and small airways narrow as a result of sporadic bronchial wall thickening brought on by granulomas inside the bronchial walls. Lobular air trapping is more noticeable when the small airways are involved in expiratory CT scans. Certain HRCT characteristics that are specific to sarcoidosis may be present, facilitating a safe diagnosis and avoiding additional invasive procedures. However, sarcoidosis can also manifest with less common symptoms (Table 9.4).

Table 9.4. *Predictors of Systemic Involvement Among Patients with Cutaneous Sarcoidosis in a Single-Center Study*

	Patients with systemic involvement (*n* = 23)	**Patients with exclusively cutaneous disease (*n* = 14)**	**OR (95% CI) [*P* value]**
Age < 54.0 years	15/23 (65%)	3/14 (21%)	**6.88 (1.48–32.01) [0.010]**
Female sex	17/23 (74%)	4/14 (29%)	**7.08 (1.60–31.33) [0.007]**
Acute disease course	11/23 (48%)	0/14	**1.92 (1.30–2.84) [0.002]**
Morphological features			
Plaques and nodules	4/23 (17%)	5/14 (36%)	0.38 (0.08–1.76) [0.208]

Papules	9/23 (39%)	8/14 (57%)	0.45 (0.08–2.67) [0.375]
Laboratory measures			
Elevated ACE	7/23 (30%)	0/10	**1.44 (1.10–1.88) [0.049]**
Elevated soluble IL-2 receptor	13/14 (93%)	3/7 (43%)	**17.33 (1.39–216.60) [0.011]**
Hypercalcemia	1/14 (7%)	0/4	1.08 (0.93–1.25) [0.582]
Elevated CRP	11/17 (65%)	1/7 (14%)	**11.00 (1.06–114.09) [0.025]**
Management			
Systemic corticosteroids	9/23 (39%)	0/14	**1.64 (1.18–2.28) [0.007]**
Topical corticosteroids	14/23 (61%)	14/14 (100%)	**0.61 (0.44–0.85) [0.007]**
NSAID	5/23 (22%)	0/14	1.28 (1.03–1.59) [0.061]
Immune-modulating drugs [a]	5/23 (22%)	1/14 (7%)	3.61 (0.38–34.69) [0.243]

Source: Boch K, Langan EA, Zillikens D, Ludwig RJ and Kridin K (2022). Evaluation of clinical and laboratory characteristics of patients with cutaneous sarcoidosis: A single-center retrospective cohort study. Front. Med. 9:980507. doi: 10.3389/fmed.2022.980507.

Especially in advanced disease with fibrosis, the differential diagnosis between sarcoidosis and other fibrosing diseases can be challenging. Table 9.5 summarizes imaging findings helpful for differentiating diseases.

Table 9.5. *Common Causes of Airflow Obstruction in Sarcoidosis (That Could Induce Wheezing)*

Cause	Form of Pulmonary Sarcoidosis
Endobronchial deposition of granulomas	Active pulmonary sarcoidosis
Cough reflex hypersensitivity granulomatous inflammation of airways	Active pulmonary sarcoidosis
Bronchospasm from granulomatous inflammation of airways	Active pulmonary sarcoidosis
Airway fibrosis from previous granulomatous inflammation of airways	Fibrotic pulmonary sarcoidosis
Development of bullous disease/ emphysema *	Fibrotic pulmonary sarcoidosis

Cause	Form of Pulmonary Sarcoidosis
Airway compression from mediastinal lymphadenopathy *,†	mediastinal lymphadenopathy from sarcoidosis

* Rare; † This manifestation most commonly occurs in patients with significantly calcified mediastinal lymphadenopathy.

Source: Judson MA. The Symptoms of Pulmonary Sarcoidosis. Journal of Clinical Medicine. 2023; 12(18):6088. https://doi.org/10.3390/jcm12186088.

Pulmonary hypertension and the growth of an aspergilloma are among the complications. A common side effect of stage IV sarcoidosis is mycetomas, which occur in patients with fibrotic sarcoidosis and manifest as a soft tissue mass inside an already-existing cavity. When hemoptysis becomes life-threatening, prompt interventional therapy (bronchial artery embolization) may be necessary. End-stage fibrosis patients experience pulmonary hypertension; however, other possible causes include mediastinal fibrosis, intrinsic sarcoid vasculopathy, which includes characteristics of pulmonary veno-occlusive disease, and extrinsic compression of the pulmonary arteries by lymphadenopathy. Before the widespread use of CT, decades ago, the staging system based on chest radiography (Siltzbach classification) was developed. It is purely descriptive and does not indicate disease activity (Oppedal et al., 2007; Laghi et al., 2009; Spagnolo et al., 2015; Dursunoglu et al., 2016; Farag, 2017) (Table 9.6).

Table 9.6. *Common and Uncommon Neurological Sarcoidosis Findings and Their Evolution*

Common	Cranial nerves	• VII (24%), II (21%) (see Table 9.2), V (12%), VIII (3–10%), oculomotor nerves, (2–6%), XI, XII (1%). • Underlying mechanisms could be either epineural/perineural granulomatous inflammation of the nerve itself or granulomatous inflammation of the leptomeningeal compartment compressing the cranial nerves. • Facial palsy is usually unilateral, but both sides can be affected at the same time in up to 30%. Prognosis is usually good, with complete recovery in about 90% of patients under corticosteroids. • Hearing loss is bilateral and asymmetrical in 75% of patients. Half of the patients have abnormal vestibular testing and most of them have additional features of neurosarcoidosis (81%). Recovery occurs in most patients (70%).

	Meningeal	• Clinical symptoms of meningeal irritation are seen in only 10% to 20% of patients with neurosarcoidosis. • Many patterns of meningeal involvement have been described, but there is a tendency to basilar meninges involvement. • Leptomeningeal disease is a more severe disorder, with a risk of hydrocephalus and tissue destruction. Hydrocephalus is due to the obstruction of the ventricles by an inflammatory or granulomatous mass or infiltration of the meningeal spaces. • CSF usually reveals mild monocyte pleocytosis (64%) and a protein elevation >1g/L (70%). Low glucose level (one-fifth of cases) and oligoclonal bands (30–42% of cases) are correlated with disability.
	Brain parenchyma	• Intraparenchymal granulomatous lesions could be either a solitary mass or multiple nodules and may cause focal neurologic deficits, seizures, or increased intracranial pressure. • Multiple non-enhancing white matter lesions are the most common imaging findings in sarcoidosis patients on MRI. These lesions are hyperintense on T2-weighted sequences and may be indistinguishable from those of multiple sclerosis.
Uncommon	Spinal cord	• Most patients present with insidious, progressive, but non-specific sensory disorders, sphincter dysfunction and weakness over months before diagnosis. • Cervical (59%) > thoracic (29%) > conus (12%) involvement. • On MRI, spinal cord sarcoidosis appears as heterogeneous patchy intramedullary lesions, a longitudinally extensive transverse myelitis with cord swelling and spinal cord atrophy in the late stages. • 80% of patients will develop neurologic sequelae and 40% to 61% with a moderate to severe handicap.
	Pituitary	• Hypogonadism is the most frequent endocrine disorder followed by TSH deficiency, diabetes insipidus and hyperprolactinemia. • MRI reveals infundibulum involvement (36.3%), pituitary stalk thickness (52%) and involvement of the pituitary gland (64%). • MRI abnormalities can improve or disappear under corticosteroid treatment, but most endocrine defects are irreversible and require long-term substitutive opotherapy.

	Peripheral neuropathy	• The most common form is chronic axonal sensory and/or motor neuropathy polyneuropathy. • Other forms include multiplex mononeuropathy, radiculopathy, brachial/lumbar plexitis, subacute demyelinating polyneuropathy mimicking Guillain-Barré syndrome, chronic demyelinating inflammatory neuropathy • Epineural and perineural granulomas, as well as granulomatous vasculitis can cause ischemic axonal degeneration and demyelination resulting from local pressure. • The prognosis is good for most patients after treatment, especially when there is a less severe presentation and a recent onset of symptoms. • Small-fiber neuropathy: patients usually present with pain, burning sensation and paresthesia. These symptoms can be migratory and fluctuant. Dysautonomia causing orthostatic hypotension, palpitations, hyperhidrosis, gastrointestinal dysmotility, or bowel/bladder dysfunction is also observed in approximately half of patients. The diagnosis of small fiber neuropathy requires skin biopsy showing decreased intraepidermal nerve fiber density of lower than 5% of the population reference mean or quantitative sudomotor axonal reflex testing showing reduced sweat output.
	Stroke	• Strokes which are thought to be related to sarcoidosis are ischemic (69%) or hemorrhagic (31%). • The main pathophysiological mechanism seems to be a granulomatous invasion of the vessels rather than cerebral vasculitis. • Cardioembolic events (e.g., atrial fibrillation associated to cardiac sarcoidosis) and atherosclerotic lesions have to be excluded

Abbreviations: MRI: Magnetic Resonance Imaging.

Source: *Sève P, Pacheco Y, Durupt F, Jamilloux Y, Gerfaud-Valentin M, Isaac S, Boussel L, Culender A, Androdias G, Valeyre D, et al. Sarcoidosis: A Clinical Overview from Symptoms to Diagnosis. Cells. 2021; 10(4):766. https://doi.org/10.3390/cells10040766.*

For instance, FDG-PET can be used to precisely measure inflammatory activity in patients who do not exhibit serological inflammatory activity but still have persistent, incapacitating symptoms. Additionally, PET has been reported to be useful in tracking therapy response and forecasting pulmonary deterioration at one year. suppression of the natural FDG uptake in the heart, e.g., allows for the identification of active cardiac sarcoidosis lesions through suitable diets. A new integrated clinicoradiological staging system has been proposed to identify patients at risk of mortality (50% in five years) and with poor prognosis. Patients were initially divided into two prognostic groups based on a weighted combination of lung function parameters; further separation was obtained if the main pulmonary and ascending aorta pathological diameter ratio (>1) was observed, or if the extent of fibrosis on CT exceeded 20%.

9.4.2. Connective Tissue Disease

The main clinical criteria used to characterize connective tissue diseases (CTDs) are typical clinical complaints and physical examination findings. The presence of specific autoantibodies also helps to narrow down the diagnosis. Although imaging plays a significant role in identifying the pattern and presence of lung disease, its role in diagnosis is limited. It is crucial to remember, however, that lung abnormalities can occasionally occur more than five years before other clinical manifestations. When a patient does not meet the criteria for a particular type of CTD, imaging may still suggest the possibility of one in these cases. Several thoracic compartments, including the lung, pleura, pericardium, lymphatics, vasculature, and heart, are susceptible to CTD involvement. Usually, multiple compartments are involved. CTDs frequently affect the respiratory system, significantly increasing morbidity and mortality. Many of the lung manifestations associated with CTD can be classified using the same system as idiopathic interstitial pneumonias. Lung biopsies are rarely performed on patients with a specific CTD, so high-resolution CT scans are often used to identify the predominant pattern of injury present. The prognosis and course of treatment depend on this pattern. Each unique CTD is associated with a wide range of potential injury patterns, though some patterns are more common than others. For example, polymyositis or dermatomyositis are most frequently associated with organizing pneumonia. It is also important to remember that a patient may exhibit multiple patterns of injury.

9.4.2.1. Rheumatoid Arthritis

High-resolution chest CT scans show abnormalities in the majority of RA patients, although these patients typically show no symptoms. In the lungs, bronchial wall thickening (12–92%), bronchial dilation (30–40%), reticulation (10–20%), ground-glass opacity (15–25%), honeycombing (10%), and consolidation (5%) are the most frequent CT findings. The first sign of RA in the lungs seems to be Airways disease. Air trapping and bronchiectasis are frequent observations. Obliterative bronchiolitis (constrictive bronchiolitis), in which the bronchioles are destroyed and replaced by scar tissue, is known to be associated with radiation therapy (RA). Mosaic perfusion with expiratory air trapping, frequently linked to bronchial dilatation, is a characteristic CT finding. Another form of small airway disease associated with rheumatoid lung disease is follicular bronchiolitis. Centrilobular nodules and regions of ground-glass opacity are the main findings on CT.

Men are significantly more likely than women to have RA lung fibrosis. UIP and NSIP are the two most prevalent patterns of lung fibrosis. When it comes to CTDs, RA is the most likely to exhibit a UIP pattern. Although nodules, pulmonary arterial enlargement, or pleural abnormality are among the other findings that may hint at the underlying diagnosis, CT findings related to interstitial pneumonia associated with RA are frequently indistinguishable from those of idiopathic varieties. Both UIP and NSIP frequently show a basilar and subpleural distribution of findings. When this distribution exhibits honeycombing and reticulation, a definitive diagnosis of UIP can be made. The presence of subpleural sparing and the absence of honeycombing allow for a confident diagnosis of NSIP. A new range of possible pulmonary side effects has been brought about by the new generation of biologic agents used to treat RA. The most significant of these is decreased immunity due to the use of anti-TNFα antibodies (adalimumab, infliximab, and etanercept). This leads to a markedly higher incidence of nontuberculous mycobacterial infection and tuberculosis (occasionally extra-articular or disseminated). In 2.5% of cases, subacute hypersensitivity pneumonitis may be linked to low-dose methotrexate. Patients with RA are likely more susceptible to developing methotrexate pneumonitis if they have radiographic evidence of interstitial lung disease before treatment. Pneumocystis pneumonia is one example of an infection that can arise during treatment.

9.4.2.2. Scleroderma (Progressive Systemic Sclerosis)

In individuals with scleroderma, parenchymal lung involvement is highly prevalent. Actually, the only CTD where lung illness is one of the defining characteristics is scleroderma. In at least 80% of cases, the lungs are abnormal at autopsy. The most prevalent pattern of abnormality is lung fibrosis, with NSIP being significantly more common (>90%) than UIP. Additionally frequent is pulmonary hypertension, which can occur either on its own or in conjunction with lung fibrosis. A higher prevalence of pulmonary hypertension is seen in individuals with limited scleroderma (CREST syndrome). On CT, esophageal dilatation is detected in as many as 80% of cases. Scleroderma-related CT findings show the predominant NSIP histology. Ground-glass opacity is the typical presentation of cellular NSIP, with a posterior and subpleural distribution. The most common findings in fibrotic NSIP are traction bronchiectasis and irregular reticulation. Although it is rarely seen, honeycombing is rarely present and is only partially present. Because fibrotic and cellular NSIP frequently coexist, results may be similar. An NSIP pattern is especially suggested by subpleural sparing.

The prognosis for scleroderma-related lung fibrosis is significantly better than that of idiopathic lung fibrosis, most likely because of the predominance of NSIP histology. For many years, fibrotic changes might not change. On a chest radiograph or CT scan, pulmonary arterial hypertension is typically associated with enlargement of the main and proximal pulmonary arteries. Nevertheless, the diagnosis of pulmonary arterial hypertension is not ruled out in patients with normal-sized pulmonary arteries, and echocardiographic pulmonary hypertension is also strongly predicted in patients with scleroderma. With a relative risk of malignancy ranging from 1.8 to 6.5, lung cancer is more common in people with scleroderma. People with lung fibrosis are frequently affected by lung cancer in this condition.

9.4.2.3. Systemic Lupus Erythematosus (SLE)

The most prevalent pleuropulmonary symptom of SLE is pleuritis, which affects 40–60% of patients and may or may not be connected to pleural effusion. Compared to the other CTDs, fibrotic interstitial lung disease is less common in SLE patients. Although the most frequent pulmonary complication of sickle cell disease (SLE) is thought to be pulmonary infection, acute pulmonary hemorrhage is also a significant pulmonary complication of this illness, as evidenced by diffuse or patchy consolidation and ground-glass opacity on radiological examination. Acute lupus pneumonitis, which affects patients with lupus, is an ill-defined condition marked by varying degrees of respiratory impairment and focal or diffuse pulmonary consolidation. The majority of cases that were previously thought to be lupus pneumonitis are now thought to have actually involved diffuse alveolar damage, either with or without pulmonary hemorrhage. Diaphragmatic dysfunction, pulmonary hypertension, and pulmonary thromboembolism are additional lupus complications that may be associated with antiphospholipid antibodies. The symptoms of diaphragmatic dysfunction, which are thought to be caused by a diaphragmatic myopathy, include platelike atelectasis and reduced lung volumes, or "shrinking lungs."

9.4.2.4. Polymyositis/Dermatomyositis (PM/DM)

Anti-Jo-1 is strongly correlated with interstitial lung disease (ILD) in patients with PM/DM. ILD affects roughly 50–70% of patients who test positive for anti-Jo-1; in contrast, if antibodies are not present, the frequency of ILD drops to roughly 10%. Anti-Jo-1 antibody-positive patients may have ILD before myositis. The most frequent pathologic findings are OP and NSIP, which frequently coexist. Similar to other CTDs, interstitial pneumonia may occur before clinical myositis manifests. A distinctive CT appearance is frequently linked to lung disease associated with PM/DM or the antisynthetase syndrome, a closely related condition. Confluent ground-glass opacity and lower lobe consolidation are superimposed upon traction bronchiectasis as a background. The distinctive histologic combination of NSIP and organizing pneumonia is reflected in this pattern. Following treatment, consolidation frequently demonstrates a notable resolution or improvement on serial evaluation; fibrosis, which is characterized by traction and reticulation bronchiectasis, typically persists.

Another pattern that may be observed in PM/DM patients is diffuse alveolar damage. Unlike the subacute or chronic symptoms of NSIP and/or organizing pneumonia, patients present with acute symptoms. Distinctive bilateral ground-glass opacity and/or consolidation are common CT characteristics associated with diffuse alveolar damage. Up to 20% of patients have an increased risk of concurrently diagnosed malignancy within a year of follow-up, with breast, lung, ovarian, and stomach malignancies being the most common causes.

9.4.2.5. Sjögren Syndrome

Regarding the pattern of pulmonary involvement in Sjögren syndrome, CT offers a wealth of information. The patterns can be further subdivided into lymphoid interstitial pneumonia, pulmonary hypertension, interstitial fibrosis, and abnormalities of the airways. The most common abnormalities related to the airways are tree-in-bud opacities, bronchiectasis, bronchiolectasis, and thickening of the bronchial wall. Air trapping on expiratory CT and mosaic attenuation on inspiratory CT are two possible signs of small airway disease. In parenchymal lung disease, nonspecific (NSIP) and lymphoid (LIP) interstitial pneumonia are the most prevalent patterns. NSIP is similar to that previously observed in scleroderma. Ground-glass opacity, a result of homogenous lymphocytic infiltration, is a characteristic of LIP. Centrilobular or perilymphatic nodules can also be observed. Cysts ranging in size from 5 to 30 mm can be observed alone or in conjunction with other findings. Based on lymphocytic wall infiltration, bronchiolar obstruction is the cause of these alterations. Cysts are useful in differentiating lymphoma from lymphoplasma. If there are effusions, consolidation, large nodules (>1 cm), or mediastinal lymphadenopathy, lymphadenopathy should be suspected. However, similar large "pseudo-alveolar" nodules can be found in combined amyloidosis and LIP. In contrast to other cystic lung diseases such as lymphangioleiomyomatosis, the cysts of LIP are fewer in number and show a peribronchovascular and lower lung predominance.

9.4.2.6. Mixed Connective Tissue Disease

The overlap syndrome known as mixed connective tissue disease (MCTD) is a separate clinicopathological entity. The main features are the following: (1) SLE, scleroderma, and PM/DM features, either coexisting or developing in turn throughout observation; and (2) antibodies to an extractable nuclear antigen (RNP). As many as two-thirds of patients with MCTD have infiltrative lung disease, which is a common cause of pulmonary involvement. Many people with the condition have no symptoms. The pulmonary anomalies are similar to those observed in PM/DM, SS, and SLE. Pleural thickening as well as pericardial and pleural effusions are therefore frequent. The most prevalent abnormality in parenchyma is ground-glass attenuation. The CT pattern and NSIP match the most closely. Consolidation, honeycombing, and poorly defined centrilobular nodules are less frequent findings. Pulmonary arterial hypertension and esophageal dysmotility with recurrent lung aspiration sequelae are two other significant complications of MCTD.

Patients with interstitial lung disease who possess some, but not all, of the characteristics of a CTD are receiving more and more attention in the literature. Many studies that looked back at patients with histologically proven UIP or NSIP who were initially diagnosed as idiopathic because they didn't meet the criteria for one of the established CTDs found subgroups of patients with one or more serological features of an autoimmune process. These subgroups have been referred to by many names, such as lung-dominant CTD, undifferentiated CTD (UCTD), and interstitial pneumonia with autoimmune features. For a subset of patients with findings suggestive but not diagnostic of a CTD, the term interstitial pneumonia with autoimmune features (IPAF) has been proposed. Patients must exhibit particular characteristics in two of the three domains—clinical, serologic, or anatomic—to meet IPAF requirements. Pathology or typical CT patterns can both satisfy the anatomic domain. Nonspecific interstitial pneumonia (NSIP), organizing pneumonia (OP), an overlap of NSIP and OP, or lymphoid interstitial pneumonia are among the CT patterns suggestive of CTD. Multi-compartmental findings are also suggestive, such as the co-occurrence of interstitial pneumonia and any of the following conditions: pericardial effusion or thickening, airways disease, pulmonary vasculopathy, or an unexplained pleural effusion or thickening.

9.4.2.7. Pulmonary Vasculitis/Diffuse Alveolar Hemorrhage

Disorders characterized by inflammation of the blood vessel walls are referred to as "vasculitis." Pathology includes leucocytes and fibrinoid necrosis in the vessel wall, which compromises the vessel's integrity and causes bleeding; it also includes necrosis and vessel lumen narrowing, which causes ischemia downstream. Systemic vasculitis classification (Table 9.7) is still up for debate. The current classification, which dates back to the 2012 Chapel Hill Consensus Conference (CHCC), divides large-, medium-, and small-vessel vasculitis (LVV, MVV, or SVV, respectively) based on the predominant vascular size involved. Antineutrophil cytoplasmic antibody, or ANCA, was added to the classification for the first time.

Table 9.7. *Main Clinical Symptoms of Particular Primary Systemic Vasculitides and their Possible Urological Manifestations*

Type	Main Symptoms	Urological Manifestations
Large Vessel Vasculitis		
Takayasu arteritis (TA)	Arthralgia, myalgia, carotidynia, absent or weak peripheral pulse, limb claudication, arterial bruit, discrepant blood pressure between arms, hypertension, angina, gastrointestinal symptoms (abdominal pain, diarrhea, gastrointestinal hemorrhage) skin lesions (erythema nodosum, pyoderma gangrenosum), respiratory symptoms (chest pain, dyspnea, hemoptysis, pulmonary hypertension), neurologic symptoms (light headedness, vertigo, syncope, orthostasis, headaches, convulsions, and strokes), visual impairment	Obstructive nephropathy
Giant cell arteritis (GCA)	Jaw claudication, ocular symptoms (transient visual loss, permanent vision loss, diplopia, Charles Bonnet syndrome), musculoskeletal symptoms (proximal polyarthralgias and myalgias, peripheral synovitis, distal extremity swelling with pitting edema), large vessel involvement (aneurysms and dissections of the aorta, stenosis, occlusion, and ectasia of large arteries), strokes	Epididymitis, orchitis, testicular masses
Medium Vessel Vasculitis		
Polyarteritis nodosa (PAN)	Skin lesions (tender erythematous nodules, purpura, livedo reticularis, ulcers, bullous or vesicular eruption), neurologic symptoms (mononeuropathy multiplexor asymmetric polyneuropathy affecting, e.g., radial, ulnar, peroneal nerves), gastrointestinal symptoms (abdominal pain, nausea, vomiting, melena, bloody or non-bloody diarrhea, life-threatening gastrointestinal bleeding), coronary artery disease (myocardial ischemia, heart failure, cardiomyopathy), myalgia, and muscle weakness, ocular symptoms (ischemic retinopathy with hemorrhages, retinal detachment, ischemic optic neuropathy), glomerulonephritis	Orchitis, scrotal necrosis, bladder, and testicular masses, ureteric stricture, spontaneous ureteric rupture, renal artery aneurysms, perirenal hematomas, spontaneous retroperitoneal hemorrhage
Kawasaki disease (KD)	Conjunctivitis, mucositis, skin lesions (rash, perineal erythema, redness or crust formation at the site of Bacille Calmette–Guérin inoculation), extremity changes (indurated edema of the dorsum of their hands and feet, diffuse erythema of their palms and soles), arthritis, lymphadenopathy (cervical lymphadenopathy), cardiovascular involvement (coronary arteries inflammation, formation of microaneurysms, myocarditis, pericarditis, valvulitis)	Sterile pyuria, hydrocele testis
Small Vessel Vasculitis		
Anti-neutrophil cytoplasmic antibody (ANCA) associated vasculitis		

Type	Main Symptoms	Urological Manifestations
Microscopic polyangiitis (MPA)	Elevated purpura, alveolar hemorrhage, glomerulonephritis	Prostatitis
Granulomatosis with polyangiitis (GPA)	Upper airways, eye, and ear disease (conductive hearing loss, sensorineural hearing loss, strawberry gingivitis, underlying bone destruction with loosening of teeth, non-specific ulcerations throughout the lining of the mouth and nasal septum), renal involvement (rapidly progressive glomerulonephritis), subglottal stenosis, lower respiratory tract involvement (pulmonary nodules, cavitary lesions, bleeding in the lungs, bronchial stenosis), arthritis, skin lesions (subcutaneous nodule on the elbow, purpura), neurologic symptoms: (sensory neuropathy, mononeuritis multiplex)	Prostatitis, epididymitis, orchitis, ureteric stricture, penile ulceration, necrotizing urethritis, large renal and bladder granulomas, vesicovaginal fistula
Eosinophilic granulomatosis with polyangiitis (EGPA)	Respiratory symptoms (asthma, allergic rhinitis, nasal polyps, pulmonary bleeding), neurologic symptoms (mononeuropathy multiplex, symmetrical polyneuropathy), renal involvement (glomerulonephritis, hypertension), cardiovascular involvement (myocarditis, pericarditis), skin lesions (elevated purpura, subcutaneous nodules, livedo reticularis), gastrointestinal symptoms (eosinophilic gastroenteritis, diarrhea, gastrointestinal bleeding, colitis)	Prostatitis, cystitis, ureteric stricture, vesicovaginal fistula
Immune complex small vessel vasculitides		
IgA vasculitis (IgAV)	Skin lesions (symmetrical erythematosus petechial or purpuric rash that almost exclusively starts on the lower limbs and buttocks), arthritis, gastrointestinal symptoms (nausea, vomiting, colicky abdominal pain, transient paralytic ileus, gastrointestinal hemorrhage, bowel ischemia and necrosis, intussusception, bowel perforation), glomerulonephritis	Epididymitis, orchitis, ureteric stricture, cystitis, priapism, spermatic vein thrombosis
Variable Vessel Vasculitis		
Bechet's disease (BD)	Oral ulcerations, skin lesions (acneiform lesions, papulo-vesiculo-pustular eruptions, pseudofolliculitis, nodules, erythema, palpable purpura), ocular disease (uveitis, secondary cataracta, glaucoma, macular edema), neurologic symptoms, arterial disease (hemorrhage, stenosis, aneurysm formation), venous thrombosis, cardiac disease, gastrointestinal symptoms (abdominal pain, diarrhea, gastrointestinal ulcerations, bleeding)	Genital ulceration, epididymitis, sterile urethritis, bladder wall ulceration, cystitis, vesicovaginal fistula, urethrovaginal fistula, priapism

Source: Nowak Ł, Krajewski W, Krajewska J, Chorbińska J, Kiełb P, Małkiewicz B, Szydełko T. Urological Manifestations of the Systemic Vasculitides—A Scoping Review. Uro. 2021; 1(4):209–221. https://doi.org/10.3390/uro1040023.

9.4.2.8. ANCA-Associated Granulomatous Vasculitis with Polyangiitis (GPA, Former Wegener's Disease)

Small-vessel vasculitis usually manifests as pulmonary involvement (SVV). Arterioles, venules, and capillaries are all impacted by SVV. It is subdivided into three types: Wegener-like granulomatosis with polyangiitis, eosinophilic granulomatosis with polyangiitis, and microscopic polyangiitis caused by antineutrophil cytoplasmic antibody (ANCA)-associated vasculitis (AAV) (formerly Churg-Strauss). The only immune complex SVV that is frequently observed to involve the lungs is the second group, which includes, among other things, antiglomerular basement membrane disease (Goodpasture). Behcet disease, also classified as immune complex-mediated vasculitis, is characterized by varying vessel sizes. Diffuse alveolar hemorrhage (DAH), acute glomerulonephritis, upper airway disease, lung nodules or cavitary nodules, mononeuritis multiplex, and palpable purpura are among the radiologic signs and clinical symptoms suggestive of pulmonary vasculitis. Pulmonary-renal syndrome is another term for some of these conditions that involve both the kidneys and the lungs.

Multiple nodules or masses of varying sizes, with or without a CT halo sign (perinodular hemorrhage), are the most common pulmonary abnormalities observed. There is no preference for the upper or lower lung zones; they usually affect the subpleural areas. Lesions range in size from 1 to 10 cm, though most are smaller. Lesions frequently have thick walls and are cavitary. wedge-shaped areas of consolidation in the periphery that resemble infarcts and may also cave in. Patients with pulmonary hemorrhage have diffuse consolidation or ground-glass opacity. Diffuse lung fibrosis (primarily UIP pattern) may occasionally be observed, but focal fibrotic changes are a reflection of previous episodes of active disease. Cavitating nodule superinfection is not unusual. Additionally visible is a reverse halo sign, which denotes organizing pneumonia. The quick temporal evolution of the nodules and airspace opacities is a crucial aspect of GPA. Furthermore, approximately 70% of cases may show a concentric thickening of the tracheal or bronchial walls along with a decrease in luminal diameter and atelectasis (15% of cases). Segmental and subsegmental bronchi are the principal sites of bronchial abnormalities. The most common involvement is with the subglottic trachea. The predominate manifestation determines the differential diagnosis. When nodules predominate, neoplasms (adenocarcinoma, metastases, and lymphoma) and specific infections (fungal and mycobacterial infections) are included in the differential diagnosis. Infection is taken into account when consolidating airspace. Other factors to take into account when there is thickening of the airways are granulomatous disease, amyloidosis, and relapsing polychondritis for airway disease.

9.4.2.8.1. Eosinophilic Granulomatosis with Polyangiitis (EGPA, Former Churg-Strauss)

The SVV that causes eosinophilic granulomatous disease with polyangiitis, also known as Churg-Strauss syndrome, almost exclusively affects asthmatic patients and is characterized by a significant increase in serum eosinophilia. It combines the clinical, radiological, and pathological characteristics of eosinophilic pneumonia (allergic granulomatosis and angiitis) with those of GPA. Numerous other organs could also be affected, such as the musculoskeletal system (up to 50%), the skin (up to 40%), and the heart (up to 47%). Peripheral nerve involvement is more common (up to 75%), whereas renal involvement and pulmonary hemorrhage are less common than in GPA. ANCA positivity is higher in active disease; up to 30% are positive, primarily MPO-ANCA. In cases of ANCA negativity (which can occur in up to 40% of cases) and the presence of readily accessible lesions (e.g., skin). Histology shows eosinophilic infiltrates, vascular, and extravascular granulomas, and small-vessel (veins and arteries) vasculitis. 50% of deaths are associated with cardiac involvement, and up to 80% of patients have a 5-year survival. Asthmatic, eosinophilic, and vasculitis phases are the three distinct clinical phases of EGPA, though they are not always observed in that sequence. Eight to 10 years separate the asthmatic phase from the vasculitic phase.

Up to 70% of patients with EGPA have upper airway disease and pulmonary abnormalities. Transient, multifocal, non-segmental consolidations or ground-glass opacifications without zonal predilection are the most frequent pulmonary findings. There have also been reports of diffuse reticular opacities and small nodules that are not cavitating. The consolidations resemble eosinophilic pneumonia if they are subpleural. About one-third of patients have pleural effusions as a result of eosinophilic pleuritis or cardiomyopathy. About 50% of patients have interlobular thickening, which is secondary to mild fibrosis, eosinophilic septal infiltration, or cardiogenic pulmonary edema. A significant thoracic symptom is abnormalities of the airways, which include mosaic perfusion, wall thickening, dilatation, and tiny centrilobular nodules. The term "bronchial wall thickening" describes the infiltration of the airway wall by eosinophils and lymphocytes (the diagnosis of asthma requires the presence of this clinical symptom at some point during the disease's course). Expanded interlobular septa could be a sign of edema from renal and/or cardiac involvement, or it could be the result of eosinophilic septal infiltration. Up to 50% of patients experience eosinophilic pleural effusions. Most patients have tree-in-bud, bronchial wall thickening, and bronchial dilatation; these airway abnormalities are probably related to asthma; eosinophilic involvement may also contribute to the thickening of the bronchial wall. In airspace disease, the differential diagnosis consists of simple eosinophilic pneumonia (Löffler syndrome), organizing pneumonia, and chronic eosinophilic pneumonia. The list is longer for airway-dominant disease and includes asthma, infectious bronchiolitis, SLE, MPA, and EAA.

9.4.2.8.2. Microscopic Polyangiitis (MPA)

A systemic necrotizing small-vessel vasculitis without granulomatous inflammation is known as microscopic polyangiitis (MPA). Clinically, it is typified by a protracted prodromal phase that is marked by fever, weight loss, and glomerulonephritis that progresses quickly. The most common cause of pulmonary-renal syndrome is microscopic polyangiitis; up to 90% of cases show rapidly progressive glomerulonephritis, and up to 30%–50% show pulmonary involvement. Over 75% of patients have ANCA positivity during their illness, with MPO ANCA accounting for 35–65% of cases. Diffuse Alveolar Hemorrhage (DAH) and glomerulonephritis together define microscopic polyangiitis. Diffuse, bilateral, or patchy airspace opacities are among the imaging findings. The opacity can display characteristics of both ground glass and consolidations, depending on the degree of blood filling in the alveoli. DAH usually affects the perihilar regions more extensively, sparing the costophrenic angles and lung apices. The characteristic of bleeding is highlighted by a halo encircling a consolidation or nodule. Interlobular lines, sometimes known as "crazy paving," may show up more during the resorption phase. Reticulation, traction bronchiectasis, and honeycombing are symptoms of fibrosis brought on by recurrent bleeding. In MPA patients, interstitial lung disease is more common than in GPA patients (Oppedal et al., 2007; Laghi et al., 2009; Spagnolo et al., 2015; Dursunoglu et al., 2016; Farag, 2017).

9.4.2.9. Antiglomerular Basement Membrane Disease (Anti-GBM Disease)

The immune complex SVV group includes anti-GBM disease, which is defined by circulating antibodies against an antigen that is intrinsic to the glomerular basement membrane. Necrotizing glomerulonephritis and acute renal failure are the outcomes. Renal biopsy is typically used to make the diagnosis. About 40–60% of cases involve diffuse alveolar hemorrhage (DAH); isolated pulmonary involvement is incredibly uncommon. While the term "Goodpasture disease" is limited to the combination of DAG, glomerulonephritis, and anti-GBM antibodies, the term "Goodpasture syndrome" is used to refer to patients with both pulmonary hemorrhage and glomerulonephritis, regardless of the underlying cause. 30% of the samples have c-ANCA or p-ANCA positivity, and more than 90% have anti-basement membrane antibodies. The incidence is higher in young men than in women (M:F = 9:1), though it can also occur in older women. Treatment will improve the prognosis. underlying lung damage, e.g., it is believed that lung involvement is predisposed by smoking or cocaine inhalation. Pulmonary fibrosis is the result of repeated episodes. Due to alveolar hemorrhage, imaging features include diffuse or patchy ground glass or consolidation, which usually goes away in a few days. Usually, the perihilar regions in the mid-zones and lower lung zones predominate and the subpleural space is spared. Rarely does pleural effusion occur. Reticular opacities, honeycombing, and traction bronchiectasis may develop following recurrent episodes.

9.4.3. Miscellaneous Systemic Disorders

9.4.3.1. Inflammatory Bowel Disease

Various respiratory issues can be linked to ulcerative colitis and Crohn's disease. These complications can either manifest before the diagnosis of inflammatory bowel disease or years after the initial diagnosis, even following complete colectomy for ulcerative colitis. It has been suggested that pulmonary complications may be more prevalent post-surgery, possibly due to the discontinuation of anti-inflammatory treatment. Tracheobronchitis and airway stenosis are common in both Crohn's disease and ulcerative colitis. Additionally, bronchiectasis, and thickening of the bronchial walls are frequently seen. Inflammatory bowel disease can also lead to parenchymal abnormalities such as organizing pneumonia, pulmonary hemorrhage, and granulomatous infiltration in Crohn's disease.

9.4.3.2. Amyloidosis and Light Chain Deposition Disease

Extracellular protein deposition in one or more organs is a feature of rare disorders such as amyloidosis and light chain deposition disease. Clinical, radiographic, and pathologic characteristics are shared by both. The primary distinction between these two entities can be seen in the fibrillar structure and Congo red staining observed in amyloidosis electron microscopy. These two things could be connected to a dyscrasia of the plasma cells. Three radiographic signs of amyloidosis are explained: diffuse alveolar septal, tracheobronchial, and nodular parenchymal. Radiographically, the nodular parenchymal form appears as one or more solid lung nodules, which are frequently discovered by accident. These could be mistaken for cancer, especially if there are spiculated borders. There may be calcification and a typical slow growth rate. Widespread deposits in the lungs are a characteristic of the diffuse alveolar septal form. Small nodules (usually distributed perilymphatically), consolidation, ground-glass opacity, and reticulation are the most frequently observed findings. Particularly suggestive may be the presence of calcification connected to these abnormalities. The tracheobronchial form exhibits calcification or widespread thickening of the bronchi and/or trachea. Less is known about the imaging results of light chain deposition disease. The two varieties are diffuse and nodular. The nodular type is characterized by sporadic, solid nodules that are frequently connected to cysts. Usually, the nodules are found inside the cysts or close to their walls. Similar to the diffuse alveolar septal type of amyloidosis, the diffuse type may exhibit diffuse small nodules.

9.4.3.3. Erdheim-Chester Disease

The infiltrative disorder known as Erdheim-Chester disease is characterized by the presence of non-Langerhans' cell histiocytes in one or more organ systems. The brain, kidneys, heart, and bones are the main organs that are impacted. Men in their middle years are most frequently impacted. Even though pathology is useful in ruling out lymphoproliferative malignancies, typical radiographic features are crucial to making the right diagnosis because pathologic findings may not be specific. Periadventitial aortic soft tissue thickening is a characteristic finding in chest imaging. The phrase "coating" of the aorta refers to this thickening, which may affect the aorta and its major branches diffusely. The most typical finding in the lungs is the thickening of the smooth interlobular septa, which is similar to pulmonary edema. The most distinctive finding outside of the chest is soft tissue circumferential to the perinephric region, which bears similarities to lymphoma.

9.4.3.4. IgG4-Related Sclerosing Disease

Once named lymphoplasmacytic sclerosing pancreatitis, IgG4-related sclerosing disease was first believed to be confined to the pancreas. It is now understood to be a systemic order connected to fibrosclerosis in several organ systems and IgG4 plasma cells. The pancreas, hepatobiliary system, salivary glands, and lymph nodes are the main organs that are affected. The chest can show a variety of findings, such as thickening of the airways, lymphadenopathy, nodules, and pleural abnormalities. It's also possible that some idiopathic interstitial pneumonia cases are caused by sclerosing disease associated with IgG4 (Oppedal et al., 2007; Laghi et al., 2009; Spagnolo et al., 2015; Dursunoglu et al., 2016; Farag, 2017).

A Closer Look

Chronic Obstructive Pulmonary Disease (COPD)

Chronic Obstructive Pulmonary Disease (COPD) is a progressive respiratory condition characterized by airflow limitation that is not fully reversible. This disease primarily affects the lungs, leading to symptoms such as chronic cough, excessive sputum production, dyspnea (shortness of breath), and wheezing. COPD encompasses two main conditions: chronic bronchitis and emphysema, often occurring together in affected individuals.

Chronic bronchitis is characterized by inflammation and narrowing of the airways, leading to increased mucus production and cough. This chronic inflammation damages the bronchial tubes, impairing their ability to clear mucus and causing persistent coughing, particularly in the morning. Over time, the airways become scarred and thickened, further obstructing airflow and contributing to respiratory symptoms.

Emphysema, on the other hand, involves the destruction of the lung alveoli, the tiny air sacs responsible for gas exchange. Exposure to irritants such as cigarette smoke or environmental pollutants triggers an inflammatory response, which, over time, leads to the breakdown of the alveolar walls. As a result, the lungs lose their elasticity and ability to recoil, impairing their ability to expel air. This results in air trapping within the lungs, leading to hyperinflation and dyspnea.

The primary risk factor for COPD is cigarette smoking, although long-term exposure to other respiratory irritants such as air pollution, occupational dust, and indoor biomass fuel combustion can also contribute to its development. Genetic factors, such as alpha-1 antitrypsin deficiency, can predispose individuals to the development of COPD, particularly at a younger age.

Diagnosis of COPD typically involves a combination of medical history, physical examination, pulmonary function tests (spirometry), and imaging studies (such as chest X-rays or CT scans). Spirometry is crucial for assessing airflow limitation and determining the severity of the disease based on parameters like forced expiratory volume in one second (FEV1) and the ratio of FEV1 to forced vital capacity (FVC). Management of COPD focuses on relieving symptoms, improving quality of life, and preventing disease progression. Smoking cessation is the most critical intervention, as it can significantly slow the decline in lung function and reduce mortality risk. Medications such as bronchodilators (inhaled beta-agonists and anticholinergics) and corticosteroids are commonly prescribed to alleviate symptoms and reduce exacerbation risk. Pulmonary rehabilitation programs, which include exercise training, education, and psychosocial support, play a vital role in improving exercise capacity and overall well-being in COPD patients. In severe cases of COPD, where medical therapy alone is insufficient, supplemental oxygen therapy or surgical interventions such as lung volume reduction surgery or lung transplantation may be considered. Despite advances in treatment, COPD remains a leading cause of morbidity and mortality worldwide, underscoring the importance of early detection, smoking cessation, and comprehensive management strategies in improving outcomes for affected individuals.

Summary

- Lung diseases associated with systemic disorders refer to a group of respiratory conditions that are interconnected with underlying systemic or whole-body diseases.
- Autoimmune diseases like rheumatoid arthritis, systemic lupus erythematosus (SLE), and scleroderma are among the primary systemic disorders associated with lung manifestations.
- Diabetes, for instance, can predispose individuals to respiratory infections, impair lung function, and increase the risk of developing conditions like chronic obstructive pulmonary disease (COPD) and asthma.
- Lung disease refers to several types of diseases or disorders that prevent the lungs from functioning properly. Lung disease can affect respiratory function, or the ability to breathe, and pulmonary function, which is how well the lungs work.
- A nagging cough or slight wheeze may barely register in the course of our busy days, but it's critically important to pay attention to even mild symptoms. Sometimes people think having trouble breathing is just something that comes with getting older.
- The pleura is the thin lining that surrounds your lung and lines the inside of your chest wall. A tiny layer of fluid lets the pleura on your lung's surface slide along the chest wall with each breath.
- Common endocrine disorders may affect the respiratory system in a variety of ways, from an increased risk of specific infections in patients with diabetes to upper airway compression in patients with goiter.
- Cardiovascular and end-organ dysfunction develops in many patients with diabetes because of its chronic metabolic derangements. Cardiovascular factors appear to contribute more than pulmonary factors to impaired physical performance in patients with diabetes.
- The incidence of multinodular goiter is declining in the United States due to the routine use of iodized salt; nevertheless, neglected goiters are still detected. Because of the thyroid's ability to expand easily in the anterior space, bound only by skin, thin muscle, and connective tissue, even large goiters may not cause tracheal impingement.
- Hypothyroidism has been associated with dyspnea on exertion, alveolar hypoventilation, respiratory failure, obstructive, and central sleep apnea, and pleural effusions. Lung volumes are generally normal or mildly decreased in mixed populations of obese and nonobese hypothyroid patients.

References

1. Cavailles, A., Brinchault-Rabin, G., Dixmier, A., Goupil, F., Gut-Gobert, C., Marchand-Adam, S., et al. (2013). Comorbidities of COPD. *European Respiratory Review*, *22*(130), 454–475. https://doi.org/10.1183/09059180.00008612.
2. Chen, S. J., Liao, W. C., Huang, K. H., Lin, C. L., Tsai, W. C., Kung, P. T., et al. (2015). Chronic obstructive pulmonary disease and allied conditions is a strong independent risk factor for osteoporosis and pathologic fractures: A population-based cohort study. *QJM*, *108*(8), 633–640. https://doi.org/10.1093/qjmed/hcv012.

3. de Lucas-Ramos, P., Izquierdo-Alonso, J. L., Rodriguez-Gonzalez Moro, J. M., Frances, J. F., Lozano, P. V., Bellon-Cano, J. M., et al. (2012). Chronic obstructive pulmonary disease as a cardiovascular risk factor: Results of a case-control study (CONSISTE study). *International Journal of Chronic Obstructive Pulmonary Disease, 7*, 679–686. https://doi.org/10.2147/COPD.S36222.

4. Dursunoglu, N., Kokturk, N., Baha, A., Bilge, A. K., Borekci, S., & Ciftci, F., et al. (2016). Comorbidities and their impact on chronic obstructive pulmonary disease. *Tuberk Toraks, 64*(4), 289–298. https://doi.org/10.5578/tt.2245.

5. Farag, A. M. (2017). Head and neck manifestations of endocrine disorders. *Atlas of Oral and Maxillofacial Surgery Clinics of North America, 25*(2), 197–207. https://doi.org/10.1016/j.cxom.2017.04.011.

6. Fouda, M. A., Alhamad, E. H., Al-Hajjaj, M. S., Shaik, S. A., Alboukai, A. A., & Al-Kassimi, F. A. (2017). A study of chronic obstructive pulmonary disease-specific causes of osteoporosis with emphasis on the emphysema phenotype. *Annals of Thoracic Medicine, 12*(2), 101–106. https://doi.org/10.4103/atm.ATM_357_16.

7. Graat-Verboom, L., Wouters, E. F., Smeenk, F. W., van den Borne, B. E., Lunde, R., & Spruit, M. A. (2009). Current status of research on osteoporosis in COPD: A systematic review. *European Respiratory Journal, 34*(1), 209–218. https://doi.org/10.1183/09031936.50130408.

8. Inoue, D., Watanabe, R., & Okazaki, R. (2016). COPD and osteoporosis: Links, risks, and treatment challenges. *International Journal of Chronic Obstructive Pulmonary Disease, 11*, 637–648. https://doi.org/10.2147/COPD.S79638.

9. Laghi, F., Adiguzel, N., & Tobin, M. J. (2009). Endocrinological derangements in COPD. *European Respiratory Journal, 34*(4), 975–996. https://doi.org/10.1183/09031936.00103708.

10. Lopez-Otin, C., Blasco, M. A., Partridge, L., Serrano, M., & Kroemer, G. (2013). The hallmarks of aging. *Cell, 153*(6), 1194–1217. https://doi.org/10.1016/j.cell.2013.05.039.

11. Mannino, D. M., Thorn, D., Swensen, A., & Holguin, F. (2008). Prevalence and outcomes of diabetes, hypertension and cardiovascular disease in COPD. *European Respiratory Journal, 32*(4), 962–969. https://doi.org/10.1183/09031936.00012408.

12. Mullerova, H., Agusti, A., Erqou, S., & Mapel, D. W. (2013). Cardiovascular comorbidity in COPD: Systematic literature review. *Chest, 144*(4), 1163–1178. https://doi.org/10.1378/chest.12-2847.

13. Naik, D., Joshi, A., Paul, T. V., & Thomas, N. (2014). Chronic obstructive pulmonary disease and the metabolic syndrome: Consequences of a dual threat. *Indian Journal of Endocrinology and Metabolism, 18*(5), 608–616. https://doi.org/10.4103/2230-8210.139212.

14. Oppedal, R. J., Khan, D. A., & Brown, E. S. (2007). Hypothyroidism in patients with asthma and major depressive disorder. *Primary Care Companion for CNS Disorders, 9*(6), 467–468. https://doi.org/10.4088/PCC.v09n0611d.

15. Raghu, G., Amatto, V. C., Behr, J., & Stowasser, S. (2015). Comorbidities in idiopathic pulmonary fibrosis patients: A systematic literature review. *European Respiratory Journal, 46*(4), 1113–1130. https://doi.org/10.1183/13993003.02316-2014.

16. Sarinc Ulasli, S., Bozbas, S. S., Ozen, Z. E., Ozyurek, B. A., & Ulubay, G. (2013). Effect of thyroid function on COPD exacerbation frequency: A preliminary study. *Multidisciplinary Respiratory Medicine, 8*(1), 64. https://doi.org/10.1186/2049-6958-8-64.

17. Schols, A. M. (2015). Nutritional advances in patients with respiratory diseases. *European Respiratory Review, 24*(135), 17–22. https://doi.org/10.1183/09059180.00010914.

18. Soriano, J. B., Visick, G. T., Muellerova, H., Payvandi, N., & Hansell, A. L. (2005). Patterns of comorbidities in newly diagnosed COPD and asthma in primary care. *Chest, 128*(4), 2099–2107. https://doi.org/10.1378/chest.128.4.2099.

19. Spagnolo, P., Tzouvelekis, A., & Maher, T. M. (2015). Personalized medicine in idiopathic pulmonary fibrosis: Facts and promises. *Current Opinion in Pulmonary Medicine, 21*(5), 470–478. https://doi.org/10.1097/MCP.0000000000000187.

20. Terzano, C., Romani, S., Paone, G., Conti, V., & Oriolo, F. (2014). COPD and thyroid dysfunctions. *Lung, 192*(1), 103–109. https://doi.org/10.1007/s00408-013-9537-6.

21. Walter, R. E., Beiser, A., Givelber, R. J., O'Connor, G. T., & Gottlieb, D. J. (2003). Association between glycemic state and lung function: The Framingham Heart Study. *American Journal of Respiratory and Critical Care Medicine, 167*(6), 911–916. https://doi.org/10.1164/rccm.2203022.

Chapter

TREATING AND MANAGING PULMONARY DISEASE

10

Contents

Introduction

Pulmonary disease treatment and management is a complex process that calls for a multimodal strategy that is adapted to the unique circumstances and requirements of each patient. Asthma, pneumonia, pulmonary fibrosis, lung cancer, and chronic obstructive pulmonary disease (COPD) are just a few of the conditions that fall under the umbrella of pulmonary diseases. The goals of effective management and treatment plans are to reduce symptoms, strengthen lung function, stop the disease from getting worse, and improve the patients' overall quality of life. Medication therapy is one of the mainstays of treating pulmonary diseases. Different medications may be prescribed, depending on the nature and severity of the condition. Breathing becomes easier for people with conditions like asthma and COPD when bronchodilators, such as anticholinergics and beta-agonists, relax the muscles surrounding the airways. Inhaled corticosteroids are frequently used as maintenance therapy in the treatment of asthma and COPD because they help reduce airway inflammation. Furthermore, bacterial infections may also be treated with antibiotics, and fungal infections that can harm the lungs are treated with antifungal drugs. Pulmonary rehabilitation is essential for enhancing the functional ability and quality of life of people with long-term respiratory disorders when combined with medication therapy. Programs for pulmonary rehabilitation usually include nutrition counseling, breathing exercises, education on lung health and disease management, and exercise training. These programs aim to provide patients more control over their symptoms, improve their physical stamina, and lessen the influence of their illness on day-to-day activities.

Supplemental oxygen therapy may be required for several pulmonary diseases, including severe COPD and pulmonary fibrosis, to guarantee that the body's tissues and organs receive enough oxygen. Oxygen therapy can help patients with symptoms like exhaustion, shortness of breath, and cognitive decline, making it easier for them to go about their everyday lives. Surgical options may be taken into consideration in situations where medical intervention is not able to stop the progression of the disease or where conservative treatments are failing. For those with end-stage lung disease who have not responded to previous treatments and who fit certain criteria for transplant candidacy, a lung transplant may be advised. In cases like bronchiectasis, surgical resection may also be necessary to remove damaged lung tissue or treat localized lung cancers.

In addition, lifestyle changes like giving up smoking, keeping a healthy weight, and avoiding pollution from the environment are crucial for managing lung diseases. In cases like COPD and lung cancer, quitting smoking is especially important for halting the progression of the disease and preventing additional lung damage. A comprehensive strategy that incorporates medication therapy, pulmonary rehabilitation, supplemental oxygen therapy, surgical interventions, and lifestyle modifications is necessary for the treatment and management of pulmonary diseases. Healthcare professionals can improve outcomes and improve the quality of life for people with pulmonary conditions by attending to the various needs of their patients and maximizing their respiratory health.

Orientation and Directional Terms

Term	Definition	Illustration
Respiratory system	Respiratory system is made up of your lungs, airways (trachea, bronchi, and bronchioles), diaphragm, voice box, throat, nose, and mouth.	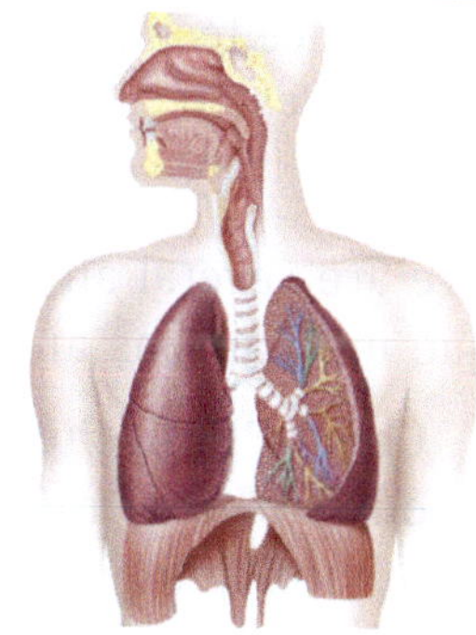
Mucociliary clearance	Mucociliary clearance (MCC) is the primary innate defense mechanism of the lung.	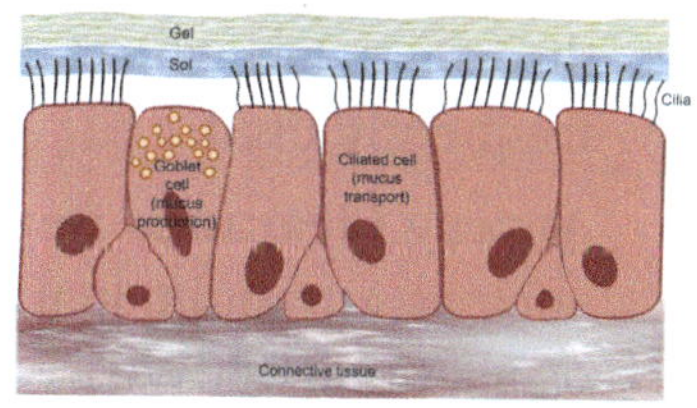
Glycopyrronium	Glycopyrronium is an anticholinergic agent used to treat hyperhidrosis, severe drooling, and COPD, used with other medications to treat ulcers, and used in anesthesia.	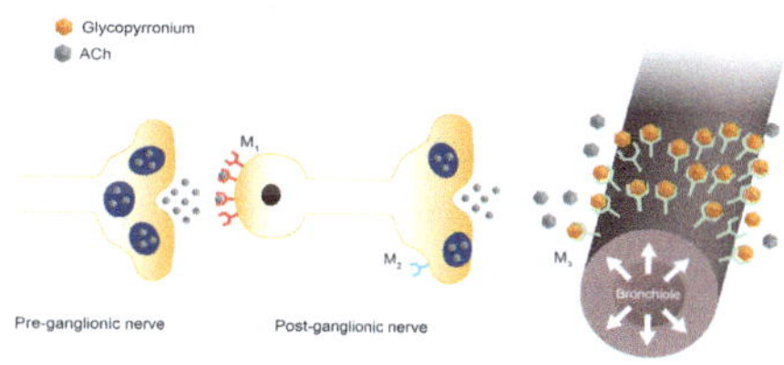
Broncholytic	It is a substance that dilates the bronchi and bronchioles, decreasing resistance in the respiratory airway and increasing airflow to the lungs.	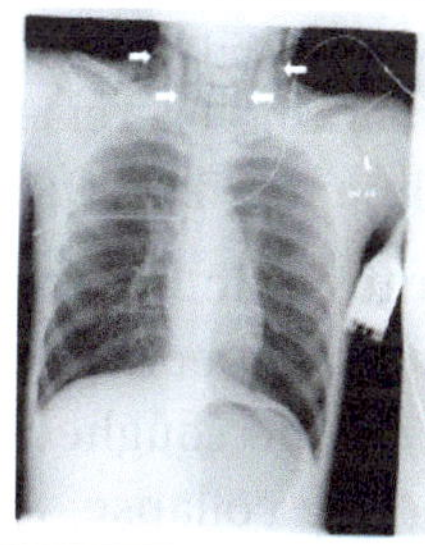
Anticholinergics	Anticholinergics are substances that block the action of the acetylcholine neurotransmitter at synapses in the central and peripheral nervous system.	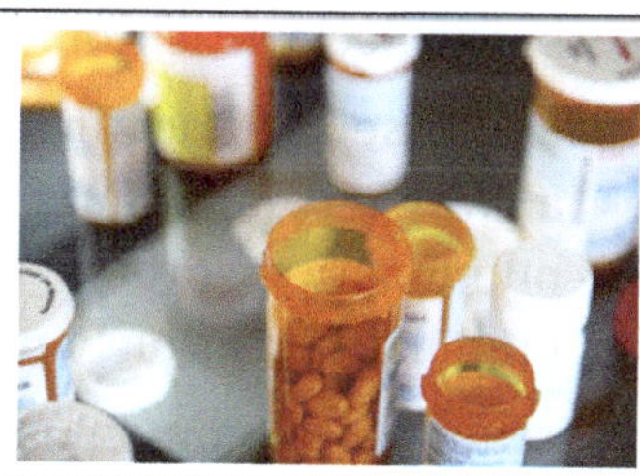

10.1. Airway Clearance Techniques

The management of a variety of pulmonary conditions, especially those marked by increased mucus production, airway inflammation, and compromised mucociliary clearance, requires the use of airway clearance techniques (ACTs). By making it easier to remove secretions such as mucus from the airways, these techniques hope to improve lung function overall, lower the risk of respiratory infections, and improve ventilation.

There are several airway clearance techniques commonly used in clinical practice, each with its unique mechanisms and indications:

- **Chest Physiotherapy (CPT)**: CPT uses manual methods to help clear mucus, carried out by a respiratory therapist or other qualified caregiver. These methods could involve breathing exercises, postural drainage (arranging the body to promote drainage), percussion (gentle tapping) and vibration over the chest wall. Neuromuscular disorders, bronchiectasis, and cystic fibrosis are among the conditions for which CPT is frequently used.
- **Airway Clearance Devices**: There are several tools available to help clear the airways, such as intrapulmonary percussive ventilation (IPV) devices, high-frequency chest wall oscillation (HFCWO) vests, and oscillatory positive expiratory pressure (PEP) devices. These gadgets produce vibrations or oscillations to help loosen mucus and make it easier to expel from the respiratory tract. They are appropriate for people with diseases like COPD, bronchiectasis, and non-cystic fibrosis bronchiectasis. They can be used alone or in combination with other therapies.
- **Active Cycle of Breathing Technique (ACBT)**: Thoracic expansion exercises, forced expiratory techniques, and breathing control are all combined in ACBT, an organized breathing method that helps to facilitate mucus clearance. It consists of multiple breathing exercise cycles followed by clearing secretions with huffing or coughing. For ailments like COPD, bronchiectasis, and asthma, ACBT is frequently used.
- **Autogenic Drainage (AD)**: Using deliberate breathing techniques, AD is a self-drainage method that moves mucus from the peripheral to the central airways, where it can be coughed up or expectorated. To maximize mucus clearance without causing airway collapse, AD uses varying breathing volumes and airflow rates. People with bronchiectasis, chronic bronchitis, and cystic fibrosis are frequently prescribed it.
- **Exercise**: By boosting mucociliary clearance, increasing cough efficacy, and lowering airway inflammation, regular exercise can also aid in airway clearance. For people with pulmonary disorders, aerobic activities like walking, cycling, and swimming can help mobilize secretions and enhance general lung function.

The treatment of pulmonary disorders marked by increased mucus secretion and compromised clearance mechanisms heavily depends on the use of airway clearance techniques. These methods are intended to maximize lung function, lower the chance of respiratory complications, and enhance the quality of life for those who have long-term respiratory disorders. To maximize therapeutic results, the choice of an appropriate airway clearance technique should take into account the patient's unique diagnosis, clinical status, and preferences. This may necessitate continuing evaluation and modification. The goal of airway clearance therapy is to remove secretions and mucus from the respiratory airways using a variety of airway clearance techniques. Many respiratory conditions impair the regular mucociliary clearance mechanism, which leads to a mucus buildup that impedes breathing and interferes with the cough reflex. Infection and inflammation can also be brought on by mucus accumulation, and recurrent infections can harm lung tissue and the airways.

Coughing and puffing are methods used in all airway clearance therapies, and they must be combined with other airway clearance techniques. The advice and recommendations for suitable airway clearance therapies are provided by respiratory therapists. They also provide training on how to employ different airway clearance methods (Hristara-Papadopoulou et al., 2008; Brunetta and Kroon, 2022).

10.1.1. Clearance Techniques

To preserve respiratory health and stop the harmful effects of inflammation, airway clearance therapy (ACTs) is used in many respiratory disorders, such as cystic fibrosis, bronchitis, bronchiectasis, and chronic obstructive pulmonary disease. Breathing, manual, and mechanical techniques are used. All of them must be used in conjunction with coughing or huffing to clear the large airways of mucus. It takes the use of an additional ACT to clear mucus from the small airways.

10.1.1.1. Breathing

Breathing techniques include the active cycle of breathing which includes huffing; and autogenic drainage, a technique that requires concentrated effort.

10.1.1.2. Huffing

The forced expiration technique, also known as huffing or a huff cough, aids in moving mucus away from the lung wall so that it can eventually be coughed out. It is necessary to huff while seated, with the mouth left open and the chin lifted slightly. After taking a deep breath that fills the lungs to about 75%, hold it for two or three seconds. The mucus is moved from the smaller to the larger airways when exhaling forcefully and slowly. At this point, one should suppress the natural urge to cough and repeat the breathing pattern a few times. To get rid of the mucus, a severe cough then ensues. Part of the active breathing cycle is huffing. Huffing as a clearing technique is not the same as the term used for inhaling substances.

10.1.1.3. Active Cycle of Breathing

There are three stages to the active cycle of breathing technique. In phase one, the airways are relaxed; in phase two, the inhaled air is moved to behind the mucus to help clear it; and in phase three, the mucus is helped to exit the lungs.

10.1.1.4.Phase One

Phase one involves relaxing the airways with gentle, effortless breathing in through the nose and out through the mouth. Maintain a relaxed upper chest and set of shoulders. The pursed lips method is advised when exhaling. When exhaling, pursed lips—as in, kissing someone—create back pressure that maintains the airways open for a longer period of time. One suggestion is to start phase two of the cycle with six breaths of control.

10.1.1.5. Phase Two

The second phase consists of chest expansion exercises. Deep breathing may be necessary to force air into the smaller airways and behind the mucus, requiring a three-second breath hold. The exhale is spontaneous and could involve some vibration or clapping in time with the beat.

10.1.1.6. Phase Three

The mucus is transferred from the smaller to the larger airways by huffing while coughing; huffing must be repeated until all of the mucus is expelled.

10.1.1.7. Autogenic Drainage

Using varying depths of inhalation and speeds of exhalation, autogenic drainage is a controlled airway clearance technique that allows mucus to be moved up the airway and causes a voluntary cough. Although this method doesn't require any equipment, it can be difficult to execute and requires the right training.

10.1.1.8. Manual

Postural drainage and manual airway clearance techniques such as clapping and vibration are used in chest physiotherapy. However, mechanical devices are frequently used in their place because they require a lot of labor and time.

10.1.1.9. Mechanical

Positive expiratory pressure (PEP), intrapulmonary percussive ventilators, mechanical insufflation-exsufflation, sometimes referred to as mechanically assisted cough, and airway oscillatory devices are examples of mechanical devices that are used. A variety of mechanical methods are employed to loosen mucus and promote expectoration. In addition to being carried out manually, chest percussion can also be carried out with the aid of specialized equipment that uses intrapulmonary percussive ventilation or chest wall oscillation. Short bursts of air are delivered through a mouthpiece by devices known as intrapulmonary percussive ventilators (IPVs), which aid in the clearing of mucus. The air can be used with nebulized medication and is delivered at a rate of about 150 pulses per minute. A passive system that doesn't require user effort is chest wall oscillation. It makes use of a specialized vest that uses a compressor to rhythmically inflate and deflate at predetermined intervals. This causes high-frequency oscillations in the chest wall that are transmitted to the lungs. These oscillations thin the mucus in the airways, making coughing easier to remove. The air supply to the vest can be manually adjusted.

Other techniques include a cough assistance phase and a vibration phase to loosen secretions. Biphasic cuirass ventilation and its related clearance mode are available in such devices. These can be used at home and are portable. Giving the airways back pressure as they exhale is known as positive expiratory pressure physiotherapy. Devices that consist of a mask or mouthpiece with a resistance applied only during the expiration phase provide this effect. The method appears to work by temporarily increasing functional residual capacity and raising gas pressure behind mucus through collateral ventilation, which delays the early collapse of small airways during exhalation.

10.1.2. Management of Chronic Obstructive Pulmonary Disease

The illness known as chronic obstructive pulmonary disease (COPD), which causes airway blockage and is treatable and preventable, is typified by enduring respiratory symptoms. In the US, an estimated 16 million adults suffer from COPD. Patients who smoke or have a history of tobacco use, those over 40, and men have the highest incidence of COPD. Up to 71% of patients in a Medicare population did not receive maintenance therapy, despite recommendations that patients with moderate-to-severe COPD should use maintenance pharmacotherapy. This underscores opportunities for better patient management and care.

When pulmonary decline is minimized and symptoms are adequately controlled, COPD is considered "stable." In contrast, managing "unstable" COPD—in patients who have frequent or severe exacerbations and a quicker decline in pulmonary function—can be more difficult. COPD flare-ups can lead to hospital stays and ED visits, depending on how severe they are. They also significantly increase the financial burden associated with COPD. Additionally, there is a direct link between more expensive treatment and the severity of the illness. The need for improved management to lower recurrent hospitalizations and readmissions linked to severe disease has been brought to light by the 2014 expansion of the Affordable Care Act Hospital Readmissions Reduction Program to include COPD.

10.1.3. Impact of Exacerbations on Patients

It has been demonstrated that increases in the frequency, intensity, and duration of exacerbations considerably lower patients' health-related quality of life with COPD. In a prospective study, the average amount of time it took for symptoms to return to baseline after an exacerbation event was about 14.5 days, but for approximately 7% of exacerbations, peak expiratory flow did not return to baseline levels in less than 99 days. This implies that after an exacerbation, lung function may experience an accelerated decline and may not fully recover. Additionally, it was discovered that with every extra year of illness, the return of lung function and symptoms to baseline levels after an exacerbation happened more slowly, making it more difficult for patients to recover from exacerbations over time. Frequent exacerbations were found to be associated with a long-term decline in lung function (as measured by forced expiratory volume in 1 second, or (FEV_1) in patients with moderate-to-severe COPD in two different studies. In a different study, patients with moderate to severe COPD showed a strong correlation between their health-related quality of life and their symptom burden and frequency of exacerbations. These findings imply that therapies aimed at lowering the frequency of exacerbations may have a major effect on both the state of health and the course of the disease. It's interesting to note that in patients with acute exacerbation of chronic bronchitis who probably also had COPD, even a single exacerbation could cause a significant increase in the rate of decline in lung function and a sustained worsening of health status.

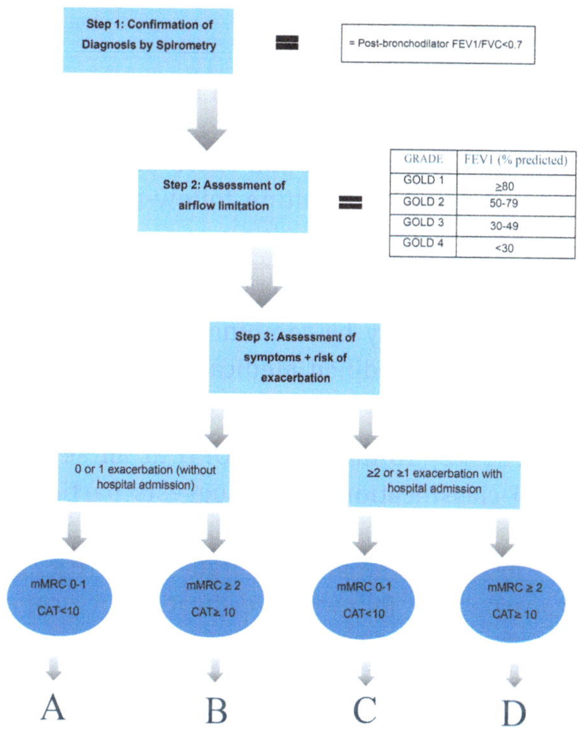

Figure 10.1. *Updated GOLD classification of COPD severity. FEV1: Forced expiratory volume in one second; FVC: forced vital capacity; GOLD: Global Initiative for Chronic Obstructive Lung Disease; CAT: COPD Assessment Test; mMRC: modified Medical Research Council score.*

Source: *Mangold V, Boesing M, Berset C, Bridevaux P-O, Geiser T, Joos Zellweger L, Kohler M, Lüthi-Corridori G, Maier S, Miedinger D, et al. Adherence to the GOLD Guidelines in Primary Care: Data from the Swiss COPD Cohort. Journal of Clinical Medicine. 2023; 12(20):6636. https://doi.org/10.3390/jcm12206636.*

A significant factor in the advancement of the disease is exacerbations, which cause patient lung function to decline more quickly. Patients with milder forms of the disease experience the biggest decline in lung function. The primary objective of COPD management is to prevent exacerbations because they are linked to a notable rise in mortality. Additionally, using the updated ABCD disease risk stratification tool, the Global Initiative for Chronic Obstructive Lung Disease (GOLD) recommendations heavily emphasize the role of exacerbations in determining treatment options (Figure 10.1).

10.1.4. Management of COPD

10.1.4.1. Stable COPD

The foundation of the current COPD management approach is symptom management in conjunction with a decrease in the risk of exacerbation. Appropriate medication (which addresses both symptom management and exacerbation prevention), encouragement to quit smoking, pulmonary rehabilitation, and routine follow-up monitoring for disease progression are the mainstays of managing COPD.

The GOLD ABCD tool classifies patients into disease "risk stratification" groups ABCD to guide pharmacotherapy by combining symptom severity, as determined by the COPD Assessment Test score or the modified Medical Research Council scale, with exacerbation risk, as determined by either spirometry-defined airflow limitation or exacerbation history.

The key to managing COPD at all severity levels is bronchodilators. Based on the patient's ABCD classification, GOLD suggests particular treatment options for the first course of therapy after a diagnosis of COPD. The follow-up treatment is different from the initial therapy because it is based on the most treatable trait (e.g., the medication(s) currently being taken), dyspnea or exacerbation) following verification of proper inhaler technique and compliance with the first treatment plan (Table 10.1).

Table 10.1. *Recommended Treatment for Stable COPD According to the 2011 and 2017 GOLD Guidelines*

Guidelines	GOLD 2011		GOLD 2017
GOLD Group	**First Choice**	**Second Choice**	**Recommended**
A	SABA or SAMA, or SABA/SAMA	LABA or LAMA	SABA or SAMA, or SABA/SAMA or LABA, or LAMA
B	LABA or LAMA	LABA/LAMA	LABA or LAMA or LABA/LAMA
C	ICS/LABA or LAMA	LABA/LAMA	LAMA or LABA/LAMA or ICS/LABA

Guidelines	GOLD 2011		GOLD 2017
GOLD Group	**First Choice**	**Second Choice**	**Recommended**
D	ICS/LABA or LAMA	ICS/ LABA/ LAMA, LABA/ LAMA, or LAMA/ ICS	LAMA or LABA/ LAMA or ICS/LABA, or ICS/LABA/ LAMA, or LAMA/ICS

SABA: short acting beta-agonist; SAMA: short-acting muscarinic-antagonist; LABA: long-acting beta-agonist; LAMA: long-acting muscarinic antagonist; ICS: inhaled corticosteroid.

Source: *Mangold V, Boesing M, Berset C, Bridevaux P-O, Geiser T, Joos Zellweger L, Kohler M, Lüthi-Corridori G, Maier S, Miedinger D, et al. Adherence to the GOLD Guidelines in Primary Care: Data from the Swiss COPD Cohort. Journal of Clinical Medicine. 2023; 12(20):6636. https://doi.org/10.3390/jcm12206636.*

Evidence from multiple studies supports the preference for combinations of long-acting muscarinic antagonist (LAMA) and long-acting β_2-agonist (LABA) over regimens containing inhaled corticosteroids (ICS). Glycopyrronium/indacaterol (LAMA/LABA) reduced the incidence of pneumonia in patients with moderate-to-severe COPD and significantly improved lung function when compared to salmeterol/fluticasone (LABA/ICS) in the LANTERN and ILLUMINATE studies. Similarly, in patients with moderate-to-severe COPD, a LAMA/LABA combination of tiotropium/olodaterol improved lung function more than salmeterol/fluticasone. In patients who had a history of COPD exacerbations within the previous year, glycopyrronium/indacaterol was found to be more effective than salmeterol/fluticasone in decreasing the rate of exacerbations and lengthening the time to the first exacerbation in the FLAME study. Notably, in patients with moderate-to-severe COPD who had either up to 1 or at least 1 exacerbation in the previous year, LAMA/LABA combination therapy significantly reduced the rate of COPD exacerbations by 31% and 11%, respectively, in comparison with LABA/ICS.

In cases where patients do not respond to ICS or where concerns arise about the risks associated with ICS, a switch from LABA/ICS to LAMA/LABA is advised. LAMA/LABA/ICS triple therapy should be taken into consideration if patients continue to experience exacerbations while following the LABA/ICS or LAMA/LABA treatment regimens. To transition from LAMA/LABA to a triple therapy, the biomarker assessment, i.e., eosinophil counts of at least 100 cells/μL indicates a higher likelihood of benefit from triple therapy in patients. Patients with eosinophil counts <100 cells/μL who have chronic bronchitis with severe airflow limitation (FEV_1<50%) and who were previously smokers should be evaluated for roflumilast and azithromycin, respectively.

Studies evaluating the combination of LAMA/LABA/ICS triple therapy have demonstrated better bronchodilator effects when compared to LAMA and LABA/ICS alone. Additionally, compared to LABA/ICS alone, triple therapy was demonstrated to reduce exacerbations by 23–35% in patients who had experienced exacerbations in the preceding year. The GOLD strategy document recommends escalation to triple therapy for patients who, despite their ABCD assessment at diagnosis, experience further exacerbations on LAMA/LABA or LAMA/ICS. The GOLD recommendations, however, point out that there is a lack of direct evidence to show whether triple therapy will benefit LAMA/LABA in the absence of a biomarker assessment. Since the 2017 update, the GOLD guidelines have included recommendations for de-escalation of treatment if additional therapies do not yield incremental benefits. This is especially relevant when it comes to stopping ICS treatment if no benefit is observed, if pneumonia is detected, or if a doctor determines that ICS was prescribed for an inappropriate original indication. This is new because, due to the progressive nature of the illness, previous COPD treatment methods have tended to be long-term and cumulative. Patients respond differently to different therapies, so it is important to always treat each patient as an individual.

10.1.4.2. Acute Exacerbation

For the treatment of exacerbations, short-acting bronchodilators—in particular, short-acting β_2-agonists—are advised. They can be taken in conjunction with short-acting anticholinergics. For moderate-to-severe COPD exacerbations or those that do not respond to short-acting bronchodilators, a systemic corticosteroid may need to be added to the treatment plan. Oral corticosteroids are preferred over intravenous corticosteroids by the European Respiratory Society/American Thoracic Society (ERS/ATS) guidelines for patients who are hospitalized due to an exacerbation. While oral corticosteroid therapy helps treat exacerbations, it is best to minimize the amount of time that corticosteroid use is employed to prevent adverse effects, such as pneumonia. While GOLD suggests a shorter duration of 5 days, ERS/ATS guidelines recommend corticosteroid treatment for up to 14 days. Shorter courses (5 days) of systemic corticosteroids were noninferior to longer courses (14 days) for patients going through an exacerbation, according to the REDUCE trial. The outcomes of both treatments were similar in terms of lung function recovery times and re-exacerbation rates within 6 months. Patients with increased sputum purulence, a sign of bacterial infection, should consider antibiotics as an adjunctive treatment. The only recommendation made by GOLD on antibiotic selection is to take local patterns of bacterial resistance into account.

Following the start of an exacerbation, symptoms such as acute respiratory failure, severe dyspnea, and/or a failure to respond to initial treatment can indicate the need for an inpatient admission.

10.1.5. Opportunities for Transitional Care Management

Hurst and colleagues claim that exacerbations in COPD are not sporadic occurrences but rather take place during an 8-week window of high risk for subsequent exacerbations. For preventative interventions, this finding offers healthcare providers a therapeutic window. One of the main objectives of managing COPD is lowering the risk of exacerbations in the future. After an exacerbation, patients should begin the appropriate maintenance medication. It is advised that all patients schedule follow-up appointments within 1 to 4 weeks of hospitalization for acute exacerbation and 12 to 16 weeks after discharge. These consultations ought to center on topics like symptom measurement, inhaler technique, and treatment regimen (Hristara-Papadopoulou et al., 2008; Brunetta and Kroon, 2022). Patients with COPD frequently have inadequate inhaler technique, which is linked to a higher risk of ED visits and hospital stays. To effectively manage COPD, patient education regarding inhaler technique must be reinforced both initially and repeatedly. Because patient satisfaction with the inhaler is thought to influence adherence, choosing an appropriate inhaler is also important for managing COPD. Medication adherence should be covered in follow-up visits and patient education. Patients with COPD frequently experience poor adherence to maintenance therapies, which is frequently multifactorial. COPD usually requires more than one medication as the disease worsens, and these medications may not be supplied with the same inhalers. Patients may become confused by using multiple inhalers, which may result in improper inhaler technique. Lack of generic inhaled options may also have an adverse effect on cost, which in turn may harm adherence.

Higher adherence is linked to fewer hospitalizations, while poor adherence is linked to higher death rates. Furthermore, mishandling of inhalers is linked to a higher frequency of severe exacerbations of COPD. As a result, the GOLD 2019 report emphasizes for the first time how crucial it is to evaluate inhaler technique and adherence in patients who have trouble controlling their symptoms before modifying their medication or treatment plan. Pharmacists in community, clinical, and hospital settings can instruct patients with COPD on medication-related matters, such as the need and benefit of taking maintenance drugs, the significance of adhering to a regimen, how to use an inhaler correctly, and how to maintain and troubleshoot it.

10.1.6. Implications for the Health System and Managed Care Community

When compared to stable COPD, COPD exacerbations result in higher doctor visits, ED visits, hospital stays, and pharmacy usage, which makes them a significant contributor to the use of healthcare resources. According to data from extensive prospective and retrospective studies, ~37 and 71% of COPD patients experience at least one exacerbation per year. Although they go unreported, patients with mild COPD can also experience exacerbations. Roughly ~9 to 31% of patients who experience a COPD exacerbation need to visit the ED, and roughly ~14 to 35% need to be admitted to the hospital.

More moderate to severe exacerbations may require ED visits or hospitalization, which increases treatment costs and increases the frequency and severity of exacerbations. Milder exacerbations are frequently treated as outpatients. Treatment for a severe exacerbation that necessitates hospitalization can cost anywhere between $7000 and $39,200 on average, with costs significantly higher for those who need mechanical ventilation. Patients with COPD frequently have coexisting conditions such as cardiovascular disease and lung cancer, which are strongly linked to higher expenses and a higher death rate after being admitted to the hospital for a COPD exacerbation. Five years following a hospital stay due to a COPD exacerbation, survival rates are thought to be as low as 45%.

Hospital readmissions within 30 days of discharge after an acute COPD exacerbation occur in ~20% of patients. Studies have shown that factors associated with re-exacerbation and readmission include longer duration of hospital stay, low FEV_1, comorbidities, high modified Medical Research Council dyspnea score, and previous admissions. A study of 90-day readmission rates following acute exacerbations found that readmission was ~35% and was significantly associated with increased mortality (13.4% in readmitted versus 2.3% in non-readmitted patients).

Patients who are readmitted frequently may exhibit a pattern known as the "frequent exacerbator" phenotype. It is believed that these patients have changes in their adaptive immune system that diminish the body's ability to control inflammation, making them more susceptible to exacerbations of COPD. This phenotype is not exclusive to patients with severe airflow obstruction; in fact, a significant percentage of patients with moderate airflow obstruction also display these characteristics.

The ECLIPSE study revealed that a considerable number of patients with varying levels of airflow obstruction were classified as frequent exacerbators. This is concerning as COPD exacerbations can lead to a decline in lung function, decreased quality of life, and an increased risk of hospitalization and death. The implementation of the Affordable Care Act Hospital Readmissions Reduction Program further emphasizes the importance of finding ways to prevent readmissions and enhance overall patient care.

Many studies have examined the factors contributing to readmissions after patients are discharged following an acute exacerbation, as well as tested methods to lower readmission rates. One study focused on a disease management program for individuals with COPD, which involved post-discharge follow-up in the community. The program successfully decreased 60- and 90-day readmission rates related to COPD and other causes. It featured home visits, clinical evaluations, medication reviews, inhaler training, and educational sessions about the disease. The care team for this program typically consisted of a nurse practitioner, a registered nurse, and a respiratory therapist. Patients discharged to skilled nursing facilities were found to be less likely to be readmitted to a hospital within 30 days of discharge than those discharged home, with or without home care (18.8%, 27.7%, and 31.1% readmission rates, respectively). In a prospective, observational study, a COPD care bundle, involving a multidisciplinary team of respiratory therapists, pulmonologists, pharmacists, critical care physicians, general internists, and nurses, was also found to improve the care of patients with COPD exacerbations. This bundle included standard nursing protocols, patient education on inhaler use and medication, and post discharge referrals to pulmonologists and was found to significantly reduce 30- and 60-day readmissions compared with control (9.1% versus 54.4% for 30-day and 22.7% versus 77.0% for 60-day). Length of hospital stay was also reduced following implementation of the care bundle, as were the total aggregate hospital costs at 90 days post-discharge, which were reduced from $19,954 to $7,652.

On the other hand, some studies have shown that the implementation of care bundles did not lead to a decrease in readmission rates for patients with acute exacerbations of COPD. One randomized study conducted at a single center found that a care bundle consisting of smoking cessation counseling, patient education, and telephone follow-up did not result in lower 30- and 60-day readmission rates. Additionally, a Medicare Bundled Payments for Care Improvement Initiative, which included services such as telephone follow-up, pulmonary rehabilitation, pulmonologist appointments, and home care, did not significantly reduce readmissions at 30 or 90 days and was not deemed cost-effective.

Multidisciplinary pulmonary rehabilitation programs, including exercise therapy and patient education, have been proven to enhance the quality of life for COPD patients. A study conducted over 5 years demonstrated that incorporating negative pressure ventilation into a pulmonary rehabilitation program led to increased exercise capacity and a decrease in lung function decline. Patients receiving this combined treatment also experienced a significant reduction in exacerbations requiring emergency department visits or hospitalization, as well as lower annual medical costs compared to those in an exercise-only program. ERS/ATS guidelines recommend initiating pulmonary rehabilitation within 3 weeks of hospital discharge, but limited accessibility to these programs remains a challenge for many patients who would benefit from them.

Initiating maintenance therapy within 30 days of discharge following an acute COPD exacerbation is crucial in reducing hospitalizations and improving outcomes. Patients who delay starting maintenance therapy have a significantly higher risk of COPD-related hospitalizations or emergency department visits. Studies have shown that starting maintenance therapy early can lead to decreased ED visits, office visits, and outpatient costs in the following year. Despite the benefits, a large number of patients are not prescribed maintenance therapy after a moderate exacerbation, highlighting the importance of adherence to maintenance medication in reducing hospitalizations and mortality. Data from the TORCH trial supports the significance of maintenance medication therapy in managing COPD (Hristara-Papadopoulou et al., 2008; Brunetta and Kroon, 2022).

10.2. Aerosol Delivery of Medication

The delivery of medication through aerosols, known as inhalation therapy, is essential for treating respiratory conditions like asthma, COPD, cystic fibrosis, and respiratory infections. This method allows drugs to be delivered directly to the lungs, where they can work quickly and effectively. Different inhalation devices, such as metered-dose inhalers (MDIs), dry powder inhalers (DPIs), and nebulizers, offer unique benefits and considerations for drug delivery efficiency, patient convenience, and ease of use.

Metered-dose inhalers (MDIs) are small, portable devices that release a controlled amount of medication in aerosol form when activated. They contain a canister with the medication and a valve that delivers the right dose. Patients need to inhale at the same time they press on the MDI to ensure the medicine reaches the lungs efficiently. Following the correct technique and dosage instructions is crucial for getting the most benefit from the medication and avoiding potential side effects. Using a spacer with MDIs can help improve drug delivery to the lungs by making it easier to coordinate inhalation and take deeper breaths.

Dry powder inhalers (DPIs) provide medication in powder form without requiring propellants or coordinated actuation and inhalation. DPIs are activated by the patient's breath, using their own inspiratory flow to disperse the medication powder into the lungs. This makes DPIs ideal for individuals with coordination issues or difficulties with hand-lung coordination. However, DPIs may need a specific level of inspiratory flow for optimal drug delivery, which can be a challenge for patients with severe airflow limitations or weakened inspiratory muscles.

Nebulizers are devices that transform liquid medication into a fine mist that can be easily inhaled through a mask or mouthpiece. They are especially useful for those who struggle to use MDIs or DPIs effectively, such as young children, elderly individuals, and those with severe respiratory issues. Nebulizers have the advantage of delivering high doses of medication over a longer time, which makes them ideal for treating conditions like bronchodilators, corticosteroids, and mucolytic agents in both acute and chronic respiratory management. However, using a nebulizer requires more time for both administering and cleaning, and they are not as portable as handheld inhalers.

Choosing the right inhalation device depends on many factors such as age, cognitive, and physical abilities, severity of the disease, medication schedule, and personal preferences of the patient. It is important for healthcare providers to evaluate each patient individually to determine the most suitable device and provide thorough education on how to use and maintain the inhaler correctly in order to achieve the best therapeutic results.

In addition to selecting the appropriate inhalation device, it is crucial to optimize medication formulations and delivery techniques to ensure that the drug reaches the lungs effectively and reduces potential side effects. Factors like particle size, inhalation flow rate, breath-hold time, and device priming can impact the efficiency of drug delivery and overall therapeutic effectiveness. Healthcare providers should work together with patients to create customized inhalation therapy plans that meet their specific needs and preferences, and regularly assess and follow up to track treatment progress, inhaler technique, and adherence.

Proper delivery of medication through aerosol is crucial in respiratory care as it allows for targeted treatment to the lungs with minimal side effects elsewhere in the body. Healthcare providers are responsible for selecting the best inhalation device, adjusting medication formulations and delivery methods, and educating patients on how to use their inhalers correctly to improve treatment results and overall quality of life for those with respiratory conditions.

10.2.1. Bronchodilators

A bronchodilator is a substance that helps to widen the bronchi and bronchioles to reduce resistance in the respiratory airway and improve airflow to the lungs. These substances can be naturally produced within the body or administered as medications, typically through inhalers, to treat breathing difficulties. Bronchodilators are most effective in obstructive lung diseases like asthma and chronic obstructive pulmonary disease, and there is some debate about their efficacy in conditions like bronchiolitis and bronchiectasis. While they are frequently prescribed, their effectiveness in restrictive lung diseases is not well-established.

Bronchodilators come in short-acting and long-acting forms. Short-acting bronchodilators provide quick relief from acute bronchoconstriction, while long-acting bronchodilators help control and prevent symptoms. There are three types of prescription bronchodilating drugs: beta-2 adrenergic agonists (short- and long-acting), anticholinergics (short- and long-acting), and theophylline (long-acting).

Bronchodilators are medications used to treat lung diseases like asthma and COPD by relaxing the muscle bands in the airways, allowing for easier breathing. They also help remove mucus from the lungs by widening the airways, making it easier to cough up.

10.2.2. Types of Bronchodilators

The two main kinds of bronchodilators that are marketed are inhalers and nebulizer solutions, which are battery-operated devices that produce a thin spray.

Two types of bronchodilators are available:

- **Short-acting bronchodilators:** Acute asthma symptoms can be promptly relieved or stopped with the help of short-acting bronchodilators. They work for a duration of three to six hours. An additional term for a rescue inhaler is a short-acting bronchodilator. Inhalers are medication canisters with a mouthpiece enclosed in a plastic holder. A steady dosage of medication is delivered by an inhaler when sprayed.
- **Long-acting bronchodilators:**

Your airways remain open for 12 hours when using long-acting bronchodilators. You avoid asthma attacks by using these inhalers daily.

10.2.3. Classes of Bronchodilators

Bronchodilators can be divided into three main classes: beta 2-agonists, anticholinergics, and theophylline.

10.2.3.1. Beta-2-Agonists

There are both long-acting and short-acting beta 2-agonists to choose from for asthma relief. Short-acting beta 2-agonists (SABAs) provide quick relief of asthma symptoms and are often referred to as "rescue" or "reliever" medications because they are the most effective for treating sudden, severe, or unusual symptoms. SABAs typically work for four to six hours, with a half-life of 15 to 20 minutes. They can also be used as a preventive measure 15 to 20 minutes before engaging in physical exercise to avoid worsening asthma symptoms.

The following SABA medications are inhaled:

- Levofredolent.
- Albuterol.

The stimulation of beta-adrenergic receptors in the smooth muscle of the airways by beta-agonists results in bronchodilation and relaxation. These drugs are frequently used as rescue or quick-relief drugs to relieve acute bronchoconstriction symptoms like wheezing, dyspnea, and tightness in the chest quickly. Depending on how long they take to take effect, beta-agonists can be classified as long-acting (LABA) or short-acting (SABA). Temporary beta-agonists (e.g., levalbuterol) are commonly utilized as rescue inhalers to provide prompt symptom relief during acute exacerbations, whereas long-acting beta-agonists e.g., for the long-term management of asthma and COPD, maintenance medications (formoterol, salmeterol, and others) are used in conjunction with corticosteroids.

1. **Anticholinergics**: Acetylcholine is a neurotransmitter that, when released into the airways, causes bronchoconstriction. Anticholinergic bronchodilators inhibit its action. Anticholinergic drugs cause bronchodilation and increase airflow by preventing cholinergic activity. These drugs are frequently used as maintenance therapy to lower exacerbations and enhance lung function because they are especially useful in the management of COPD. Temporary anticholinergics (e.g., ipratropium bromide) are accessible for the immediate alleviation of symptoms, whereas long-acting anticholinergics (e.g., tiotropium, and aclidinium) offer long-term bronchodilation and manage COPD symptoms.
2. **Methylxanthines**: Methylxanthines, which include theophylline and aminophylline, cause bronchodilation by blocking phosphodiesterase and opposing adenosine receptors in the smooth muscle of the airways. Methylxanthines may be used as adjunctive therapy in patients with severe asthma or COPD who have not responded well to other bronchodilators, despite being less frequently used than beta-agonists and anticholinergics. However, careful monitoring of serum levels is necessary to maximize efficacy and minimize toxicity when using methylxanthines due to their limited therapeutic window, potential for side effects, and potential for drug interactions.

Some bronchodilators may also have anti-inflammatory qualities in addition to their bronchodilatory effects, which would enhance their usefulness in the treatment of asthma and COPD. In order to provide both bronchodilation and anti-inflammatory effects, combination inhalers that combine bronchodilators and corticosteroids are frequently used in the treatment of asthma and COPD. This improves symptom control and lowers the risk of exacerbations.

In general, bronchodilators are essential for treating respiratory disorders marked by airway blockage because they relieve symptoms, strengthen the lungs, and improve patients' quality of life. With customized treatment plans designed to maximize therapeutic outcomes, the type and severity of the underlying respiratory condition, the patient's preferences, and the patient's response to therapy all play a role in the selection of an appropriate bronchodilator regimen. In order to achieve effective symptom control and reduce the risk of disease exacerbations, bronchodilator therapy requires routine assessment and monitoring of lung function, symptoms, and medication adherence.

10.2.3.2. Combination of Albuterol and Ipratropium Bromide

Long-acting beta-2 agonists (LABAs) can be taken twice a day to help you maintain and manage your airways in the long run. LABAs and inhaled corticosteroids combine well to treat asthma. Corticosteroids can lessen lung and airway edema. LABAs are also useful in treating exercise-induced asthma.

Accessible as a dry powder inhaler (DPI), LABAs are. Several of these medications are:

- Salmeterol.
- formoterol.

Anticholinergic medications such as tiotropium bromide and ipratropium bromide reduce the effects of acetylcholine in the body. Ipratropium bromide is available in two forms: an inhaler and a nebulizer solution, which can be used up to four times a day. Tiotropium bromide also comes in an inhaler form, with recommended usage either once a day or four times a day as advised by a doctor. These medications are not intended for immediate relief but are effective in managing difficult asthma symptoms.

10.2.3.3. Theophylline

Taken once daily, it helps control severe symptoms of asthma. However, theophylline is no longer the suggested course of action. To ensure you are taking the recommended dosage of theophylline, blood tests are required. Depending on the kind you take, bronchodilators can have different side effects.

10.2.4. Side Effects of Bronchodilators

The following are a few side effects of beta 2-agonists:

- Shivering or unpleasant feelings.
- Over excitement.
- Increased heart rate.
- Stomach pain.
- Having trouble sleeping.

Certain beta 2-agonists, including albuterol, are available as pills or syrups. Since there is a higher dosage in these formulations, there may be more adverse effects. They enter and are absorbed in your bloodstream.

Side effects of anticholinergic medications include:

- Dry throat, eyes, and nose.

- Nausea and vomiting.
- Short-term visual impairment if the drug gets in your eyes.
- Anticholinergic drugs may make it difficult to go to the toilet. Consult your physician if you have any bladder-related conditions. These conditions could be benign bladder stones.

Among theophylline's adverse effects are:

- Nausea and vomiting.
- Stomach ache.
- Leprosy.
- Pain.
- Irregular or rapid heartbeat.
- Muscular cramps.
- Shivering.
- Unpleasant feelings.

10.2.5. How to Use Bronchodilators?

You must use your bronchodilator inhaler appropriately to get the whole recommended dosage. Use your bronchodilator inhaler as best you can by doing the following:

- Shake your inhaler 10 or 15 times. Make sure the cap is on firmly.
- Remove the cap.
- Take a deep breath, then exhale completely.
- Lips encircling the mouthpiece.
- Press the inhaler once.
- Take a calm, deep breath through your lips. If you hear something that sounds like a horn, you should slow down your breathing.
- Take 10 seconds to breathe in and out. Count slowly to aid in the drug's entry into your lungs.
- Repeat these steps for each puff that your healthcare provider has prescribed. There should be a minute or so between each puff.
- Use mouthwash or water to rinse your mouth after taking a corticosteroid inhaler. Rinsing with mouthwash reduces any bad effects.

10.2.6. Antibiotics for Pulmonary Conditions

The treatment of a number of pulmonary disorders, such as respiratory tract infections, exacerbations of long-term lung diseases, and infectious aftereffects of lung surgery, depends heavily on antibiotics. These drugs are especially made to target and eradicate the bacterial pathogens that cause lung infections, which lessens symptoms, stops the disease from getting worse, and lowers the possibility of complications.

10.2.6.1. Respiratory Tract Infections

Treatment for upper respiratory tract infections, which can impact the respiratory system as a whole, often involves the prescription of antibiotics. (e.g., pharyngitis, sinusitis) or within the lower respiratory tract (e.g., pneumonia, bronchitis, etc.). Cough, fever, sputum production, and breathing difficulties are common symptoms of acute bacterial infections of the respiratory tract. When laboratory testing, clinical presentation, and microbiological culture results point to bacterial pathogens—like *Streptococcus pneumoniae*, *Haemophilus influenzae*, or *Moraxella catarrhalis*—as the cause, antibiotics are indicated. Antibiotic stewardship principles, which minimize needless antibiotic use and stop the emergence of antibiotic-resistant bacteria, as well as the severity of the infection, the patient's age and comorbidities, and local antimicrobial resistance patterns, all influence the choice of antibiotic therapy.

10.2.6.2. Exacerbations of Chronic Lung Diseases

Exacerbations of long-term lung conditions, like bronchiectasis and chronic obstructive pulmonary disease (COPD), which are frequently brought on by bacterial infections, are commonly treated with antibiotics. Exacerbations of COPD are frequently brought on by bacterial pathogens like *Haemophilus influenzae*, *Streptococcus pneumoniae*, and *Moraxella catarrhalis* and are linked to worsening respiratory symptoms, increased sputum production, and decreased lung function. When treating moderate-to-severe exacerbations of COPD, antibiotics are advised, especially for those who have purulent sputum or other indications of systemic inflammation. In this case, the antibiotic therapy option could involve beta-lactam antibiotics (e.g., cephalosporins, amoxicillin-clavulanate), macrolides (such as clarithromycin, azithromycin), or fluoroquinolones (e.g., levofloxacin, moxifloxacin), based on variables like comorbidities, previous antibiotic exposure, and patterns of local resistance.

10.2.6.3. Infectious Complications of Lung Surgery

Infections that arise from lung surgery, such as surgical site infections, postoperative pneumonia, and empyema, must be prevented and treated with antibiotics. Lung-related surgical procedures, including lung transplants, pneumonectomies, and lobectomies, increase the risk of infection from bacteria, especially in patients with immunocompromised conditions, underlying lung diseases, or long operating times. Antibiotic prophylaxis is a standard preoperative treatment used to lower the risk of surgical site infections and complications following surgery. Broad-spectrum antibiotics covering common respiratory pathogens and possible multidrug-resistant organisms may be empirically started in cases of suspected or confirmed postoperative infections, pending the results of culture and sensitivity testing. In addition to antibiotic therapy, surgical drainage and debridement may be required in cases of empyema or abscess formation to aid in the resolution of infection.

10.2.6.4. Cystic Fibrosis

Antibiotics are essential in managing cystic fibrosis (CF), a genetic disorder characterized by ongoing respiratory infections, airway inflammation, and lung damage. CF is linked to issues with clearing mucus, increased mucus production, and recurrent flare-ups caused by bacteria like *Pseudomonas aeruginosa*, *Staphylococcus aureus*, and *Burkholderia cepacia* complex. The goal of antibiotic therapy in CF is to control bacterial growth, eliminate pulmonary pathogens, and decrease the frequency and severity of flare-ups to preserve lung function and enhance quality of life. Treatment plans may involve using inhaled antibiotics (such as tobramycin and colistin) for long-term management, oral antibiotics (like azithromycin and ciprofloxacin) for acute episodes, and intravenous antibiotics (such as meropenem and ceftazidime) for serious or difficult-to-treat infections.

Antibiotics are essential in treating a range of pulmonary conditions, such as respiratory tract infections, exacerbations of chronic lung diseases, and infections following lung surgery. To ensure the best possible outcomes and minimize resistance development, it is crucial to use antibiotics carefully based on clinical judgment, microbiological evidence, and antimicrobial stewardship principles. Collaboration among healthcare professionals, including pulmonologists, infectious disease specialists, microbiologists, and pharmacists, is vital to ensure evidence-based prescribing practices and personalized patient care. This approach helps preserve the effectiveness of antibiotics for future generations.

10.2.7. Nutritional Aspects of Pulmonary Conditions

The management of pulmonary conditions is greatly impacted by nutrition, which affects respiratory function, the course of the disease, and the general quality of life of those suffering from lung diseases like lung cancer, cystic fibrosis, pulmonary fibrosis, and chronic obstructive pulmonary disease (COPD). Maintaining immune system function, controlling inflammation, promoting the health of respiratory muscles, and averting complications linked to malnutrition all depend on optimal nutrition. As a result, treating nutritional issues is a crucial part of providing complete pulmonary care.

10.2.7.1. Energy Requirements

Due to their higher resting energy expenditure, increased work of breathing, and metabolic needs related to tissue repair and chronic inflammation, people with pulmonary conditions frequently require more energy. However, decreased food intake and inadvertent weight loss may result in malnutrition and muscle wasting. These factors include dyspnea, fatigue, systemic inflammation, and decreased appetite. In patients with pulmonary conditions, assessing energy needs and ensuring sufficient calorie intake is critical to maintaining lean body mass, preventing weight loss, and promoting respiratory muscle function.

10.2.7.2. Protein Intake

Since protein is essential for immune system performance, tissue repair, and muscle maintenance, people with pulmonary conditions—especially those who are vulnerable to malnutrition and muscle atrophy—need to consume enough of it. Patients with COPD, CF, and lung cancer may have higher protein requirements because of increased protein turnover, inflammation, and metabolic demands brought on by the underlying disease process. Lean meats, poultry, fish, eggs, dairy products, legumes, and soy products are high-quality protein sources that can help satisfy protein requirements and promote the best possible immune system and respiratory muscle function.

10.2.7.3. Micronutrient Supplementation

Because of things like inadequate food intake, malabsorption, adverse drug reactions, and elevated metabolic demands, people with pulmonary disorders may be lacking in certain micronutrients, which include vitamins and minerals, which are crucial for immune system and respiratory health. Micronutrient supplements, such as those containing zinc, selenium, vitamin D, C, and E, may improve lung function, respiratory muscle strength, inflammation, and a patient's susceptibility to respiratory infections. Nonetheless, supplementation ought to be customized to meet the needs of each patient based on laboratory testing, clinical judgment, and nutritional assessment; potential interactions and contraindications should also be taken into account.

10.2.7.4. Fluid Intake

In particular, those with conditions like CF and COPD, which are linked to increased mucus production and thickening of respiratory secretions, need to drink enough water to maintain the hydration and viscosity of respiratory secretions, facilitate mucus clearance, and avoid dehydration. Excessive consumption of fluids, however, may make symptoms like peripheral edema and dyspnea worse in individuals suffering from heart failure or advanced lung disease. To maximize respiratory function and general health, specific fluid intake recommendations based on hydration status, renal function, and underlying disease should be given.

10.2.7.5. Weight Management

For people with pulmonary disorders, achieving, and maintaining a healthy body weight is crucial to maximizing exercise tolerance, respiratory function, and overall quality of life. The main goals of weight management techniques should be to promote sufficient nutrient intake, strike a balance between energy intake and expenditure, and address the causes of malnutrition and obesity. Nutritional therapies, including dietary counseling, oral nutritional supplements, and pulmonary rehabilitation programs, may help patients with COPD or CF feel better overall by improving their muscle strength, exercise capacity, and nutritional status.

To effectively manage pulmonary conditions and support respiratory function, immune response, and general health, it is essential to address nutritional aspects. Healthcare professionals should evaluate each patient's nutritional status, energy needs, dietary intake, and metabolic requirements before creating a personalized nutrition care plan that meets their unique requirements. To maximize nutritional support, enhance clinical outcomes, and improve the quality of life for people with pulmonary conditions, pulmonologists, dietitians, respiratory therapists, and other members of the healthcare team must work together (Hristara-Papadopoulou et al., 2008; Brunetta and Kroon, 2022).

10.3. Oxygen Therapy

The use of oxygen as a medical treatment, known as oxygen therapy or supplemental oxygen, can benefit individuals with low blood oxygen levels, carbon monoxide toxicity, cluster headaches, and during anesthesia induction. It is also helpful for maintaining blood oxygen levels in chronic conditions like severe COPD or cystic fibrosis. Oxygen can be delivered through various methods, including nasal cannula, face mask, or endotracheal intubation at normal pressure or in a hyperbaric chamber. Additionally, it can be administered through ECMO therapy by bypassing the airway.

For cells to function normally, oxygen is needed. On the other hand, oxygen toxicity brought on by abnormally high concentrations can cause lung damage and respiratory failure. Increased oxygen concentrations, especially when smoking, can also raise the risk of airway fires. Without humidification, oxygen therapy can also cause the nasal mucosa to dry out. An oxygen saturation of 94–96% is sufficient under most circumstances, but 88–92% is preferred in those who are at risk of carbon dioxide retention. Saturations should be as high as possible in cases of cardiac arrest or carbon monoxide toxicity. Although air normally contains 21% oxygen by volume, oxygen therapy can raise this percentage to 100%. In the developed world, oxygen therapy is the most widely used hospital treatment. It started to become popular around 1917. It is presently listed as an essential medicine on the World Health Organization's list. Oxygen concentrators or oxygen tanks can be used to supply oxygen at home.

10.3.1. Who Needs Oxygen Therapy

Oxygen therapy is prescribed for people who can't get enough oxygen on their own. This is often because of lung conditions that prevents the lungs from absorbing oxygen, including:

- chronic obstructive pulmonary disease (COPD).
- pneumonia.
- asthma.
- bronchopulmonary dysplasia, underdeveloped lungs in newborns.

- heart failure.
- cystic fibrosis.
- sleep apnea.
- lung disease.
- trauma to the respiratory system.

Doctors use tests to assess a person's eligibility for oxygen therapy, such as measuring the oxygen levels in their arterial blood or using a pulse oximeter. This device can determine oxygen saturation without needing a blood sample by attaching it to a body part, like a finger. Low oxygen levels may indicate that supplemental oxygen would be beneficial for the person.

Arteriole blood oxygen levels should be between 75 and 100 mmHg (millimeters of mercury). The requirement for additional oxygen is indicated by an oxygen level of 60 mmHg or less. Additionally hazardous and capable of harming lung cells is an excess of oxygen in the blood. You should not be breathing more than 110 mmHg of oxygen. While some people require oxygen therapy constantly, others only require it in specific circumstances or on rare occasions. Certain people receive oxygen therapy at their physician's office, while others have a portable oxygen system or an oxygen supply in their homes.

10.3.1.1. What Are the Symptoms of Low Oxygen?

When you aren't getting enough oxygen, you'll experience a host of symptoms, including:

- rapid breathing.
- shortness of breath.
- fast heart rate.
- coughing or wheezing.
- sweating.
- confusion.
- changes in the color of your skin.

If you experience any of these symptoms, seek immediate medical attention.

10.3.1.2. What are the Different Types of Oxygen Therapies?

There are several different types of oxygen therapies that can be used. These include:

- oxygen gas.
- liquid oxygen.
- oxygen concentrators.
- hyperbaric oxygen therapy.

10.3.1.2.1. Oxygen Gas

A transportable tank can be used to hold oxygen gas. We refer to these as compressed gas systems. A smaller oxygen tank can be used outside the house, and a larger stationary concentrator is used inside. To extend the oxygen supply, oxygen-conserving devices may be used in conjunction with the smaller tanks. Oxygen is not given continuously; it is given in bursts.

10.3.1.2.2. Liquid Oxygen

Another way to store liquid oxygen is in a transportable tank. Since liquid oxygen is more concentrated, a smaller tank can hold more of it. For those who lead busy lives, this is beneficial, but if not used promptly, it will disappear. These are refilledable tanks. Many places offer home delivery services for both liquid and gaseous oxygen.

10.3.1.2.3. Oxygen Concentrators

Compared to the other options, oxygen concentrators are less portable. An oxygen concentrator is a machine that extracts other naturally occurring gases from the air, concentrates oxygen for medical purposes, and takes it from the room. Concentrators have the advantages of being less expensive and not needing to be filled like tanks are. There are versions that are portable. However, the majority of models are too big to be genuinely portable. Through a tube, oxygen is dispersed from the tank. Via nasal tubes, a face mask, or a tube put straight into the windpipe, it enters the lungs.

10.3.1.2.4. Hyperbaric Oxygen Therapy

Compared to other oxygen therapy techniques, hyperbaric oxygen therapy is unique. People in a pressurized chamber or room will breathe in pure oxygen. The air pressure is raised to three or four times the standard levels inside the hyperbaric chambers. As a result, more oxygen is given to the body's tissues. Air bubbles in your blood vessels, severe infections, and wounds are all frequently treated with this kind of oxygen delivery. It's important to use hyperbaric therapy with caution to prevent dangerously elevated blood oxygen levels.

10.3.1.2.5. Delivery Methods

The most common delivery method is the nasal cannula, which consists of a tube that runs through both nostrils. Other delivery methods include:

- the nonrebreather mask
- the incubator (for infants)
- continuous positive airway pressure (CPAP)

10.3.1.3. What Are the Benefits of Oxygen Therapy?

Whatever the cause, oxygen therapy can be very helpful for people who frequently have low oxygen levels. By reducing dyspnea, people who regularly use oxygen therapy, if necessary, can become more mobile and active. In many cases, it can also prolong life expectancy and greatly improve quality of life.

Oxygen therapy can also reduce symptoms such as:

- headaches
- irritability
- fatigue
- swollen ankles

Oxygen therapy can help the growth and development of children who have chronic lung conditions. It can also lessen symptoms such as headaches caused by low oxygen levels, and behavioral changes or problems (Hristara-Papadopoulou et al., 2008; Brunetta and Kroon, 2022).

10.3.2. Medical Uses

In many different situations and environments, hospitals, emergency medical services, and first responders use oxygen extensively. High-flow oxygen is often necessary in certain situations, such as resuscitation, severe trauma, anaphylaxis, significant bleeding, shock, active convulsions, and hypothermia (Figure 10.2).

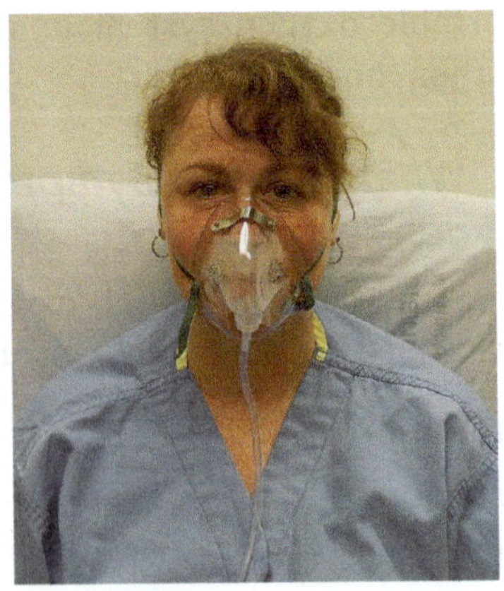

Figure 10.2. *Oxygen therapy.*

Source: https://upload.wikimedia.org/wikipedia/commons/thumb/e/e8/Simple_face_mask.jpg/479px-Simple_face_mask.jpg.

10.3.2.1. What Are the Guidelines for Using Oxygen Therapy?

To start oxygen therapy, your doctor will prescribe for you. They will instruct you on how to use it and how frequently to use it. Included in this will be the flow rate, or the amount of oxygen you require each minute. You must strictly adhere to all of your doctor's instructions. You should consult them before making any changes if you feel that the oxygen therapy isn't helping.

Some people only require oxygen when they are sleeping or exercising. Some people are always in need of oxygen. The majority of oxygen therapy options include transportable oxygen tanks, allowing you to use them outside of your house if needed. When using oxygen therapy, avoid using drugs or alcohol as these substances can cause breathing difficulties. Inform your doctor about all other prescription medications you may be taking before starting oxygen therapy.

10.3.2.2. What Are the Safety Considerations for Oxygen Therapy?

Despite not being flammable, oxygen is still required for combustion. Excessive oxygen levels cause fires to burn more quickly. Make sure to store oxygen tanks safely and exercise caution when handling them near heaters and open flames.

10.3.2.3. Acute Conditions

When dealing with acute hypoxemia, oxygen treatment should be adjusted to a target level determined by pulse oximetry (usually 94–96%, or 88–92% in COPD patients). Increasing oxygen delivery, also known as FIO2 (fraction of inspired oxygen), is one way to achieve this. The British Medical Journal advised in 2018 that oxygen therapy should not be initiated for saturations above 90 to 93% and should be discontinued for saturations greater than 96%. This could be because there is a link between higher mortality and overoxygenation in critically ill patients. Pneumothorax, sickle cell crisis, cluster headaches, and carbon monoxide poisoning are among the conditions for which these guidelines do not apply.

For many years, oxygen therapy has also been used as a last resort for treating decompression sickness. Decompression illness is typically treated with recompression in a hyperbaric chamber with 100% oxygen. Recompression therapy works best when administered four hours after resurfacing; earlier treatment is linked to fewer recompression treatments needed to resolve the condition. Literature has indicated that heliox might be a preferable substitute for oxygen therapy. As long as hyperoxic environments are avoided, oxygen therapy may be helpful in the context of stroke. Before having their prescription renewed, patients receiving outpatient oxygen therapy for hypoxemia after an acute illness or hospitalization should have a new evaluation by a doctor to determine whether they still need this kind of treatment. If the initial hypoxemia has cleared up, it might not be necessary to use more resources for further treatment.

10.3.2.4. Chronic Conditions

Emphysema, chronic bronchitis, and chronic obstructive pulmonary disease (COPD) are common conditions that may need a baseline of additional oxygen. In addition, patients may need more oxygen when experiencing acute exacerbations. Despite relatively normal blood oxygen levels, oxygen may also be prescribed for respiratory failure, advanced cancer, end-stage cardiac failure, dyspnea, or neurodegenerative disease. Physiologically, it may be indicated in people with arterial oxygen partial pressure $PaO_2 \leq 55$mmHg (7.3kPa) or arterial oxygen saturation $SaO_2 \leq 88\%$.

Patients with chronic conditions that make them more susceptible to carbon dioxide retention should have their oxygen therapy carefully titrated (e.g., emphysema, COPD). In these cases, oxygen therapy may reduce the respiratory drive, which increases the risk of acidemia, hypercapnia, and increased mortality from respiratory failure. Titrated oxygen therapy has been associated with better results, primarily because the ventilation/perfusion ratio has been gradually improved. Emergency oxygen administration is never contraindicated because the risks of not administering oxygen to a patient in need outweigh the risks of not administering it. Transferring from the field to definitive care that uses titrated oxygen usually takes place well before noticeable declines in respiratory drive are noticed.

10.3.2.5. Contraindications

There are certain situations in which oxygen therapy has been shown to negatively impact a person's condition.

- Oxygen therapy can exacerbate the effects of paraquat poisoning and should be withheld unless severe respiratory distress or respiratory arrest is present. Paraquat poisoning is rare, with about 200 deaths globally from 1958 to 1978.
- Oxygen therapy is not recommended for people with pulmonary fibrosis or bleomycin-associated lung damage.
- ARDS caused by acid aspiration may be exacerbated with oxygen therapy according to some animal studies.
- Hyperoxic environments should be avoided in cases of sepsis.

10.3.2.6. Adverse Effects

In some instances, oxygen delivery can lead to particular complications in population subsets.

- In infants with respiratory failure, administration of high levels of oxygen can sometimes promote overgrowth of new blood vessels in the eye leading to blindness. This phenomenon is known as retinopathy of prematurity (ROP).
- In rare instances, people receiving hyperbaric oxygen therapy have had seizures, which have been previously attributed to oxygen toxicity.
- There is some evidence that extended HBOT can accelerate the development of cataracts.

10.3.2.7. Alternative Medicine

Alternative medicine practitioners have been promoting "oxygen therapy" as a cure for various illnesses such as AIDS, Alzheimer's disease, and cancer. The American Cancer Society states that there is no scientific evidence to support the effectiveness of putting oxygen-releasing chemicals into the body to treat cancer and warns that some of these treatments can be harmful.

10.3.3. Physiologic Effects

The human body responds to oxygen supplementation in many physiological ways. The clinical context determines whether or not a patient will suffer negative consequences from these effects. Hyperoxia is the term for situations in which organs have an excessive amount of oxygen available to them. While using noninvasive high-dose oxygen therapy, the following side effects could be seen (i. e. higher pressure oxygen delivery—not ECMO—is linked to an aggravation of the subsequent side effects.

10.3.3.1. Absorption Atelectasis

According to certain theories, oxygen therapy may hasten the onset of atelectasis, or partial or total lung collapse, and also encourage the denitrogenation of gas cavities (e.g., pneumocephalus, pneumothorax). This theory is predicated on the notion that oxygen enters the body more quickly than nitrogen does, causing oxygen-rich, poorly ventilated regions to absorb oxygen more quickly and develop atelectasis. Higher fractions of inhaled oxygen (F_IO_2) are hypothesized to be linked to rising atelectasis rates in the clinical setting. When treated appropriately, absorption atelectasis is thought to usually have no major consequences in clinically healthy adults.

10.3.3.2. Airway Inflammation

Regarding the airway, high oxygen delivery levels (usually >40% O2) have been associated with both tracheobronchitis and mucositis. These higher oxygen concentrations have been linked to increased alveolar toxicity in the lungs (a phenomenon known as the Lorrain-Smith effect). Elevated oxygen concentrations and atmospheric pressure have been shown to increase mucosal damage, which could lead to the development of ARDS and even death.

10.3.3.3. Central Nervous System Effects

Decreased cerebral blood flow and intracranial pressure (ICP) have been reported in hyperoxic conditions, with mixed results regarding impact on cognition. Hyperoxia has also been associated with seizures, cataract formation, and reversible myopia.

10.3.3.4. Hypercapnia

Excessive oxygen exposure in the context of the Haldane effect reduces the binding of deoxyhemoglobin to CO2 in the blood among CO2 retainers. The associated increase in PaCO2 (hypercapnia) that results from this unloading of CO2 may play a role in the development of acid-base disorders. The extra CO2 produced by this effect may be too much for patients with underlying lung diseases like COPD to expel, making their condition worse. Furthermore, it has been demonstrated that oxygen therapy lowers respiratory drive, which increases the risk of hypercapnia.

10.3.3.5. Immunological Effects

In certain human conditions, hyperoxic environments have been shown to reduce granulocyte rolling and diapedesis. Regarding anaerobic infections, it has been noted that patients treated with hyperbaric oxygen therapy for necrotizing fasciitis require fewer debridement procedures and have improved mortality rates. This could be the result of otherwise anaerobic microorganisms becoming oxygen-intolerant.

10.3.3.6. Oxidative Stress

Prolonged exposure to oxygen can exceed the body's ability to handle oxidative stress. The rate of oxidative stress seems to be affected by both the concentration of oxygen and the duration of exposure, with potential toxicity noted to occur within hours under certain high oxygen conditions.

10.3.3.7. Reduction in Erythropoiesis

It has been noted that hyperoxia lowers serum erythropoietin levels, which lessens the stimulus for erythropoiesis. It doesn't seem that hyperoxia in normobaric settings can totally stop erythropoiesis.

10.3.3.8. Pulmonary Vasodilation

Hypoxia is known to be a strong pulmonary vasoconstrictor in the lungs because it causes pulmonary vascular muscular contraction by activating an inward sodium current and inhibiting an outward potassium current. From the few studies done on patients with pulmonary hypertension, the effects of hyperoxia do not appear to have a particularly strong vasodilatory effect. As a result, a slight but apparent effect is seen.

10.3.3.9. Systemic Vasoconstriction

Oxygen acts as a vasoconstrictor in the systemic vasculature, raising blood pressure slightly while lowering heart rate and cardiac output. These general physiological effects do not appear to be significantly affected by hyperbaric conditions. Clinically, in some patient populations, such as those with atrial septal defect, this may result in increased left-to-right shunting. One theory suggests that increased reactive oxygen species from oxygen therapy speed up the breakdown of endothelial nitric oxide, a vasodilator, although the exact mechanism of the vasoconstriction is unknown. Cluster headaches are thought to be prevented by the underlying mechanism of these vasoconstrictive effects.

10.3.4. Storage and Sources

Oxygen can be separated by several methods (e.g., chemical reaction, fractional distillation) to enable immediate or future use.

The main methods utilized for oxygen therapy include:

- Liquid storage – Liquid oxygen is stored in insulated tanks at low temperatures and allowed to boil (at a temperature of 90.188 K (−182.96 °C)) during use, releasing gaseous oxygen. This method is widely utilized at hospitals due to high oxygen requirements.
- Compressed gas storage – Oxygen gas is compressed in a gas cylinder, which provides a convenient storage method (refrigeration is not required). Large oxygen cylinders hold a volume of 6500 liters (230 cu ft) and can last about two days at a flow rate of 2 liters per minute (LPM). A small portable M6 (B) cylinder holds 164 or 170 liters (5.8 or 6.0 cu ft) and weighs about 1.3 to 1.6 kilograms (2.9 to 3.5 lb). These tanks can last 4–6 hours with a conserving regulator, which adjusts flow based on a person's breathing rate. Conserving regulators may not be effective for patients who breathe through their mouths.
- Instant usage – The use of an electrically powered oxygen concentrator or a chemical reaction-based unit can create sufficient oxygen for immediate personal use. These units (especially the electrically powered versions) are widely used for home oxygen therapy as portable personal oxygen. One particular advantage includes continuous supply without the need for bulky oxygen cylinders (Figure 10.3).

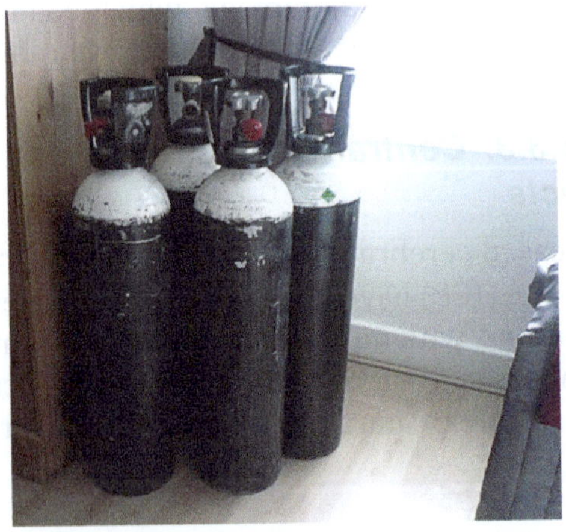

Figure 10.3. *Oxygen cylinders.*

Source: https://upload.wikimedia.org/wikipedia/commons/thumb/3/37/Home_oxygen_canisters.jpg/800px-Home_oxygen_canisters.jpg.

10.3.4.1. Hazards and Risk

The risk of rapid combustion is also increased by highly concentrated oxygen sources. Although oxygen by itself is not flammable, adding concentrated oxygen to a fire can intensify it significantly and help burn materials that would normally burn relatively inertly. Concentrated oxidants and fuels near present a risk of fire and explosion, even though an ignition event (e.g., a spark or heat source) is required to start combustion.

Combustion can proceed quickly and vigorously in the presence of concentrated oxygen. To minimize ignition sources, special training is required during the design and manufacture of oxygen systems because steel pipes and storage vessels used to store and transmit both gaseous and liquid oxygen will act as fuel. Hydrocarbons like oil and grease can spontaneously ignite in a high-pressure environment with highly concentrated oxygen, causing an explosion or fire. The ignition source is the heat generated by the quick pressurization. To guarantee that there are no possible fuels present, storage containers, regulators, pipes, and other equipment used with highly concentrated oxygen must be oxygen-clean before usage. This is not limited to pure oxygen; there is a risk of ignition at any concentration much greater than atmospheric (roughly 21%).

No-smoking guidelines have been implemented by certain hospitals, which can assist in separating sources of ignition from medically supplied oxygen. These regulations do not completely remove the possibility of harm to patients using portable oxygen concentrators, particularly those who smoke. Aside from candles, aromatherapy, medical equipment, cooking, and intentional vandalism, these are other potential sources of ignition.

10.3.5. Nicotine and Tobacco

The highly addictive chemical nicotine, which is present in tobacco products, has a significant impact on one's physical and mental health. Worldwide, tobacco use—mainly in the form of smoking—remains a major public health concern because it can lead to a wide range of illnesses, such as cancers, cardiovascular diseases, and respiratory ailments. Nicotine addiction endures despite a general understanding of the dangers of tobacco use, which encourages tobacco use and undermines initiatives to encourage quitting smoking.

The use of nicotine and tobacco greatly affects respiratory health. Smoking is the main cause of preventable respiratory diseases such as COPD, lung cancer, and asthma. Inhaling toxic chemicals and carcinogens found in tobacco smoke harms the airways, reduces lung function, and raises the chances of developing respiratory issues. Nicotine addiction sustains smoking habits, causing ongoing exposure to harmful substances and worsening respiratory symptoms. Furthermore, exposure to secondhand smoke puts nonsmokers at risk of respiratory infections, asthma attacks, and other negative respiratory effects.

The use of tobacco and nicotine also has a significant impact on the cardiovascular system. In addition to constricting blood vessels and raising heart rate, blood pressure, and cardiac output, nicotine also raises the risk of atherosclerosis, endothelial dysfunction, and thrombosis. Smoking exposes people to nicotine over time, which increases their risk of cardiovascular illnesses like heart attacks, strokes, and coronary artery disease. Tobacco use has a wide range of effects on cardiovascular health; for example, secondhand smoke exposure raises the risk of cardiovascular events in nonsmokers. The main components of using tobacco and nicotine are addiction and dependence. Nicotine produces feelings of pleasure, euphoria, and increased alertness by acting on the reward pathways in the brain. Long-term nicotine exposure builds tolerance and dependence, necessitating higher doses of the drug to produce the same effects and resulting in withdrawal symptoms when stopped. Genetic, environmental, and behavioral variables all play a role in the intricate and multidimensional nature of nicotine addiction. It can be difficult to overcome nicotine dependence and stop smoking; comprehensive cessation interventions, such as behavioral counseling, medication, and support groups, are necessary.

In addition to its many health advantages, quitting smoking lowers the risk of smoking-related illnesses, improves respiratory health, and improves one's general quality of life. Interventions for quitting smoking try to treat nicotine addiction, control symptoms of withdrawal, and encourage people to change to healthier lifestyles. Healthcare professionals are essential in encouraging smoking cessation and offering tools, direction, and support to those who are trying to give up the habit. Even though nicotine addiction presents difficulties, it is possible to stop smoking if you have the willpower, support, and resources to help you find evidence-based cessation techniques.

The use of tobacco and nicotine has a great deal of negative effects on one's physical and mental well-being, leading to a variety of illnesses and health issues. Developing comprehensive public health strategies that target youth tobacco initiation, reduce tobacco consumption, and promote smoke-free environments is necessary to combat tobacco use and nicotine addiction. Through heightened awareness of the dangers of tobacco use, encouragement of quitting, and the implementation of efficient tobacco control policies, society can lessen the harmful effects of nicotine and tobacco on health, thereby improving the well-being of both individuals and communities (George, 2024).

A Closer Look

Mucociliary clearance

Mucociliary clearance is a vital mechanism in the respiratory system that helps maintain lung health by removing inhaled particles, pathogens, and mucus from the airways. It involves the coordinated action of mucus-producing cells and cilia, tiny hair-like structures lining the respiratory tract.

The process begins with the secretion of mucus by goblet cells and submucosal glands in the airways. This mucus serves as a sticky trap for inhaled particles, such as dust, bacteria, and viruses. The cilia, which are constantly in motion, beat in a coordinated rhythm, moving the mucus along the airway surface toward the throat. The mucus, along with trapped particles, is then either swallowed or expelled through coughing.

Effective mucociliary clearance is essential for preventing respiratory infections and maintaining clear airways. Several factors can affect this process, including smoking, which can damage cilia, or conditions like cystic fibrosis, where thickened mucus is harder to clear. Inflammatory diseases such as chronic bronchitis or asthma can also impair mucociliary function.

Enhancing mucociliary clearance is a therapeutic goal in conditions where mucus buildup is problematic. This can be achieved through hydration, chest physiotherapy, inhaled medications (like mucolytics), or bronchodilators, which help improve mucus mobility and airway patency.

Summary

- Treating and managing pulmonary diseases is a multifaceted endeavor that requires a comprehensive approach tailored to the specific conditions and needs of each patient.
- Airway clearance techniques (ACTs) are vital components of the management of various pulmonary conditions, particularly those characterized by excessive mucus production, airway inflammation, and impaired mucociliary clearance.
- Autogenic drainage is a controlled airway clearance technique using different depths of inhalation, and different speeds of exhalation that enables mucus to be moved up the airway producing a voluntary cough.
- Chronic obstructive pulmonary disease (COPD) is a preventable and treatable disease with airway obstruction and is characterized by persistent respiratory symptoms.
- Aerosol delivery of medication, also known as inhalation therapy, is a cornerstone of treatment for various respiratory conditions, including asthma, chronic obstructive pulmonary disease (COPD), cystic fibrosis, and respiratory infections.
- Dry powder inhalers (DPIs) deliver medication in powder form without the need for propellants or coordination of actuation and inhalation.
- A bronchodilator or broncholytic (although the latter occasionally includes secretory inhibition as well) is a substance that dilates the bronchi and bronchioles, decreasing resistance in the respiratory airway and increasing airflow to the lungs.
- Antibiotics play a vital role in the management of various pulmonary conditions, including respiratory tract infections, exacerbations of chronic lung diseases, and infectious complications of lung surgery.
- Antibiotics play a central role in the management of cystic fibrosis (CF), a genetic disorder characterized by chronic respiratory infections, airway inflammation, and progressive lung damage.
- Oxygen therapy, also referred to as supplemental oxygen, is the use of oxygen as medical treatment. Supplemental oxygen can also refer to the use of oxygen enriched air at altitude.
- Common conditions that may require a baseline of supplementary oxygen include chronic obstructive pulmonary disease (COPD), chronic bronchitis, and emphysema.

References

1. Atkinson, D. L., Minnix, J., Cinciripini, P. M., & Karam-Hage, M. (2020). Nicotine. In B. A. Johnson (Ed.), *Addiction Medicine: Science and Practice* (2nd ed., chap. 23). Philadelphia, PA: Elsevier.
2. Brunetta, P. G., & Kroon, L. (2022). Smoking cessation. In V. C. Broaddus, J. D. Ernst, T. E. King, et al. (Eds.), *Murray and Nadel's Textbook of Respiratory Medicine* (7th ed., chap. 66). Philadelphia, PA: Elsevier.
3. Burnham, P., Stanford, G., & Stewart, R. (2021). Autogenic drainage for airway clearance in cystic fibrosis. *The Cochrane Database of Systematic Reviews, 2021*(12), CD009595.

4. Cystic Fibrosis Foundation. (n.d.). Active Cycle of Breathing Technique (ACBT). Retrieved from: https://www.cff.org (accessed on 22 October 2024).
5. George, T. P. (2024). Nicotine and tobacco. In L. Goldman & K. A. Cooney (Eds.), *Goldman-Cecil Medicine* (27th ed., chap. 363). Philadelphia, PA: Elsevier.
6. Gotts, J. E., & Benowitz, N. L. (2022). Smoking hazards: Cigarettes, vaping, marijuana. In V. C. Broaddus, J. D. Ernst, T. E. King, et al. (Eds.), *Murray and Nadel's Textbook of Respiratory Medicine* (7th ed., chap. 65). Philadelphia, PA: Elsevier.
7. Homnick, D. N. (2007). Mechanical insufflation-exsufflation for airway mucus clearance. *Respiratory Care, 52*(10), 1296–1305, discussion 1306–1307.
8. Hristara-Papadopoulou, A., Tsanakas, J., Diomou, G., & Papadopoulou, O. (2008). Current devices of respiratory physiotherapy. *Hippokratia, 12*(4), 211–220.
9. McIlwaine, M., Button, B., & Nevitt, S. J. (2019). Positive expiratory pressure physiotherapy for airway clearance in people with cystic fibrosis. *The Cochrane Database of Systematic Reviews, 2019*(11).
10. Volsko, T. A. (2013). Airway clearance therapy: Finding the evidence. *Respiratory Care, 58*(10), 1669–1678.

INDEX

C

D

E

F

G

M

N

O

Printed and bound by CPI Group (UK) Ltd, Croydon, CR0 4YY
27/07/2026
02178136-0001